Enabling Independence
A Guide for Rehabilitation Workers

In loving memory of
Iris Tatton,
who traced the rainbow through the rain

Enabling Independence
A Guide for Rehabilitation Workers

Edited by

Hazel Mackey
Occupational Therapy Services Manager
Bucknall Hospital
Stoke-on-Trent

and

Susan Nancarrow
Primary Care Research Coordinator
Trent RDSU
The University of Sheffield

Photography by Julie Brookes
Illustrations by Diane Hand

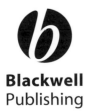

Blackwell
Publishing

Editorial Offices:
Blackwell Publishing Ltd, 9600 Garsington Road, Oxford OX4 2DQ, UK
    Tel: +44 (0)1865 776868
Blackwell Publishing Professional, 2121 State Avenue, Ames, Iowa 50014-8300, USA
    Tel: +1 515 292 0140
Blackwell Publishing Asia, 550 Swanston Street, Carlton, Victoria 3053, Australia
    Tel: +61 (0)3 8359 1011

First published 2006 by Blackwell Publishing Ltd

ISBN-13: 978-14051-3028-8
ISBN-10: 1-4051-3028-8

Library of Congress Cataloging-in-Publication Data
Enabling independence : a guide for rehabilitation workers / edited by
    Hazel Mackey and Susan Nancarrow ; photography by Julie Brookes
    ; illustrations by Diane Hand. – 1st ed.
        p. ; cm.
    Includes bibliographical references and index.
    ISBN-13: 978-1-4051-3028-8 (pbk. : alk. paper)
    ISBN-10: 1-4051-3028-8 (pbk. : alk. paper)
    1. Rehabilitation. 2. Medical rehabilitation. I. Mackey, Hazel.
II. Nancarrow, Susan A.
    [DNLM: 1. Rehabilitation–methods. 2. Recovery of Function.
3. Rehabilitation–psychology.   WB 320 E564 2006]
RM930.E52 2006
671'.03–dc22

                                                            2005030636

A catalogue record for this title is available from the British Library

Set in 10/12 pt Stone Sans
by Newgen Imaging Systems (P) Ltd. Chennai, India
Printed and bound in India
by Replika Press Pvt, Ltd, Kundli

For further information on Blackwell Publishing, visit our website:
www.blackwellpublishing.com

Contents

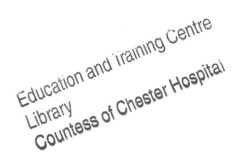

Foreword

Rehabilitation workers come in all shapes and sizes! They may be profession-specific or work with a broad range of health and social care professionals; they may be more or less experienced and may undertake prescribed activities or be left to use their own initiative. Whilst rehabilitation workers are given many different titles, job descriptions and responsibilities, one thing unites them all: that rehabilitation workers are not only essential, but frequently central to health and social care provision. This will increasingly become the case with the changing demography leading to more dependent older people, and fewer younger people entering related professions. This book acknowledges the talents and skills of many rehabilitation workers and formalises fundamental and practical information, which will assist them in undertaking and extending their role constructively and safely.

Rehabilitation workers support and assist a profession or a team of professionals. Increasing the shared knowledge of principles and fundamental practice of rehabilitation should go a long way in replacing the often well-intentioned, but ad hoc approach to rehabilitation, enabling coherent and integrated management of impairment, disability and social participation.

This book, which adopts a problem-solving approach bolstered by sufficient theory and principles and illustrated with case histories, can be used as a resource by teams to guide team learning and working, as well as being an individual resource to assist with personal development. Whole-team learning, true interprofessional learning, will inevitably lead to more effective and efficient involvement with patients as well as to a more satisfactory work experience for all staff.

This book takes a client-centred approach, considering functions in appropriate environments, thus making the text unique amongst those that were written for this audience. It does not just simplify a professional perspective but stimulates new ways of thinking and working, breaking down the boundaries that separate professional roles.

Pam Enderby

Acknowledgements

The editors are grateful for the valuable advice and feedback from rehabilitation workers Janet Fletcher, Marie Cross, Tracy Amos, Jackie Higham, Heather Forrester, Julie Dawson, Peter Nash, Karen Rogers and Nicola Weston. In addition, we would like to thank Professor Mark Doel, Research Professor of Social Work at Sheffield Hallam University, for his contribution, and Jo Adlard for his support with the production of the manuscript.

List of contributors

Sue Ball

Sue is a community occupational therapist, working in Stoke-on-Trent, England. After many years working as an occupational therapy support worker, she gained her professional qualification in occupational therapy in 2004, after completing a part-time in-service BSc (Hons). She has experience in rheumatology, elderly care and many community settings. Currently, she is working within a community setting with adults aged sixteen and over. Sue has special interests in manual handling, and teaching.

Hannah Barratt

Assistant psychologist, older adult speciality, North Staffordshire Combined Healthcare Trust, Bucknall Hospital, Stoke-on-Trent.

Hannah graduated from Staffordshire University in 2001 and has worked as an assistant psychologist in North Staffordshire Combined Healthcare with a number of client groups, including older adults.

Sandi Carman

Sandi has recently taken up the general manager post for the Women's and Children's Services at Barnsley Hospital NHS Foundation Trust, where she was previously the training and development manager. Her move into management came after an eight-year career in occupational therapy; a career which started with a BSc in the profession at Liverpool University and progressed to an MSc in health care practice at Sheffield Hallam University. As an occupational therapist, Sandi became a specialist in burns and plastic surgery, an area of the profession which requires expert technical skills and knowledge. Her interest in the field led her to focus on work rehabilitation for clients with upper limb injuries and this culminated in a dissertation for her Master's. On secondment to the now named Workforce Development Confederation she worked closely with students and staff at hospitals in Trent and South Yorkshire, looking at placements and how they could best be improved in occupational therapy and physiotherapy. In her management roles at Barnsley, Sandi has been able to use the experience and skills she gathered during her earlier career and build upon them through further studies in human resource management.

■ Lindy Clemson

Doctor of Philosophy (epidemiology), Master of Applied Science (Occupational Therapy), Bachelor of Applied Science (Occupational Therapy). Senior Research Fellow, School of Occupation and Leisure Sciences, Faculty of Health Sciences, the University of Sydney.

Lindy has over 30 years' experience as an occupational therapist and a recently completed PhD in epidemiology. She has a background in consultancy and research in the areas of physical and cultural environments, adaptation and ageing, functional assessment, and the independence of older persons at home and in the community. She has over 30 publications, with 17 of these being in the area of falls prevention assessment and management, in particular aspects of home and community safety. Recently completed research included a randomised trial of the effectiveness of a community-based falls prevention programme (Stepping On) in which she was the principal chief investigator. This multifaceted programme, based on principles of self-efficacy and social cognitive learning, was successful, reducing falls by 31%.

■ Maureen Coulthard

Maureen obtained her degree in occupational therapy from the University of Manitoba in 1987 and is currently pursuing a Master's degree in gerontology at the University of Regina. Her clinical focus has included paediatrics, adult neurology and injured worker rehabilitation. Her career has spanned both health and post-secondary education sectors in management, project management and clinical streams. She developed a 40-week occupational therapist assistant/physical therapist assistant programme, and was programme head and instructor. She has served on, or chaired, several committees, programme advisory boards, working groups and task forces on a departmental, regional, provincial and national level. The focus of such committees, working groups, forums and panels has included the training and use of support personnel, development of position papers and guidelines for supervision of support personnel, revision of the CAOT Profile of Occupational Therapy, education of occupational therapists in Canada and, most recently, primary health care. She published an article in the *Canadian Journal of Occupational Therapy* entitled Preparing occupational therapists for practice today and into the future.

▪ Keith David Hill

Bachelor of Applied Science (Physiotherapy), Graduate Diploma of Physiotherapy, Doctor of Philosophy. Senior Research Fellow, National Ageing Research Institute, and Co-director, Falls and Balance Clinic, Melbourne Extended Care and Rehabilitation Service, Parkville, Victoria, Australia.

Keith has almost 25 years' experience as a physiotherapist involved in rehabilitation and aged care. He completed his PhD in 1998 entitled 'Balance studies in older people'. Keith currently coordinates a number of falls prevention related projects and research initiatives, as well as running falls prevention training programmes for general practitioners, health professionals and home care workers. He has published 30 papers and six book chapters in the areas of balance and mobility assessment and treatment, and falls prevention in older people, including the first effective randomised trial of a falls prevention programme in a hospital setting. He has conducted falls prevention programmes in the community, hospital and residential care settings.

▪ Peter Hudson

Peter Hudson is an Associate Professor and Deputy Director of the Centre for Palliative Care (St Vincent's Health and University of Melbourne, Australia). He has been an investigator on National Health and Medical Research Council projects researching palliation issues associated with nausea and neurological disorders and pain. He was an investigator on a Commonwealth project focusing on developing palliative care guidelines, competencies and a training programme for staff in residential aged care facilities. Peter is also involved in research projects associated with the management of diabetes at the end of life, an evaluation of a day hospice and the attitudes of nurses toward evidence based practice. He is a working party member for two national projects regarding the 'Respecting patient choices programme' and the 'Social impact of caring for the terminally ill'. Peter coordinates palliative care nursing education (postgraduate Diploma/Masters) at the University of Melbourne and is vice-president of the Board of Directors of Palliative Care Victoria.

▪ Angela Knisely-Marpole

Angela qualified in 1971 as a physiotherapist and then spent the next ten years working in an NHS rehabilitation and rheumatology hospital, having done a six-month hydrotherapy course. She then worked for Possum® Controls for four years as a regional assessor for equipment for the severely disabled. Twenty years ago she came back into the NHS, working in a psychiatric hospital. This included working closely with liaison psychiatry with chronic fatigue clients and other multi-pathology conditions. She has completed a postgraduate diploma in acupuncture and is about to start her dissertation entitled 'Does acupuncture improve the quality of life of chronic fatigue patients?'

■ Hazel Mackey

Hazel qualified as an occupational therapist in 1985. Since then she has worked as a clinician, academic and manager. She is currently the Occupational Therapy Services Manager for North Staffordshire Combined Health Care NHS Trust, in England.

She has many years of experience working in rehabilitation settings, first within elderly care and latterly in various primary care settings. For the last ten years she has been involved in the education and training of therapy support workers through National Vocational Qualifications at levels 3 and 4. She is currently studying for a PhD at Keele University. Her research topic looks at role redesign in the health service.

■ Kelly McPhee

Kelly completed a Bachelor of Science (major in Psychology) at the Australian National University in 1991. She worked as a care assistant and auxiliary nurse with children and adults with profound physical and intellectual disabilities in Canberra, and as an auxiliary nurse in rehabilitation hospitals in Sydney before qualifying as a speech pathologist from the University of Sydney in 1995. She has had varied experience within her professional career within the acute hospital and community setting. She has worked with children and adults with intellectual disabilities, acquired neurological conditions and head and neck cancer in Australia and the UK. She is currently employed by the National Health Service (NHS) as a speech and language therapist in Sheffield, working with older people requiring rapid support to facilitate safe, early discharge from hospital.

■ Anna Moran

Community rehabilitation research associate/physiotherapist.

Anna qualified as a physiotherapist in 2000 and has worked in a variety of clinical areas in Australia and the UK. Since 2002 she has worked in primary care settings in Yorkshire, UK, providing rehabilitation to older people in their homes. Her interest in social and health care in the community led her to take a research position with the University of Sheffield where she is currently employed on a three-year Department of Health project to evaluate older people's community and intermediate care services. She has a particular interest in the workforce that serves older people's community services.

■ Gail Mountain

Gail Mountain qualified as an occupational therapist in 1976. She then spent approximately ten years working with people with mental health problems and older people as a practitioner and manager of various occupational therapy services in West Yorkshire. In 1987, Gail went to work at the University of Leeds as a research assistant on a project looking at the relationship between environment and the behaviour of older people with severe dementia on long-stay wards. This marked the beginning of a research career. A range of other projects at the universities of Leeds and York followed, mainly concerned with older people. Gail returned briefly to the NHS from 1991–1994 to manage occupational therapy services in a range of services in Leeds Community and Mental Health NHS Trust. This was followed by three years working at the Nuffield Institute for Health, University of Leeds, in community care research. As part of her research portfolio, Gail obtained a Master of Philosophy degree in 1990 and a Doctorate in 1999, both from the University of Leeds. Employment by the College of Occupational Therapists from 1998 to 2001 helped to marry her previously parallel research and occupational therapy careers. Gail now works at Sheffield Hallam University as Director of the Centre for Health and Social Care Research, where she is responsible for research within and across eight professional groups including allied health, nursing and social work.

■ Susan Nancarrow

Susan is a senior research fellow and primary care research coordinator with Trent Research and Development Support Unit, based at the University of Sheffield. Her research interests include workforce development and workforce flexibility, especially for allied health professions. Within this, she is interested in the introduction of new roles through the growth of support workers. Susan trained as a podiatrist in Australia and has worked in a range of clinical roles, including aboriginal health, private practice, primary health care delivery in northern India, chief podiatrist and multidisciplinary service manager for a community health service. As a podiatrist, Susan was particularly interested in the lower limb complications associated with diabetes. She completed her PhD in health services research at the Australian National University before moving to the UK in late 2001 to work as a senior lecturer at Sheffield Hallam University.

■ Beverly Palin

Bev is a Registered General Nurse and is currently a community nurse coordinator/caseload holder for the intermediate care service in Staffordshire, England.

Intermediate care is a rehabilitation service that supports discharge from hospital and prevents admission to hospital. It is a multidisciplinary service which supports the client to reach their optimum independence, within their own home. Bev is responsible for the assessment, care allocation, evaluation and discharge of all clients within her own caseload. She supports rehabilitation workers during their national vocational qualifications. She has devised a self medication training programme for staff, and has also been a nutritional link nurse.

■ Darren Perry

Darren Perry is a clinical psychologist working in north Staffordshire. As an integral member of a multidisciplinary stroke team, he contributes to the psychological care of stroke survivors and their carers in acute and rehabilitation ward settings as well as in the community. He has a special interest in psychological adjustment to illness, neuropsychological impairment and ageing. He provides regular teaching and training to nursing and therapy staff on the provision of non-specialist psychological care for hospital in-patients. In addition, he contributes to local training programmes for rehabilitation support workers, physiotherapists, clinical psychologists and psychiatrists. He is currently studying a post-doctoral qualification in clinical neuropsychology at the University of Nottingham and is involved in research and audit projects to examine psychological and neuropsychological aspects of stroke rehabilitation.

■ Martin Ridgeway

Martin's career in occupational therapy began in 1998. He was employed by Stoke-on-Trent Social Services Disability Resource Team as an occupational therapy assistant. This role and the work environment helped him to develop the valuable self-management, communication, professional and interpersonal skills necessary to work effectively, confidently and competently in this specialised area of occupational therapy. In 2000, following some independent study covering social welfare and human biology, he secured a place on the BSc (Hons) in Occupational Therapy training course at the University of Derby as a part-time student. In 2004 he qualified as an occupational therapist and has continued to practice occupational therapy in a community multidisciplinary team for Staffordshire Social Services.

■ Bob Spall

Bob Spall is an experienced clinical psychologist with a special interest in loss issues and he has extensive experience of staff training in relation to palliative care. He has worked with a wide range of adults with psychological difficulties, in recent years focusing more on older clients with psychological problems relating to physical ill health and their carers. Also, he has wide experience of teaching various professional groups and of supervising trainee clinical psychologists from university courses in the Midlands and the north-west of the UK. Currently he leads a small team specialising in work with older adults, and the team, in addition to providing a clinical service, provides training, for example in relation to psychological care for staff from various disciplines. Team members also carry out applied research relating to helping older people and their carers overcome psychological difficulties.

■ Christine Sutton

Christine qualified as an occupational therapist in 1979. Since then she has worked within various hospital and community settings in Sheffield, Cheshire and Staffordshire, UK. Since 1992 she has worked within the primary care setting in north Staffordshire, working in the community and providing rehabilitation to young adults and the elderly who present with a wide range of physical disabilities. Since 2002, she has been a head occupational therapist, managing the primary care occupational therapy service in Stoke-on-Trent. She developed a special interest in continence, undertaking study in the subject, and organised a local conference for the occupational therapy service to raise awareness and increase knowledge of the therapist's role in promoting continence and managing incontinence issues with the client. Christine has presented at the Association for Continence Advice Annual Conference (2003) and represented the occupational therapy service at meetings and training sessions to promote the therapist's role. Currently, she is undertaking a secondment one day a week with the local Continence Advisory Service to investigate and develop the occupational therapist's role within this area.

■ Julie Vickerman

Clinical specialist/research occupational therapist.

Julie qualified as an occupational therapist in 1983 and has worked in a variety of clinical areas including learning disability, acute medicine, cardiac rehabilitation, and community equipment and adaptation. In 2000 she became the first clinical specialist occupational therapist in the UK to work in the field of continence care. She is a member of the multiprofessional continence team in Chorley, Lancashire, UK. This team consists of a nurse, physiotherapist and occupational therapist working within a dedicated continence service. They were winners of the Department of Health Primary Care Award in July 2003. Julie also has a part-time seconded post with PromoCon, Disabled Living, Manchester, UK. This research post focuses on raising the national profile of the occupational therapist's role in continence promotion. One aspect of this work involves delivering teaching packages to under- and postgraduate occupational therapists. She has presented at several national conferences and has published papers on the subject. Her particular interest is in the impact of functional impairment on the ability to maintain continence.

■ Claudia von Zweck

Claudia von Zweck is the Executive Director of the Canadian Association of Occupational Therapists (CAOT), a national voluntary professional association representing over 7100 members across Canada. Claudia has published papers on a broad range of topics relating to occupational therapy practice, including evidence based practice, health human resource planning and the role of support workers.

Before coming to CAOT in 1995, Claudia worked in health care administration as a quality improvement specialist. Claudia also worked as an occupational therapist in a variety of settings, including rehabilitation centres, home care and a regional children's treatment centre. Claudia's educational background includes a Master of Science in Community Health and Epidemiology from Queen's University, Ontario, and a Bachelor of Science in Occupational Therapy from the University of Toronto. She is currently pursuing her doctorate in rehabilitation sciences at Queen's University.

■ Freda Vrantsidis

Bachelor of Behavioural Science, Graduate Diploma in Information Services. Research Fellow, National Ageing Research Institute, Parkville, Victoria, Australia.

Freda has worked for the National Ageing Research Institute for over five years as a project officer, mainly in the falls prevention area. She has worked with a range of health professionals, been involved in falls prevention activities in the sub-acute hospital and residential aged care settings, and participated in an evaluation of four acute hospital falls prevention projects. In 2004 she was involved in updating a literature review of the effectiveness of falls prevention interventions for the Australian Government, Department of Health and Ageing and the development of a community based falls prevention guide.

Glossary of terms

Activity analysis is a detailed examination of an activity, breaking it down into sequences of component tasks and identifying the skills required to perform these tasks.

Adaptation is the process by which the individual adjusts to changes in their environment in a way that allows them to continue to function.

Aim: a brief statement of the general purpose of the rehabilitation programme.

Anxiety is a feeling of apprehension, worry, unease, fear of the future or dread.

Aphasia is language impairment where the client is unable to communicate and/or comprehend speech and/or the written word.

Apraxia is a problem with planning and coordinating the muscles for movement patterns.

Assessment is the critical appraisal of a client's interests and capabilities using subjective and objective data, which is relevant to the preparation of an intervention plan.

Assumption: an acceptance that something is true without testing the evidence for it.

Case management is a collaborative process which assesses, plans, implements, coordinates, monitors and evaluates the options and services required to meet an individual's needs to promote cost effective outcomes.

Case manager: individual assigned to the role of case management. See also key worker.

Chaining is a technique in which an activity is broken down into segments for the client to learn sequentially. Forward chaining is carrying the task from the first step until completion. Backward chaining starts with the last step in the task and works backwards in sequence to the first step.

Client: the individual who seeks the services of the rehabilitation worker.

Cognition is the mental activity of perceiving, thinking, understanding and reasoning.

Compensatory techniques are used to compensate for physical or cognitive deficits in performance, for example the provision of assistive equipment, or the teaching of a new technique.

Competence is the ability to perform skills to a level that allows the satisfactory performance of roles.

Compliance: adherence to a treatment regime.

Confidentiality is the principle of only sharing information about clients with those who have a need to know it in order to benefit the client, or when the safety of others may be at risk.

Culture: the collective attitudes, beliefs and behaviour that characterise a particular social group over time. The group may range from racial groupings, to a social class, a locality or a particular workforce.

Depression is a mood disorder characterised by feelings of hopelessness and sadness.

Development is the progressive and continuous change in shape, function and integration of the body from birth to death.

Disability is any restriction or lack of ability to perform an activity in the manner or within the range considered normal for a human being.

Disease is a matter of pathology and medical diagnosis that may or may not lead to physical or mental impairment. The presence of disease does not necessarily cause symptoms, illness, disability or incapacity.

Dysarthria is difficulty speaking due to damage or weakness of the muscles used to make the sounds for speaking.

Dysfunction is the inability to maintain the self at a satisfactory level because of a lack of the necessary skills.

Empowerment is the process that enables people to take control and responsibility for their own lives, to enjoy the rights and responsibilities of active citizenship, and to fulfil a social role that contributes to their own and also to other people's wellbeing.

Enabling is a facilitation process through which people have the means and opportunity to be involved in solving their own problems, or is an action by the rehabilitation worker to assist an individual to perform activities more easily.

Energy conservation is the technique used to enable a client to achieve maximum function with limited energy expenditure.

Environmental adaptation is changing the physical or social features of an environment to enhance performance.

Feedback is information about the consequences of the actions taken by a person performing a skill.

FIP notes: a type of progress note which documents findings, interpretation, plan. See also SOAP notes.

Function is the possession of the skills necessary for successful participation in the range of roles expected of the individual.

Goal is a concise statement of a defined outcome to be attained at a particular stage in the rehabilitation programme. Goals may be short or long-term.

Group dynamics is the study of the factors and conditions that affect the actions in a group.

Impairment is any loss or abnormality of physiological, psychological, or anatomical structure or function.

Incoherence is incomprehensible speech or thinking.

Interdisciplinary team comprises individuals from different disciplines who work cooperatively to achieve the client's treatment goals.

Intervention refers to the application of treatments, techniques, methods, drugs or surgery to improve the client's condition.

Isometric exercise: contraction of muscles without moving a joint.

Isotonic exercise: contraction of muscles which involves movement of a joint.

Joint protection involves instructing clients in ways to manage personal, domestic and work activities in a manner which reduces or eliminates potentially damaging stresses on vulnerable joints.

Key worker: the person who has the main responsibility for relating to a client and is the main point of contact.

Monitoring is the process of keeping a regular check to ensure that any significant changes are noticed.

Motivation is the force that causes people to act.

Multidisciplinary team comprises professionals from various disciplines who assess and treat clients autonomously and meet regularly to coordinate treatment.

Occupation is the culturally and personally meaningful activity that an individual engages in over a period of time.

Orthotics is the assessment for, design of, production and fitting of orthoses (splints) for functional or supportive purposes.

Pacing involves techniques which enable the individual to perform activities or tasks in a preplanned manner involving timed activity and rest periods, in order to maximise effective performance and minimise undesirable consequences.

Perception is the capacity to recognise sensory stimuli (visual, tactile, auditory and proprioceptive) in a meaningful way.

Peripheral neuropathy: damage to the peripheral nerves (commonly the feet and hands) causing loss of sensation.

Physiology is the science of functions and phenomena of living organisms and their parts.

Problem solving is the set of cognitive strategies used to resolve difficulties.

Prognosis is a clinical forecast of the probable course of an illness and the eventual outcome of the disease or condition.

Re-enablement: a comprehensive programme of activities delivered by a team which aims to work with a client and their family or carers to maximise the client's wellbeing and help them adapt to changing life circumstances.

Relaxation consists of various methods of voluntary physical or mental control designed to produce physical and mental relaxation and relieve the effect of stress or anxiety.

Role-play involves the use of drama techniques and improvisation to enable clients to act out roles or situations which they wish to explore.

Self-efficacy is the individual's perception of being able to perform a functional task or occupation.

Self-esteem is the individual's appraisal of his/her competencies and abilities to master situations which confront them.

SOAP notes: a system for documenting client progress notes using the headings subjective, objective, assessment, plan.

Social skills training consists of educational programmes designed to improve skills in interaction and acceptable social behaviour.

Vocational rehabilitation: the process whereby clients are helped to access, maintain or return to employment or other useful occupation.

Section 1
The tools of enabling independence

- Introduction
- Agreeing and reaching goals
- Teaching for rehabilitation

Introduction

Susan Nancarrow & Hazel Mackey

In the developed world, people are living longer and enjoying more extended periods of active life than ever before. At the same time, there is a growing trend to keep people out of hospitals and, where possible, avoid admission to long-term residential care. This means that more and more people are returning to the community following acute and sometimes disabling illnesses like strokes, or remaining at home for longer periods after a diagnosis with a progressive or terminal disease.

As a society, we are altering the way we manage many conditions, as well as changing our expectations after illness. We no longer expect that an 80-year-old woman who has a fall and fractures her hip will stay in bed for the rest of her life. Instead, she is likely to be discharged from hospital within two weeks and resume relatively normal activities within a few months. Advances in technology mean that people can be helped to regain much of the function they had before a bad fall, fractured hip, or a stroke. Many people now expect to be able to return to their pre-illness level of functioning.

Some people will regain full function after an acute or disabling illness or accident. However, in some instances they will never recover their previous level of function. Instead, they might need to learn a new way of doing the things that they did previously, change their approach to what they do, or have their environment altered in a way that simplifies their activity. These changes mean that people need to have the skills and ability to remain independent in their chosen environment.

This book is for workers who are involved with clients during the phase of their care when they are starting to regain some of their previous skills, confidence and abilities. It is also designed to help clients who have developmental delay who might be learning some of these skills for the first time. This book aims to provide you, as a rehabilitation worker, with the skills that you need to help the client become more independent in their functioning, as well as working with families and carers to help them support the client to achieve their goals.

We have chosen to use the term 'client' in this book, rather than patient, consumer or service user. The term 'patient', whilst clear, was felt to imply dependence rather than reinforce the enabling philosophy of rehabilitation and enablement. The word 'service user' could become confused with the other beneficiaries of the service, including carers or the client's family. The rehabilitation workers and clients we consulted were generally uncomfortable with the term 'consumer'. So, for the purpose of consistency, we have adopted the term client to refer to the main recipient of the care of the rehabilitation worker.

It was easier to reach consensus on the term 'rehabilitation worker' to describe the person delivering care, as this reflects the role of the worker, and can encompass a wide range of disciplines. However, it is important to acknowledge that rehabilitation workers can have a number of different titles, and may include support workers, therapists, social workers, therapy assistants, re-enablement support workers, pharmacists, counsellors and psychologists, to mention only a few. In many cases, the work of a rehabilitation worker will include components of all of these roles, and more. As a result, this book has been written with input from a range of different disciplines to provide an interdisciplinary perspective on the diversity of roles and tasks delivered by rehabilitation workers.

■ Who are rehabilitation workers?

For the purpose of this book, rehabilitation workers include any staff member involved in the delivery of rehabilitation or re-enablement that is designed to optimise the functioning of clients within their chosen environment. This could include all of the members of a multidisciplinary team involved in providing rehabilitation, including allied health practitioners, social care providers, assistant practitioners, support workers, nurses and medical practitioners. However, the book is primarily designed for workers with an interdisciplinary role who spend a great deal of time working closely with the client in a rehabilitation environment.

Rehabilitation workers are not new, and have existed in many different guises for at least two decades in some areas. However, there has been a recent rapid growth in the numbers of rehabilitation workers in Australia, Canada, the USA and the UK. In the UK, for instance, it is now rare to find a community rehabilitation team that does not employ at least one rehabilitation worker. The increase in rehabilitation workers appears to be the result of a number of factors. There is a growing interest in interdisciplinary working as a way of improving client-centred care, and rehabilitation workers are ideally placed to provide an interprofessional role within these teams. Additionally, with shortages in doctors, nurses and allied health professionals, there is recognition that some of the tasks that have traditionally been performed by these workers can be carried out by other staff.

This book is designed to help workers involved in the rehabilitation process whose roles fall across a number of traditional boundaries. As a rehabilitation worker, you are likely to be in a position where you spend quite a lot of time with each client, so you have time to get to know them and their family, and possibly understand their needs and environment in a way that other types of workers may not. You may work with a number of different types

Introduction

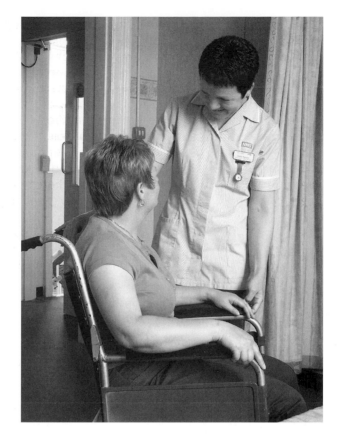

Figure 1 Rehabilitation worker with a client.

of staff, such as physiotherapists, occupational therapists, speech and language therapists, social workers, dieticians, podiatrists, general practitioners, psychologists and nurses. Sometimes, any or all of these workers might leave instructions for you to carry out with the client. Sometimes, you might identify a need for the client to see one of these workers.

Stop and think

Mrs Maloney lives alone and suffers from frequent falls. She is referred to a rehabilitation team that includes a physiotherapist, occupational therapist, podiatrist, nurse, social worker, general practitioner and a rehabilitation worker. What role do you think each team member will contribute to Mrs Maloney's rehabilitation?

Because of your relatively unique position, working so closely with the client and a variety of staff, you need to have a wide range of different types of skills. Possibly the most important of these are your communication skills, and an ability and willingness to contact the right person at the right time, and to ask questions.

This book aims to prepare you to work within an interdisciplinary team, identify appropriate goals for a client and work within a team to help deliver those goals. It presents a range of scenarios that you are likely to encounter when you are delivering rehabilitation support.

One of the challenges that we had preparing this book was the wide range of different perspectives and philosophies of each member of the rehabilitation team. Each of those perspectives is important and valuable. For instance, in the above example of Mrs Maloney, the roles of the different workers might include the following:

■ The occupational therapist may examine the environmental risks that contribute to falling.
■ The physiotherapist could look at the client's strength and balance.
■ The podiatrist might treat any foot problems and advise on footwear.
■ The nurse could undertake a medication review to identify any drugs that the client is taking that may decrease their stability.
■ The rehabilitation worker may be involved in delivering the intervention plan on a regular basis.
■ The general practitioner (GP) may look for any underlying pathology that could be causing the frequent falls, such as a urinary tract infection.
■ The social worker may be involved in assessing Mrs Maloney for a care package to provide meals on a regular basis.

These are stereotypical examples of the roles of the different team members, and it is likely that many of the different team members' roles will overlap. However, it is true that each of those team members will have received different training and will perceive the needs and possible intervention for Mrs Maloney differently. Given current approaches to health provider training that focus on bodies of knowledge that reflect professional philosophies, rather than holistic approaches to the treatment of specific conditions, it is unlikely that one single health care provider could treat all of the factors that contribute to the client's risk of falling.

This is not to devalue the importance of the professional input. But the added value that you bring to the multidisciplinary team is often a broad understanding of the client's needs. Part of the approach we have used in this book is a problem-solving approach that lets you use your own experience, knowledge and values to work with the client to understand their needs, and then consider a wide range of possibilities for the management of those needs, rather than seeing the problem as a 'physiotherapy problem' or an 'occupational therapy problem' or a 'podiatry problem'.

It is important to reinforce the point that whilst rehabilitation workers may work under the direction of a range of other professionals, you play a vital role in the team in ensuring that the client is viewed holistically. As a member of a rehabilitation team, you are responsible for the outcomes of your work with the client. As a result, it is your responsibility to ensure that you have the right skills to perform your job and have the appropriate support mechanisms in place.

■ Re-enablement and rehabilitation

Case study Mr Jones

Mr Jones was referred to a therapist by his GP after he was discharged from hospital following a stroke. The therapist identified that one of his goals was to be able to tie up his shoelaces so that he could go walking. The therapist decided that Mr Jones' main problem was that he did not have enough flexion in his spine and decided that the treatment should focus on increasing his spinal range of motion. After six episodes of therapy and some home exercises, his spinal range of motion had increased significantly. The therapist deemed that the treatment was successful and that Mr Jones could be discharged. However, Mr Jones could still not tie his shoelaces.

The World Health Organization has been credited as describing rehabilitation as the combined and coordinated use of medical, social, educational and vocational measures for training or retraining the individual to the highest possible level of functional ability.

Re-enablement is a relatively new concept which describes a comprehensive programme of activities, delivered by a team that aims to work with a client and their family or carers to maximise the client's wellbeing and help them adapt to changing life circumstances (Royal College of Nursing, 2000).

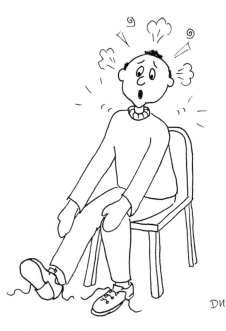

Figure 2 Mr Jones attempting to tie his shoelaces.

The terms rehabilitation and re-enablement have very similar meanings and are often used interchangeably. The approach used in this book is a re-enabling approach to rehabilitation. Re-enablement is person centred. In other words, it is planned with the client around their goals, needs and existing circumstances. It recognises that the client is generally the person with the greatest expertise and understanding about themselves and their own needs. Re-enablement also involves those close to the client, including their families, carers and friends. In the rather extreme case study of Mr Jones, re-enablement would have focused on achieving the client's goals through the use of a holistic perspective, rather than focusing on a specific therapeutic outcome from the perspective of a single practitioner.

The purpose of re-enablement is:

■ To help people live in the community safely and efficiently.
■ To optimise the independence of the client in their own home by helping them learn or re-learn the skills they require for daily living and to restore confidence.
■ To prevent avoidable hospital admissions.
■ To reduce the level of ongoing care needed (when appropriate).

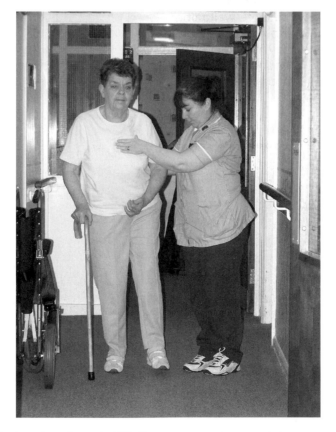

Figure 3 Client undergoing rehabilitation.

Re-enablement should include the following components (Ford et al, 2000):

▪ **Support**: the rehabilitation worker should ensure that the client's basic emotional and psychosocial support needs are met. This should be done in a culturally sensitive way, it should facilitate self-expression and take account of the client's relationships with other people.

▪ **Restore function:** re-enablement incorporates the principles of rehabilitation to help the client optimise their ability to do day-to-day tasks and prevent further deterioration. This may include adaptation of the environment, re-learning old skills, or learning new ways to undertake previous skills. This might include rehabilitation in mobility, transfers, kitchen activities and leisure activities.

▪ **Promote independence:** re-enablement promotes independence by providing education and advice to clients and their carers to promote health and safety in their home. It encourages independence by teaching the client self-care activities. This can include independence in their basic activities of daily living, such as bathing and dressing or managing their medications. It may also involve working with the client's family or carer to provide them with skills necessary to support the client in their environment.

▪ **Enhance wellbeing:** working with the client towards their own goals to improve quality of life but also to promote their basic health care. This may include providing pain relief, nutritional advice and support, and promoting safety in the home to prevent accidents. You may also be required to change health damaging habits or to prevent ill health evolving into a

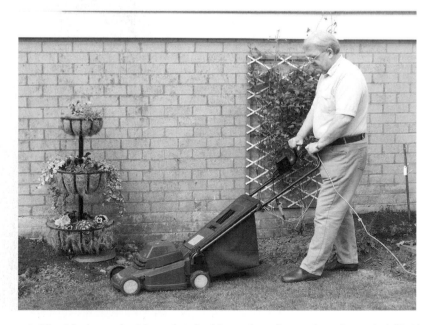

Figure 4 Client independent in caring for his garden after undergoing rehabilitation.

chronic stage. This could involve working with a range of different agencies that deal with the environment and housing.

Re-enablement should be focused around a structured care plan that is based on achieving realistic client goals within a specified timeframe. Re-enablement should emphasise the needs/desires of the client rather than the goals of the therapist and should be written and expressed in client-centred terms. For instance, the goal should be explained as 'the client is able to tie his shoelaces', rather than 'the client should be able to achieve five degrees of flexion in their spine'. The client-centred goal will orient your treatment towards a holistic way of addressing needs, rather than focusing on the discipline specific, therapeutic outcome.

Re-enablement is different from the provision of personal care in a number of ways. Personal care is normally done 'for' or 'to' a client, whereas re-enablement works closely with the client to help them help themselves. For instance, if someone has just come home from hospital following a stroke, and has difficulty using the left side of their body, a rehabilitation worker could work with that client to help them to become independent in making a cup of tea. This is different to a personal carer, who would probably make the cup of tea for the client, and possibly even prepare some meals for them.

There is a big difference between these two approaches. As you are aware, it only takes about five minutes to make a cup of tea for someone. But helping someone who may have difficulties communicating, or moving parts of their body, to make a cup of tea could be a very slow and frustrating process, and may take an hour or more. In fact, the first few times you attempt it, it may only be possible for the client to do some steps towards making the cup of tea before they become tired. Or you may recognise that it is not possible for the client to make a cup of tea at all because they cannot reach the cupboard where the tea bags are kept, or have difficulty turning on the taps.

You can see that to make that client independent in their own home could take some time, require modifications to the person's home (such as taps and storage) and might involve learning some new skills, or re-learning some old skills that have been altered by their underlying condition.

The book focuses on ensuring that individuals can function, to the best of their ability, in their chosen environment. We look at optimising function from two perspectives, by supporting the person so they have the ability to do certain physical activities designed to keep them independent and by adapting the environment to make sure it is as supportive as it can be.

Independence and interdependence

It is important to be aware of the distinction between independence and interdependence. Whilst each of our clients is a unique individual, they are also part of broader, interpersonal relationships which play an important role in rehabilitation. For example, Mr Jones is Jennifer's father and Patrick's friend. As part of her role as a 'daughter', Jennifer has always done Mr Jones' laundry, and as a 'friend' Patrick has always driven Mr Jones to the supermarket. Now that Mr Jones is undergoing rehabilitation, he could be encouraged to become more independent and learn how to make his own way to the supermarket, or learn how to do his own laundry. However, if Mr Jones, Jennifer and Patrick are happy with the current arrangements, there is little motivation to change. The relationship between Mr Jones, Patrick and Jennifer is an interdependent relationship.

Sometimes, however, you may be involved in a situation where one person wishes to renegotiate the tasks that go with their role. Jennifer still wants to be a daughter but now works full time, so has little time to do her father's laundry, or Mr Jones may want to arrange his own transport to the supermarket so that he is not tied to Patrick's routine. In this case, your role is to help the individual adapt and to integrate new roles and obligations into a daily pattern of living.

Part of the re-enablement approach to rehabilitation is to ensure that the client is integrated into their social circle or wider community in a way that is appropriate for them. Making a client fully independent may limit their social interactions and lead to isolation. It is important to negotiate with the client and their support networks the appropriate levels of independence and interdependence to enable them to achieve their goals in a sustainable way.

▦ Client-centred practice

Client-centred practice aims to create a supportive, dignified and empowering environment in which clients direct the course of their care. The terms 'person-centred' or 'patient-centred' are used frequently now to describe approaches to delivering health and social services. You might think that all services should be centred around the person or people they are designed to help; however, this is frequently not the case. Or at least, many services could be better designed to support clients.

The original approaches to person-centred care were designed to reduce inefficiencies resulting from the fragmentation and specialisation of hospital based services. Client-centred practice means that services are arranged around client needs rather than around buildings, equipment or staff requirements. The following principles distinguish client-centred practice:

- ▫ Grouping clients with similar needs.
- ▫ Bringing the services closer to the client.
- ▫ The use of staff who have a wide range of skills and who often work across professional boundaries within dedicated teams.
- ▫ The use of care protocols and integrated client records.

All over the world, health services are being rearranged to try to improve client-centred care using strategies with names like 'collaborative practice', 'flexible working', 'care management', the 'single assessment process', and 'streamlined services'. Client-centred practice is claimed to benefit clients and staff in many ways, including improvements in readmission rates, client and carer satisfaction, reduced staff absenteeism and sickness, reduced complication rates and errors.

In delivering client-centred care, staff need to listen to the client; respect their dignity and privacy; recognise individual needs; ensure clients can access information to help them make informed decisions; provide coordinated and integrated care; and involve and support carers.

■ International Classification of Functioning, Disability and Health

The World Health Organization (WHO) has developed the International Classification of Functioning, Disability and Health (ICF) as a way of describing the impact of a health condition. Instead of focusing on the diagnosis or particular health conditions, the ICF provides a way to look at the consequences of a range of conditions, including their impact on the physical, emotional and psychosocial ability of someone to function independently in their own environment. The ICF has been adopted by many different professions and in a number of different countries as a bio-psychosocial model of functioning.

This model is particularly valuable in rehabilitation, where it is rare to be treating the actual underlying disease. Instead, rehabilitation tends to focus on managing the impact of the underlying disease by improving a client's ability to perform activities and participate in society. In some cases, the limitations in activity and participation will stem from a range of different pathologies, or from underlying social circumstances. The ICF provides a way to look at the impact on the client (see Figure 5).

Case study Mandy

Mandy is an artist who used to teach painting and drawing as part of a local adult education programme. She developed cataracts which gradually reduced her eyesight to the point that she could no longer see to paint or teach painting. Her blindness also stopped her driving.

Using the ICF framework, her underlying *health condition* was the cataracts.

■ The impact on her *body function* was the impairment of her eyesight.
■ Her *activity* limitation is that she is unable do her art any more and she is unable to drive.
■ The impact on her *participation* is that she can no longer do her paid job as an artist.

■ Promoting health

Rehabilitation tends to occur after the client has experienced some sort of trauma or event that has had the effect of reducing their previous functional status. Obviously, it would be ideal to prevent the problem arising in the first place.

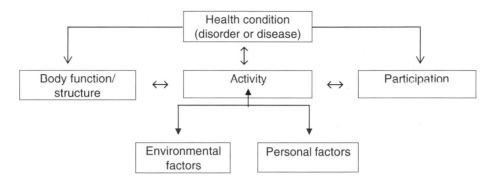

Figure 5 WHO International Classification of Functioning, Disability and Health. Adapted from the World Health Organization International Classification of Functioning, Disability and Health (WHO, 2001).

By keeping the principles of prevention in mind whilst you are enabling independence, you may be able to help keep the client independent even longer and reduce the potential for future accidents or traumatic events.

There are three commonly used levels of prevention: primary, secondary and tertiary.

■ **Primary prevention** aims to reduce the risks of ill health and disability arising in the healthy population. This includes large-scale approaches such as road traffic policies which aim to reduce the number of road traffic accidents and therefore prevent the resulting death or disability. It also includes environmental safety, for instance creating a safe environment to prevent slips, trips and falls. Ensuring that the client has a healthy, well-balanced diet is also a form of primary prevention.

■ **Secondary prevention** involves the early detection of a problem, followed by the introduction of an appropriate intervention. It is designed to reduce the risks in groups who already have risk factors for particular conditions, or to restore those people to their former state of health. An example of secondary prevention is the introduction of falls prevention classes for people who are at risk of falling.

■ **Tertiary prevention** involves working with clients who already have a chronic condition, to reduce the impact of the condition and help them make the most of their potential. This can include the provision of rehabilitation and re-enablement, which can include education and advice.

As a rehabilitation worker you are ideally placed to identify possibilities for promoting good health and preventing future accidents or illness at all three stages. Thoughts about future prevention should feature in a good intervention plan. When you are working with a client, try to consider the ways that you can contribute to their future health promotion. This could include modifications to the environment to make it safer for the client, their family, and for you as a worker in that environment. You may direct the client to appropriate health promoting courses or classes such as exercise, balance or coordination classes.

Consider the individual needs of the client and the local resources and facilities available.

■ How to use this book

This book has four sections:

- ■ Section 1 provides the background and philosophy to the process of re-enablement and rehabilitation. We talk about the specific skills that a rehabilitation worker needs to optimise independence, and the processes of assessment, goal setting and intervention planning. This section also describes the teaching skills you will need as a rehabilitation worker to enable independence in your client and their support networks.
- ■ Section 2 discusses the key activities you are likely to need to go through to improve a client's function or help to keep them independent in their own environment. These include practical activities of daily living, such as washing, dressing and eating, but also engagement in the wider social environment. We use a series of eight case studies to illustrate the key points for each of the activities, and to highlight some common conditions that you are likely to experience in your work.
- ■ Section 3 identifies some specific issues that you are likely to encounter in the enablement process, including communication issues, incontinence, the risk of falling, memory loss and psychological problems.
- ■ Section 4 provides information to support you in your role as a rehabilitation worker. We discuss the organisation and context in which you are likely to work, and discuss some of the issues you might encounter in this setting, particularly around teamworking and supervision. We examine the issues around lifelong learning, and discuss the implications of carer support.

Often, in dealing with some of the more complex aspects of rehabilitation you will need to ask 'Why?' Why is this person behaving like this? Why is this happening? Why do I feel like this? To help you reflect on key topics we have included 'Stop and think' boxes. These are designed to help you to think about the issues and decide your own views of them. We recommend that you complete these exercises as a useful way of clarifying and deepening your understanding of important issues.

To facilitate further study there is a suggested reading list at the end of each chapter. Here you will find suggestions for further reading on specific topic areas as well as details of Internet resources you may wish to explore.

Rehabilitation is complex work that relies on an extensive knowledge base and a wide range of skills. This book will, we hope, go some way towards helping you develop a much firmer grasp of that knowledge base. If you already have a lot of experience in working in rehabilitation you are likely to have developed a broad knowledge base. However, it is also possible that you have developed your understanding gradually, over time, in a piecemeal way. This book should help you link those elements of knowledge together into a more coherent and consistent framework of understanding.

It must be emphasised that this book will not provide you with all the information and knowledge you need. The knowledge base relevant to your work is far too great to be condensed into a book of this size. Therefore we have focused on what we consider to be key areas. What is offered here is an introductory foundation to your studies which should provide you with:

■ A basic introduction to the relevant subject areas.
■ The opportunity to reflect on how your experience fits in and reflects the knowledge base.
■ Exercises to help you to recognise and consolidate the knowledge base underpinning your work.
■ A set of guidelines on how to continue developing your knowledge and skills.

■ Further reading

Ford, P., McCormack, B., Willis, T. and Dewing, J. (2000) Defining the boundaries: nursing and personal care. *Nursing Standard*, 15 (3) 43–45.

Hagedorn, R. (2001) *Foundations for Practice in Occupational Therapy* (3rd edition). London, Churchill Livingstone.

Royal College of Nursing (2000) *The Role of the Nurse in the Rehabilitation of Older People*. London, Royal College of Nursing.

WHO International Classification of Functioning. Retrieved 10 November 2005 from http://www.who.int/classifications/icf

Agreeing and reaching goals

Susan Nancarrow

Introduction

This chapter provides an overview of the steps that a team will go through when planning and assessing client care, from the initial referral until discharge. It includes a discussion of the issues around the agreement of the goals with the client and their carer, the processes of documenting those goals, discharge planning and writing discharge summaries.

The process of rehabilitation

The process of rehabilitation involves working closely with a client and their family or carer to help them progress from their current state of functioning to a more optimal level of function. This requires an understanding of the current level of function of that client, as well as an understanding of what they would like to achieve, and the support available to them to make the changes. You need ways to measure when you have been successful in achieving the goals of the client, or at least made improvements.

For the purpose of this book we will describe the whole package of care, from the point of referral until discharge as an *episode of care*. The episode of care includes the input from all of the members of the multidisciplinary team whilst the client is registered with the service. If the client is discharged from the service and then readmitted, then that constitutes a new episode of care. In a rehabilitation setting, an episode of care could last anything from a single visit right up to a number of weeks or months, but it should be time limited.

Each individual session with the client by any practitioner is one *occasion of service*. An occasion of service could be very short, as little as five minutes if it is just a check-up or follow-up visit, or it could last for many hours. For instance, the initial assessment may last for a couple of hours. An episode of care is therefore made up of a number of different occasions of service that are delivered by a number of different health and social care providers.

The services designed to deliver rehabilitation can be broken down into a number of parts. Most clients will have an episode of care that includes the following components:

- A *referral* into the service.
- *Screening* to determine the appropriateness of the referral.
- An *assessment* of the client.
- *Setting goals*.
- An *intervention plan* that is designed to meet those goals.
- A *re-evaluation* to review the goals and achievement of the goals, and ensure that the intervention remains appropriate.
- *Discharge* from the service.
- *Follow-up*.

It is normal in a rehabilitation setting to have a team involved in the delivery of the intervention. The team may include the physiotherapist, occupational therapist, speech and language therapist, podiatrist, psychologist, nurse, rehabilitation assistant, social worker, dietician, pharmacist and the general practitioner. Other practitioners may be involved as well, depending on the type of service you work for, and the goals of the client. For instance, the team may include a specialist medical practitioner and/or complementary and alternative therapists. The chapter in Section 4 on Teamworking and supervision describes some of the different ways that teams may work together to help achieve the goals of the client.

▪ Referral

The referral is normally the first point of client contact with the service. Referrals can come from a number of different sources. The client may be referred by another practitioner, such as a general practitioner or physiotherapist; from another type of team or service; or sometimes from a hospital discharge planner. In some cases, the client may refer himself or herself to the service. A good referral that comes from another practitioner or service should include a letter or telephone call that provides some basic information about the client, their needs, and the reason for their referral to the service.

When you are working as part of a multidisciplinary team, there are often clear guidelines about how new referrals are managed. Some services have a single point of contact where all referrals are directed. Someone at that point of contact will decide on the most appropriate course of action for that referral. In other services, the referrals come to all members of the multidisciplinary team who decide jointly on the outcome of the referral. Some services direct the referrals to senior members of the multidisciplinary team to undertake the screening and assessment.

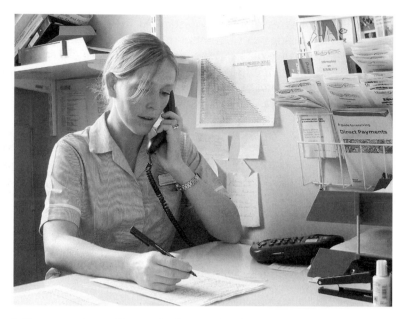

Figure 1 Team member taking a telephone referral.

The way that the referrals are managed will impact on the ability of your service to screen the referral and determine how quickly your service needs to respond to the referral.

Stop and think

Do you know what the protocol is for managing new referrals within your service?

■ Screening

Screening is the way that your service determines whether or not the referral is appropriate for the client. The types of questions that screening can answer include 'Is this the right setting to help this client?' and 'Can our service meet the needs of this client?' or 'Is there another service that could better meet the needs of this client?' In some cases, there may be eligibility criteria that clients need to meet to be able to access your service, such as geographical boundaries of the service or limits based on age, diagnosis or socio-economic status.

Screening can also have the important function of enabling the service to *prioritise* access to care. Prioritisation enables the service to dedicate resources to those clients who have the greatest or most urgent need. This is sometimes called 'triage'.

Screening is particularly important in rehabilitation services to ensure that your team can meet the needs of that client. For instance, many services that provide rehabilitation assume that the clients are medically stable, so access to medical care may be limited. It may be inappropriate to take a referral for a client who requires intravenous antibiotics if your service cannot provide access to nursing care. Clients with mental health problems may require access to a wider range of services to aid the rehabilitation process and you need to be clear about whether you have access to the right services to be able to help these clients.

Your service should have clear guidelines around what constitutes an appropriate referral, and any eligibility criteria. This will simplify the screening process, but also makes it easier for referrers to know who they can and cannot direct to your team. If you receive an inappropriate referral, you should notify the person or agency who made the referral, and explain why the referral was inappropriate and suggest a more appropriate service if you are aware of it. Your team may even provide some written guidance, such as brochures or referral proformas to help referrers know what types of clients should be referred to your service.

Stop and think

What are the eligibility criteria for your service?
Does your service have a system of prioritising or 'triaging' clients?

■ Assessment

Once the screener has determined that the service is appropriate for the client, the next stage of the process is the assessment. The assessment is used to find out more information about the client to help with the process of goal setting and intervention planning. It is important to remember that whilst an initial, detailed assessment takes place at the start of the episode of care, the assessment process is continuous and should be reviewed regularly.

A rehabilitative assessment needs to be comprehensive and consider a wide range of needs of the client. As the Introduction highlighted, the focus of rehabilitation is generally less about the medical diagnosis and more about the ability of the client to function within their different environments and participate in society. The assessment needs to take into account a wide range of issues and expectations that are likely to have an effect on what the client wants to achieve, and their ability to achieve their goals. Factors you need to consider include the client's physical, social and emotional status; their normal vocation; the financial resources they have available to support them; the level of support available from family and friends, and cultural issues (See Box 1).

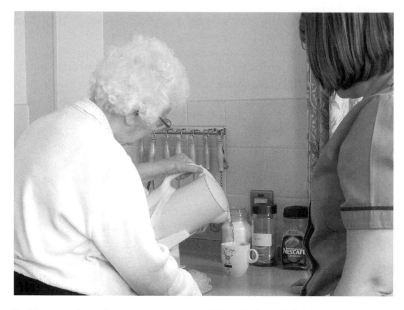

Figure 2 Client undergoing an assessment of her kitchen skills.

Box 1   Factors to consider in the assessment

Previous medical history
Medication history
Communication (level, language, ability)
Movement
Function
Nutrition
Environment (home, work, social)
Recreation
Support structures and family relationships
Goals and expectations of the client and their
  family

Initiative
Attitude towards re-enablement
Motivation levels
Mental and emotional state
Social attitudes
Cultural background
Financial status
Employment or vocational status
Ability and willingness to learn
Spiritual needs

As a rehabilitation worker, you are likely to be involved in constantly assessing and reassessing the client. As a result, your interaction with the client plays an important role in informing the rest of the team about the client's progress, the effectiveness of the intervention, and the need for new or different interventions.

There are many different types of assessment tools. Most professional groups will have their own, discipline specific assessment tool. But there is an increasing focus on 'single assessment tools' that are used by all members of the team. You can find more information about these tools in the chapter in Section 4 on Teamworking and supervision.

The comprehensive nature of the assessment has a number of implications for the way that it is undertaken. The assessment needs to be timely so that it can be performed as soon as the client requires your service. It is very difficult to put appropriate, effective and safe services into place without the information from the initial assessment.

The initial assessment is normally quite time consuming. It is important to allow time so that you can obtain a clear understanding of the needs and abilities of the client, but also to allow you to develop a relationship with that client.

You will often need to involve the family or carer of the client in the assessment process. This helps to clarify the needs and abilities of the client whilst highlighting the expectations of everyone else involved in the day-to-day care of the client.

The assessment should be performed in an environment where the client feels safe. You need to minimise distractions while the assessment takes place and ensure that the client knows that their information will be treated in accordance with the confidentiality policies of the service.

The assessment process needs to be well organised. You should ensure that you have allowed sufficient time to undertake the assessment, and have the tools you require to do the assessment. Many services now use a single assessment proforma that can be completed by one assessor who has been trained to look at a wide range of different issues.

A good assessment requires a skilled assessor. In many cases, the assessor will have to learn specific skills to provide them with the holistic approach they need to evaluate such a broad range of client needs. It is also possible that the assessor might identify specific issues that require further, specialised assessment by another practitioner. For instance, where the assessor identifies specific communication problems, they may ask a speech and language therapist to undertake further assessment. If the assessor notices that the client appears confused and/or distracted, they may refer them to their general practitioner for a more thorough medical assessment to eliminate the possibility of a medical issue such as a urinary tract infection, or to exclude a mental health problem. The assessment tells you what you have to work with. It should give you an idea of the potential of the client to be able to achieve certain rehabilitation goals.

■ Goal setting

Before you decide what intervention you are going to deliver, you need to start with a clear list of the goals of the client which have been carefully considered in light of their potential ability to achieve those goals. For instance, there is no point setting a goal of the client being able to paint the house if the client is unlikely to be able to walk. It is very important in the rehabilitation process to have a set of clear goals that the client, their carer and/or family, as well as the whole multidisciplinary team, are clear about and have agreed on. Those goals should set the target for the whole team to work towards.

We are all familiar with the physical reality of a goal in games such as football. It is a marked area where players attempt to lodge the ball and it is also the act of successfully doing this. As such, it is the focus of all the players' efforts. *Personal goals* are the desires that we hope to achieve. They are not necessarily as physical as a pair of goalposts, but to achieve success they require the same degree of focus as players in a football game.

There are many different kinds of personal goal. Consider these seven goals and think about how they are different from each other.

- Charlie wants better access from his council flat to the street.
- Vinita wants to get on with her teenage daughters.
- Phyllis wants Jack to do more about the house.
- Evelyn wants to visit the guest house where she and her husband used to holiday.
- Bob wants to feel better about his appearance.
- Judy wants a companion.
- Mick and Esther want a good night's sleep.

Some goals are *physical*. For example, Charlie's access to his council flat might entail resources such as a ramp from the street to his flat. Often these resources have *financial* implications. Evelyn's goal will require the finances to travel and pay for the guest house, and perhaps for a carer to accompany her.

Some goals are *psychological*, involving a person's state of mind. Bob's goal is concerned with his feelings about himself and a desire, perhaps, to develop greater self-confidence. Sometimes this involves *relationships*, too, for example Vinita's goal is not just about herself, but includes her daughters. Judy's desire for a companion may be rooted in the wish for a new relationship and the feelings of closeness that this will bring.

Many goals have a combination of all of these elements: physical, financial, psychological and relationship. Evelyn's visit to the guest house may have its roots in a psychological need for nostalgia and closure, to remember her husband and the happy times they had together.

There are other ways in which these goals are different. For example, Bob's goal seems to involve only himself, whilst Mick and Esther have a shared goal. Some goals are about another person: Phyllis wants someone else's behaviour to change (in this case her husband, Jack). Some goals are even about another person who is not yet on the scene, such as Judy's desire for a companion.

These differences lead us to ask questions. For example, how motivated do each of these people feel about their particular goal? For some there will be a strong desire, for others it may just be 'something that would be nice, but I can't see it happening'. Some are more in the control of the person themselves, and others will rely on other people's behaviour, attitude and actions. Some goals might take a long time to achieve, others may be just a few steps away. All in all, we might feel that some of these goals are more likely to be successful than others.

What we find ourselves needing to do is to ask further questions about each of these goals. Until we know why Judy wants a companion, why Mick and Esther are not sleeping well, and why Bob feels bad about his appearance, it is difficult to begin to know how we might help them to achieve their goal. Indeed, it is even more important that the person themself knows *why* the goal is important to them. Does Judy know *why* she wants a companion? Greater knowledge will help everybody know whether the goal is likely to be successful and, if not, in what ways it may need to be modified. The rest of this chapter explores this process in more detail.

Whose goals are important?

One of the biggest obstacles to overcome when agreeing a goal with someone is moving away from *your goal for the person* to the *person's goal for himself or herself*. Although the rhetoric is strong on needs-led assessments, empowerment and user-centred services, the practice can be rather different. The referral process often narrows rather than broadens possibilities, and agencies find ways of excluding people from access to scarce resources by applying strict eligibility criteria. All of these factors can make it difficult to put the rhetoric into reality. Nevertheless, if we are truly to enable independence we must be able to work with a person in their whole context, not just as 'a confused person', 'a deaf person', ' depressed person'. As we will discover later in this chapter, the process of agreeing goals and helping people to achieve them is a skilled one, and it takes time.

It is not just the agency's goals which may be at variance with this process. There might be conflicting goals within a family or community. Enabling independence through the achievement of goals means finding ways of reconciling conflicting goals. Vinita may want her daughters to behave in ways which do not meet their own aspirations, and her daughters may have goals of which Vinita disapproves. However, perhaps they *can* agree that their lives would be better if they could learn to respect these differences. With your help, they may be able to agree a common goal which opens up communication between them, and which gives practical assistance to Vinita when her arthritis flares up. Perhaps this shared goal can then be framed in such a way that it meets the agency's criteria for involvement, so that you can provide the kind of assistance that is necessary. Improvements in Vinita's situation may well depend on your ability to find creative ways of bringing all of these potentially competing goals together.

A process to agree and reach goals

The seven goals earlier in this chapter have been presented as though they were 'given'. However, it usually takes time to think about our goals and to shape them into something that is achievable. First, as we have seen, it is likely that a person's situation is framed in problem language. Translating problem language into goal language is a careful and skilful job, taking time to listen to the person's view of their situation and gaining their confidence in order to encourage them to begin to think in goal language. Challenging problem language directly or asking people outright 'what is your goal?' is unlikely to be effective. The time needs to be right.

Two principal methods that have been developed with goal language in mind are 'task-centred practice' and 'solution-focused therapy'. The latter is largely concerned with therapeutic contexts, such as counselling, although its principles are applicable to the wide range of situations in social care where rehabilitation workers can help. The Further reading section at the end of the chapter has more information about this. The task-centred method was first devised in the USA, but has travelled well to other countries and cultures, and has a good track record of research and development to learn from. It is this method which we will briefly consider as a way to help people to agree and reach their goals.

The task-centred method

Although it is called 'task-centred', this method is actually a very *person-centred* way of working; in other words, it takes as its starting point the needs and wants of the person or people with whom you are working. Although it provides a systematic model or blueprint, it can be adapted sensitively to different situations. It is a vehicle which helps people to achieve their goals, even though the various goals will be quite different and particular to each individual or family's situation.

Let us take one of the examples from the seven goals earlier in this chapter to see how the task-centred method can help us to help people formulate and achieve their goal. We will consider Evelyn, who wants to visit the guest house where she and her husband used to holiday. Now, that is not what Evelyn said when you first met her. At that point she was depressed and rather weepy and was referred because she didn't seem able to do much for herself, or perhaps just didn't want to do anything for herself. Her hearing and her memory are both deteriorating. To begin with, you used the problem language to which she was accustomed and asked her what she saw as the main problems. After quite a long meeting together, these were the main problems as Evelyn saw them and using her own words:

- My hearing's getter worse.
- I can't remember things.
- I miss my husband still; it's four or five years since he died, but I still don't feel I have got over it.
- I feel bad about relying on my daughter so much: she's got her own life to lead.
- The house needs a lot of work doing on it, but I can't do it myself and I can't afford to have someone in.

You asked Evelyn if she were choosing which of these problems to work on, which one would it be. Evelyn talked it over with you and decided that it was the third one, the missing her husband. Her eyes fill with tears just mentioning it. Privately you are wondering what can be done with this problem. Even so, you trust Evelyn's judgement and you ask her open questions about her feelings. You also now explain that you would like to move away from the problems and towards a goal, something that she would like to happen. You acknowledge that nothing will bring her husband back, but ask her if she can think of anything she would like to do that would help. There is quite a silence and you wonder if you should say something or perhaps she did not hear you properly. Eventually, Evelyn asks you to get a photo album from a dresser. She opens the album and flicks through, stopping at one of the pages.

'We used to go to Blackpool, you know. Every year, to the same place. He died the day before we were due to go, that last time. We never made it that year. I've not really thought about it before, and I don't know whether it's possible, but I'd do anything to go back and see the place, I really would.'

And that is how Evelyn arrived at her goal.

At this stage your mind is full of many questions. Can Evelyn actually achieve this goal: financially, physically, emotionally? What resources will she need to do this successfully? Will she be able to remember from one week to the next that this is her goal? How long would it take to achieve this goal? Is it your role to help her to do this? Is the guest house still there?

However, the task-centred method provides a framework to help you and Evelyn take the process to the next stage. You find out how motivated Evelyn is to achieve this goal (she wants to do it very much), and you ask open questions which help her to think about how feasible it is. Your questions help *her* to raise the possible obstacles, rather than you pointing to them; similarly, your questions help her to arrive at possible ways round these obstacles, without needing your suggestions. Together, you agree that the goal is possible and that it will probably take about six weeks to achieve. You agree that you will meet once a week to work out what tasks each of you need to do along the way, and that you will review your progress on these tasks from week to week.

There are two kinds of task: those that you do together when you meet (called 'session' tasks) and those that you each do between sessions ('homework' tasks). In this session, you telephone directory enquiries to find the telephone number of the guest house. Then, Evelyn says that she wants to ring the guest house there and then. You had not planned on moving so quickly because there are so many other things to check, especially who might accompany her. You gently share these reservations, but Evelyn is looking very animated and still wants to make the call. She is clear about what she wants to say, that she will find out the price for a weekend stay and find out whether they have room in about six weeks' time. In fact, during the phone call, she goes a step further and makes a provisional booking. When she finishes the call she tells you that she hasn't done anything like this since her husband died. She looks so different from when you first walked in the door.

You discuss the homework tasks which you and Evelyn will do between now and the time you meet again in a week's time. It is *not* a list of tasks that you give her to do; most of these suggestions come from Evelyn as a result of your questions and discussion together. You spend quite some time looking at each task in detail, discussing who the best person is to do each one and how it can be done. The tasks are written down so that Evelyn can remind herself. You agree these 'homework' tasks for the first week:

(1) Evelyn will write a list of reasons why she wants to go to the Blackpool guest house. When the going gets tough, or if she forgets what her goal is about, she will read the list to remind her why this goal is important to her.
(2) Evelyn will make a list of the things she will need to take with her.
(3) You will talk with Merryn, Evelyn's daughter, to let her know what the goal is, and just to test the water to see if there is any possibility of her accompanying her mother (*Evelyn wanted you to do this because she wants Merryn to be able to say 'no'*).
(4) You will make other enquiries about a possible companion through the local Council for Voluntary Service.

The work continues each week with Evelyn, and any other people who are important to achieving the goal, reviewing progress on the tasks which were agreed at the last session, working on any tasks in the session itself, then developing new homework tasks to be completed between now and the next session. In this way, you help Evelyn to move step by step from the present difficulty to a future goal, with each small success building confidence along the way. It is a very careful process and one which both you and Evelyn find interesting and rewarding.

As you will have noted, this method requires you to be open to new ways of working. Your agency and the referral sheet no doubt placed Evelyn in the 'memory loss', 'depressed', 'hearing problem' boxes, and now you find yourself helping her to achieve a goal which does not seem to be related to these referral categories. However, Evelyn's goal is the one she truly wishes to achieve and, if we look below the surface, we can see how it will have an impact on many other areas of her life, including many that are in those referral boxes. With your skilful questions and careful attention she has arrived at a goal which she feels highly motivated to achieve, and which, through discussion, you both know to have a reasonable chance of success. Undoubtedly, the experience of working towards a goal she wants to achieve will help her depression and the techniques you are using with her will aid her memory. The work on her goal does not prevent you doing any other necessary assessment, for example to refer for further investigation into her hearing loss. However, it will be important to translate the goal language which is proving so successful with Evelyn into *agency language*; that is, to help your agency understand how your work with Evelyn is helping her to be more independent, which is at the heart of your rehabilitation work and the agency's purpose.

■ The intervention plan

The intervention plan sets out the way that the team will achieve the goals. Because of the complex nature of re-enablement, and the fact that it often involves helping people to function better within their own environment, there are often numerous different ways to address the same problem. One of the

> **Box 2** Components of a good intervention plan
>
> Client details (name, gender, date of birth)
> Reason for referral
> Date of assessment
> Details of the assessment
> Precautions or contraindications
> All goals should be clearly stated
> It should clearly state who is going to achieve the goal
> It should describe the actions the client has to perform to achieve the goal
> It should describe the standards that need to be reached
> The timeframe for achieving the goal
> How you will evaluate progress towards achievement of the goal

benefits of a multidisciplinary team is that team members generally bring a range of different perspectives to help address the same problem.

Deciding on the best intervention to address a particular problem

A useful framework to determine the appropriateness of an intervention will consider the following features (Bauer, 1989):

- The resources available.
- The use of research evidence.
- The risks associated with the intervention.

Knowledge of the resources available

The rehabilitation process will depend greatly on the level of support that is already available to your client. For instance, you need to consider whether the client lives alone or lives with an able-bodied person who may be able to provide some support for the client, or even fulfil some of the important activities of daily living for that client, such as cooking and cleaning for them. If the client lives alone in a rural or remote area with limited access to other health services, then it is likely that your service may have to provide some of the intervention that would normally be delivered by someone else. For instance, if the client needs their feet cared for in order to remain independent and prevent falls, but you do not have access to a podiatrist, then you need to consider how you are going to be able to deliver that service.

One of the key aspects of being able to support clients to become independent is having knowledge of a wide range of resources within the local community, such as meals on wheels, social support groups and voluntary support agencies. If you do not already have one, it is worth establishing a resource folder for your team or service that provides information about the range of services available in your region. It is also useful to include a list of other types of services,

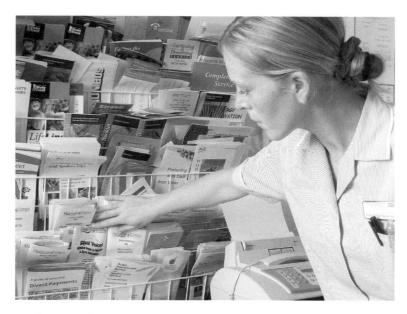

Figure 3 Selecting information leaflets to give to a client.

like a good handyman, carpenter, or plumber because you are guaranteed to
come across some of these problems in a client's home occasionally. The Internet
can be useful to help you identify some of these services.

Stop and think

Make a list of all of the supporting resources that are you aware of within your local
community, including voluntary services and social support groups.

Use the available research evidence

Good practice should be guided by research findings. There are a number
of different ways to find out what the best research evidence is. Normally,
good quality research is published in journals that have a rigorous peer review
process. However, there are literally hundreds of thousands of journals that
publish research outputs, so it can be a daunting process to find the right paper
in the appropriate journal when you need it. Many professional bodies have
newsletters that provide summaries of the most recent research evidence. It is
a good idea to find at least one good quality newsletter or journal that you can
read regularly to provide you with up-to-date information that is relevant to
your practice.

You may have heard of 'best practice guidelines' or 'clinical practice guidelines'. These are summaries of the best evidence around management of particular types of conditions or disease management. For instance, there are guidelines for the management of patients with stroke, palliative care and incontinence, to list only a few. Many of these guidelines are available on the Internet for easy and quick access. You do need to be careful when you are selecting guidelines to make sure you access the most up-to-date guidelines, and those that have used the best research evidence.

If you document your care properly, you will start to develop your own body of evidence about the effectiveness of different types of interventions for particular clients. See the chapter in Section 4 on Lifelong learning to identify other ways of accessing evidence that you can incorporate into your practice, including reflective practice and journal clubs. Good discharge summaries also help you develop your own evidence about what worked well with a particular client and what did not work well, based on the clinical experiences of your team. This is a valuable way of learning from clinical experience.

Consider the risks

No intervention is without risks. However, it is likely that different types of interventions will come with different levels of risk. You need to consider the risks associated with the interventions you are thinking of delivering, and weigh these against the benefits you perceive that the client is likely to receive. You will also need to consider the families' and carers' attitudes to different risks. In some cases, the families are more risk averse than the clients, or have a clearer idea of the types of risks the client may face when they return to their own home.

Red and yellow flags

Red and yellow flags are a useful way to highlight particular precautions or 'contraindications' in situations that may cause particular risks for the client, or mean that they may not respond well to a particular type of treatment.

Red flags highlight the physical risks to the client of performing a particular intervention. For instance, a suspected bone fracture in the leg could be a red flag for full weight-bearing and mobilisation of a client. Cancer of the spine is a red flag for spinal manipulation.

Yellow flags are psychosocial risk factors that may influence the outcomes of treatment. These may be psychological, economic, or in some cases environmental factors that may be barriers to being able to achieve a particular outcome. For instance:

■ Clients who are unable or unwilling to participate in the rehabilitation process because of expectations that they should be cared for, or negative perceptions about the possible outcomes of the process.

- Clients who require particular treatment modalities that are too expensive for them, such as expensive medication, nutritional supplements or equipment.
- Clients or carers who are unwilling to accept support and/or therapeutic interventions.
- Lack of motivation to participate in the re-enablement process.

■ Evaluating the effectiveness of the intervention

People often express their goals in rather vague terms. Consider the seven goals at the beginning of this chapter and give them each a mark out of ten for how specific they are. Although most of them score less than 5/10, a few questions would help to bring their mark up. As it stands, *Phyllis wants Jack to do more about the house* is around 4/10 on the line from vague to specific. However, if we ask Phyllis what this means, she might say, 'Well, I want him to vacuum the downstairs once a week and wash up at weekends'. That would immediately bring it nearer to a 9/10. Once a goal becomes more specific it is more likely to provoke action: Jack may feel relieved that 'doing more about the house' is not quite as bad as his worst nightmares had suggested.

You need to help people to be more specific about their goals because that helps them to know when they have been successful and to measure progress along the way. For example, if someone's goal is *to smoke less*, we need to know how much they smoke now, how many would constitute 'less' (technically just one fewer than they currently smoke would be 'less', but this would not be a meaningful success), and over what period of time this is to be achieved. So, this goal might be reframed as, *Currently I smoke 30 a day and I want to cut this down to 10 cigarettes a day, or less, in four weeks' time, then I want to maintain this level.* Each week it would be possible to see whether there was a successful downward trend from 30 a day to 10 a day. To measure the success of the final part of this goal, *to maintain this level at 10 cigarettes a day or less*, we would need to check it every so often, perhaps once a month, to see if that level of smoking was being maintained or improved even further.

All intervention plans should include some way of determining whether you have achieved the goals you set out to achieve. There are numerous ways of doing this, and goal evaluation and re-evaluation needs to become a routine part of the delivery of the intervention. These tools should help you determine quickly whether you are doing something very wrong, but if used routinely, should help you ascertain whether the intervention approaches you are using are effective across a number of clients.

Some of the more common tools for evaluating change that you might be familiar with include:

- Activities of daily living.
- Functional Independence Measure (FIM).

- Barthel's Index (including MBI (Modified Barthel Index)).
- Falls Risk Assessment Scale.
- TUG (Timed up to Go)*.
- Therapy Outcome Measure (TOMs).
- Braden Scale (skin care).
- Waterlow Scale (dietary, incontinence, medication, mobility and skin care).

You don't necessarily need to use a pre-defined tool like the ones listed above. It is important at various stages throughout the episode of care to reflect on the actual goals of the client, ascertain how far you have come in achieving those goals and describe these in the client's notes.

Documenting ongoing progress

Every occasion of service provided to a client should be recorded in some way in the client's file. These are normally called *progress notes* because they document the progress of the client through their intervention plan. The client's file should have a clearly delineated section for recording progress notes. Sometimes different professions will document their progress notes in separate parts of the file, or even separate files. However, this restricts the interprofessional learning that can take place by documenting all the progress notes in one location. Ideally, progress notes should be entered into a common section which is used by all of the practitioners involved in the care of the client. They should be clearly dated and the name and profession of the worker printed at the end of the entry. It can sometimes be useful to document the time you saw the client. The entries are made sequentially and in chronological order. This makes it easy for the last person visiting the client to see what happened most recently, but also to follow the client's progress throughout the episode of care.

There are numerous ways to document progress, but three of the most common approaches are (Sames, 2005):

(1) Narrative notes
(2) SOAP notes
(3) FIP notes

Narrative notes

As the name implies, narrative notes are unstructured notes that are used to record client progress. They are normally written in paragraph form, and do not use prescribed subheadings. You need to be quite disciplined when you use narrative notes to ensure that you cover the key components of the

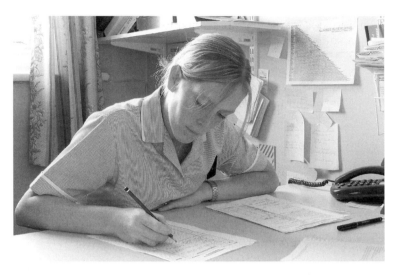

Figure 4 Updating a client's progress notes.

intervention, and capture some aspects of progress, as the example below illustrates.

Box 3   Narrative notes

Dressing – Miss Ferns' sitting balance is much improved. She is now able to sit unaided on the edge of the bed to dress. She is unable to identify items of clothing when they are folded and laid out on the bed besides her, but is able to identify items when they are held up in front of her. Miss Ferns is distressed by her inability to dress independently. She had difficulty putting on her left shoe due to swelling of her foot and ankle. Will undertake a standardised perceptual assessment. Will monitor the swelling and report to GP if it has not reduced in two days.

SOAP notes

SOAP stands for: subjective, objective, assessment, plan, because these are the headings that are used to structure the progress notes using this method.

The *subjective* component of the notes is normally what the client tells you and should reflect their view. You may even use quotes if you wish.

The *objective* notes are where you record your own observations about the client. What you write in the objective section will depend on the purpose of your component of the intervention. For instance, if you were a nurse and the client complained that he felt that he had a fever (the 'S'), then you would take their temperature and record this as your 'O'. On the other hand, if you are a rehabilitation assistant working with a client to prepare a meal, your 'O' may reflect the ability of the client to be able to reach the cupboards where the food is stored. The 'O' can also be used to record the client's progress against their goals.

The *assessment* is where you make some interpretation of the subjective and objective data.

The *plan* is what you do about it.

Box 4 SOAP notes

Dressing

S   Miss Ferns says that she is 'pathetic' and 'useless'.

O   Miss Ferns was tearful. Miss Ferns sat unaided on the side of the bed to dress. She was unable to identify items of clothing when they were laid out on the bed beside her, but was able to identify them when they were held up in front of her. Miss Ferns has a swollen left foot and ankle which caused some difficulty in putting her shoe on.

A   Miss Ferns has a loss of ability in figure–background discrimination. Miss Ferns is distressed by her inability to dress independently.

P   To carry out a standardised perceptual assessment. To monitor the swelling in the left foot. To try placing her clothes on a plain background. To give Miss Ferns regular feedback on the progress she is making.

FIP notes

FIP stands for: findings, interpretation, plan, and these notes are sometimes called DAP notes, or: description, assessment, plan. Like the SOAP notes, they use these letters as subheadings for each component of the notes. The main difference in this form of documentation is that the 'findings' section is a combination of the 'subjective' and 'objective' component of the SOAP notes. The 'interpretations' and 'findings' are exactly the same as the 'assessment' and 'plan' in SOAP note format.

Other systems of recording

If you are using a structured approach to care provision, such as a clinical pathway, you may use a proforma that instructs you on the types of assessment you should do, and gives you clear guidelines about the types of findings you should document and the way they need to be recorded.

Box 5 FIP notes

Dressing

F   Miss Ferns was tearful and upset. She is now able to sit unaided on the side of the bed to dress. She is unable to identify items of clothing when they are placed on the bed next to her, but is able to identify them when they are held in front of her. Miss Ferns has a swollen left foot and ankle which caused her some difficulties when putting her shoe on.

I   Miss Ferns has a loss of ability in figure–background discrimination. Miss Ferns is distressed by her inability to dress independently.

P   To carry out a standardised perceptual assessment. To monitor the swelling in the left foot. To try placing her clothes on a plain background. To give Miss Ferns regular feedback on the progress she is making.

■ Re-evaluation

It is important to constantly evaluate the progress of the client against their goals as you go along. This depends on having clear goals in the first place, against which you can determine the client's progress. But it is also possible that the client's goals may change throughout their care. For instance, their circumstances or their health may change, which could impact on their initial goals, or their ability to achieve the initial goals (a major shift in either health status or circumstances may call for a reassessment of the client). Good, ongoing documentation systems, such as SOAP notes have built-in ways of ensuring that you record the ongoing progress of the client.

■ Discharge

The discharge from the service marks the end of the episode of care for the client. Discharge can occur for a number of reasons. The client may have achieved all of their goals, moved to a different service or facility, or they may have decided not to continue with the programme.

It is important at the end of every episode of care to prepare a discharge summary. The discharge summary provides an overview of the whole episode of care. There is no right way to prepare a discharge summary, and some services may have a summary form, others will not. The types of items that a discharge summary could usefully include are listed in Box 6. If you use SOAP notes in your file management, then it is quite appropriate to use SOAP format to write the discharge summary.

Good discharge summaries can serve a number of purposes:

■　You can use your discharge summary as a basis to provide feedback to the referring practitioner or organisation. It will provide the information you

need to tell them exactly what you did, over what period of time, and what
you achieved.

■ It can provide a useful audit tool to show you which interventions are
effective and which ones are not, under particular circumstances.

■ It can show you variations in the type and amount of care provided to
highlight areas where you may be able to increase the efficiency of the
service, or perhaps highlight areas of unmet need.

■ It can be useful to help plan future service needs, such as workforce
numbers and service capacity.

In some cases, one member of the team might stop providing their service before the client is discharged from the team. For example, a dietician
might be called in to provide nutritional advice for the client early on in
the episode of care. The dietician may only require two occasions of service
with the client, and may complete these within the first week of the intervention taking place. In this case, the dietician will complete 'discontinuation
notes'. These can be incorporated into the regular progress notes for the client,
or may be documented in a separate part of the file. However, the discontinuation notes of the dietician should be included in the overall discharge
summary.

■ Follow-up

It is important that every episode of care has a system of follow-up built into it. At
discharge, the client should be notified that they will receive follow-up contact
by a member of the team, and the approximate date should be documented
on the care plan at discharge. Follow-up can be undertaken by telephone or
face-to-face visit. The purpose of the follow-up is to ensure that the client has
been able to maintain their level of functioning; to check that the follow-on

---

Box 6   Components of the discharge summary

Dates of admission and discharge
Reason for referral
Reason for discharge
Summary of the client's progress against their goals
Initial status of the client
Ending status of the client
Summary of effective management strategies
Summary of ineffective management strategies
Types of practitioners involved in the client's care
Number of occasions of service received by the client
Follow-on plans or referrals
Date of follow-up
Signature

services that were required have been implemented; and to ensure that there have been no changes in the status of the client since discharge. It can also provide important reassurance to the client to know that they will have some future contact with the service again. The follow-up should be documented on the care plan, and may use the same outcome measures or evaluation tools that were used during the intervention.

Conclusion

Each service will vary slightly in their approach to agreeing and reaching client goals, depending on the background of the team leader, the location of client care and the purpose of the service. However, the basic principles described in this chapter should help you develop a clear protocol for managing the goals of the client from their first point of entry into the service until after discharge.

Further reading

Bauer, D. (1989) *Foundations of Physical Rehabilitation. A Management Approach.* Melbourne, Churchill Livingstone. *This book has been around for a long time, but describes some valuable basic principles around the development of rehabilitation interventions.*

Bowling, A. (2004) *Measuring Health: A Review of Quality of Life Measurement Scales.* Milton Keynes, Open University Press. *This book describes a range of different health outcome measures and the principles of measuring changes in health status.*

Doel, M. (2002) Task-centred work In: R. Adams, L. Dominelli & M. Payne (eds), *Social Work: Themes, Issues and Debates* (2nd edition). (pp. 191–200). Houndmills, Macmillan. *This chapter gives a succinct nine-page account of the task-centred method to help people to prioritise their problems, choose their goal, and work towards the successful achievement of that goal.*

Doel, M. & Marsh, P. (1992) *Task-centred Social Work.* Aldershot, Ashgate. *This book considers the task-centred model in more detail, with a chapter devoted to each stage of the work, including ways of evaluating the success of the work. A case example runs throughout the book involving two elderly neighbours, one of whom is suffering from Alzheimer's; goals are developed which involve both neighbours, and the book helps us to understand how we can use this approach in a very difficult situation.*

Marsh, P. & Doel, M. (2005) *The Task-centred Book.* London, Routledge. *An unusual book, in using the current work of several social care workers and social workers to illustrate task-centred, goal-oriented ways of working. All of the cases are real (though anonymised for confidentiality) and the information is taken from portfolios written by the social care workers and social workers involved. The cases cover a wide range of work, including children's services, adult services, learning disability and mental health services, demonstrating that this method of working to help people to achieve their goals is possible across a wide range of social care.*

Sames, K.M. (2005) *Documenting Occupational Therapy Practice.* New Jersey, Pearson Prentice Hall. *Provides detailed explanations and descriptions of all components of documenting occupational therapy practice, including clinical records, report and even grant writing. It has relevance to other disciplines as well.*

Sharry, J. (2001) *Solution-focused Groupwork.* London, Sage. *The solution-focused approach is time-limited and moves straight into 'solution language' rather than 'problem language'. It is based on short-term therapeutic approaches and is applicable across the range, with its roots in counselling techniques. This provides a practical guide to using these approaches in groups.*

Teaching for rehabilitation

Hazel Mackey

Introduction

How many times have you found yourself repeating the same teaching method with one person after another, not sure whether the techniques you were using really suited the person you were using them with?

As someone who works in rehabilitation you will be engaged in teaching during your daily contact with clients, carers and colleagues. Teaching may be defined as the stimulation of learning. It is an active process, conducted through planning, doing and evaluating. Whether client, carer, student or colleague, the learner is an active partner. In order to be an effective teacher you need to know your subject, but this alone is not enough. Teaching involves the ability to impart this knowledge to others in a way they can understand and act upon. Some people have a natural aptitude for teaching, but most of us have to work hard to develop our teaching skills.

This chapter aims to help you choose the most appropriate way of delivering a rehabilitation programme. There is no one 'best' method. Different methods suit different situations and different people. You can mix and match methods, combining them to ensure that more is learned. Another goal of this section is to increase your competence and confidence in selecting, designing, adapting and implementing teaching methods.

Teaching opportunities arise throughout the rehabilitation worker's career. They range from:

- Individual rehabilitation sessions.
- Training carers.
- Student education.

- In-service training with colleagues.
- Public relations events such as career awareness and health promotion.

Regardless of the setting, you must have an interest in guiding and motivating the learner as they strive to acquire new skills or improve old ones.

▪ Adult learning

Malcolm Knowles coined the word 'androgogy' to refer to the art and science of helping adults to learn. There are five principles of adult learning:

(1) Adult learning is characterised by being problem centred rather than subject centred and the need for immediate rather than postponed application of knowledge.
(2) Adult learning is related to an adult's readiness to learn, which is related to life events.
(3) Adults accumulate a reservoir of experience that becomes a resource for learning.
(4) Adults become increasingly independent and self-directed as they age. This means that they can participate in diagnosing, planning and evaluating their own learning needs.
(5) Adult learners are more often motivated by internal needs than by external pressures.

Compare this approach to learning with the one you experienced at school, which you are probably more familiar with. The diagram below shows some of the main differences between using an adult approach to learning and pedagogy, the more traditionally child-oriented approach.

Table 1 Differences between children and adults as learners.

Children	Adults
Rely on others to decide what is important to be learned.	Decide for themselves what is important to be learned.
Accept the information being presented at face value.	Need to validate the information based on their beliefs and experiences.
Expect that what they are learning will be useful in their long-term future.	Expect that what they are learning is immediately useful.
Have little or no experience to draw on.	Have much past experience to draw on.
Have little ability to serve as a knowledgeable resource.	Have significant ability to serve as a knowledgeable service.
Are content centred.	Are problem centred.
Learn in an authority oriented environment.	Function best in a collaborative environment.
Planning is teachers' responsibility.	Share in planning.

An awareness of how adults learn is important, as your job is to provide well-organised experiences which speed up the learning process and enable the client to make well-informed choices in solving life's problems.

Using the principles of androgogy in your daily working practice ensures that you:

- Establish an effective learning environment where clients feel safe and comfortable expressing themselves.
- Encourage clients to set their own learning goals.
- Involve the clients in the planning of the method as well as the content of the rehabilitation programme.
- Encourage reflection, by the asking of questions and by involving the client in evaluating their own performance/learning.

■ The experiential learning cycle

Much of rehabilitation uses active methods of learning which involve transmitting information by participating in activities and by practising.

To fully learn from an experience it is not enough simply to have the experience. You need to encourage the client to reflect on their experience; determine how that experience relates or builds on their existing knowledge; and decide how they will use this knowledge to change their actions in the future (see Figure 1).

■ Interpersonal and communication skills

An effective rehabilitation worker is concerned with the general wellbeing and growth of the client. If a good relationship is to develop, the foundations for it need to be laid in the first few meetings.

The effectiveness of your teaching will depend on your communication skills. An overview of communication skills follows, but more information can be found in Section 3 under Communication.

Two important areas for effective communication are questioning and explaining. Both are underpinned by active listening, including attention to verbal and non-verbal cues and the skilful use of silence.

Active listening

It is important to allow the client to articulate areas in which they are having difficulty or which they may wish to know more about. Listening attentively requires you to take an active role, not a passive one. Not only do you need to pay attention to what is being presented, but you must also demonstrate this attention. This can be achieved through your body language, facial expression and eye contact, as well as verbal encouragements.

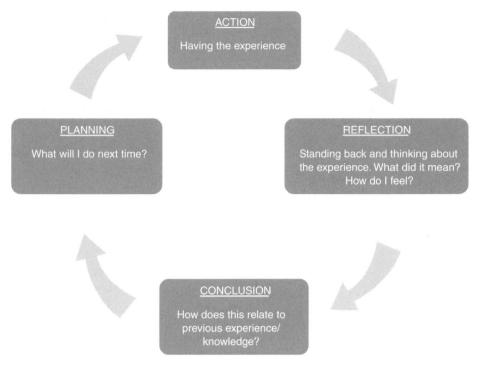

Figure 1 The experiential learning cycle.

The use of silence

Silence can be uncomfortable, especially when those present do not know one another well, but it does allow time for reflection, and, if not hurriedly filled, can communicate that you have time and interest in the client.

Questions

Asking questions can fulfil many purposes, such as to clarify understanding, to promote curiosity and to emphasise key points. Questioning stimulates interaction and can be effective and useful when thoughtfully developed, or ineffective and stifling when used carelessly. They can be classified as closed, leading, or open questions. Closed questions usually only require a 'yes' or 'no' answer. They leave little room for the respondent to open up the conversation. Leading questions are phrased in such a way as to direct the respondent into giving the answer the questioner expects. In a rehabilitation programme, questions should usually be open: that is, they cannot be answered with a simple 'yes' or 'no', so as to invite discussion and reflection. Questions beginning with 'why', 'what', 'how', 'when', 'who', and 'where' are particularly effective in opening up the discussion and helping people clarify what they are trying to express.

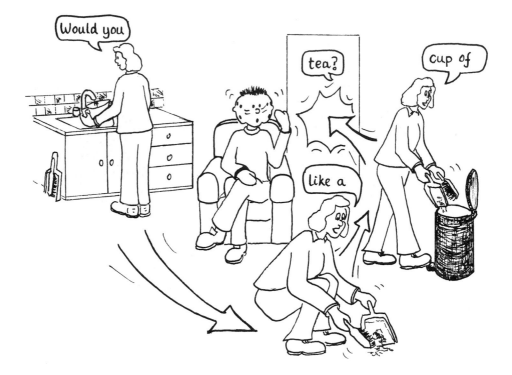

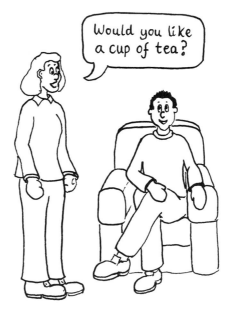

Figure 2 It is important to communicate clearly.

Stop and think

Bob, a man with a learning disability, has said that he wants to feel better about his appearance. At this stage we know no more than this, and we have choices about how we help Bob to find out more about his goal. Below are seven examples of this invitational style of questioning. Read them and consider why these kinds of questions might be especially helpful.

- What is it that you don't like about your appearance?
- How does your appearance affect how you feel?
- What would make you feel better about your appearance?
- Do you think other people notice your appearance?
- When do you feel better about your appearance?
- Putting your appearance to one side, what helps to make you feel good?
- What does 'feel better' mean to you? How would I know that you were feeling better about your appearance?

Box 1   Guidelines for asking questions

Do not ask too many questions: sometimes, clients can feel pressured and threatened when they are bombarded by questions.

Ask questions that serve a purpose: a question is a request for information. The request may be for observations, facts, thoughts, opinions or feelings. The information supplied should enable you to move forward in some way.

Restrict the use of closed questions to establishing facts: one closed question begs another and there is the danger of bombarding the client with ineffective questioning.

Use open questions: help clients talk about specific experiences.

In asking questions keep the focus on the clients and their experiences and needs.

Allow adequate time for responses: don't speak too soon.

Explanations

Explaining often goes hand in hand with questioning. Clear explanations are dependent upon knowing precisely what you wish to explain. It is important to present only as much information as people can cope with at any one time. It is often better to deliver small packages of information over several sessions rather than trying to cover a great deal in one or two sessions.

It is important to ensure that both the content and the presentation of the explanation is at the appropriate level.

There are five basic skills involved in effective explaining:

(1) **Clarity and fluency:** be clear about what you mean, speak the language of the client, allow time for absorption.
(2) **Emphasis and interest:** make good use of voice, gestures, materials and paraphrasing.
(3) **Use examples:** most people will remember information more easily if they have a relevant example to relate it to.
(4) **Organisation:** present your information in a logical sequence, and use link words and phrases, which allow the information to flow.
(5) **Feedback:** offer the chance to ask questions. Check if the message has been understood.

■ Planning

One of the most important principles of an effective rehabilitation programme is the need for planning. Planning provides structure, both for you and the client, and also provides a framework for reflection and evaluation. Planning a whole rehabilitation programme, rather than one session at a time, helps maintain uniformity and to identify progression. It is important to have some idea about the client's expected performance and the specific goals to be covered.

Planning is an active process which can use a variety of approaches to identify the client's goals and make decisions about the best way forward. Possible pitfalls should be identified so that they can be avoided. It is useful to identify a number of different ways to meet the client's goals; to have Plan B ready in case Plan A fails, and you may need to upgrade or downgrade an activity (see Activity Analysis later in this chapter).

Timing is an important element in the planning process. Sessions that are too long may overwhelm the client in terms of fatigue and attention span, but each session must be of sufficient length to allow time for active engagement. As apart of the planning process you need to know who is to be taught and where the teaching is to take place, so you can consider the learning environment. You also need to be clear about the priorities for teaching.

Motivation

From the minute we awake, we are motivated in many different ways:

- To get up for breakfast because we feel hungry is a *physical* motivator.
- To get changed from your nightwear to day wear is a *social* motivator.
- To come to work is a *financial* motivator.
- To go to the gym or night class is a *personal* motivator.
- To take your child to see the doctor is a *role* motivator.

Many factors affect our motivation and each person is motivated differently. It is vital for us to find out what motivates the clients we are working with as this will affect our teaching methods (see the previous chapter on Agreeing and reaching goals).

Heightening motivation can be done through reinforcement, as our behaviours are modified by the consequences we receive or expect. As rehabilitation workers we need to plan for positive reinforcement. This includes:

■ **Social methods:** verbal praise, gestures such as thumbs up, or facial expressions such as smiles.
■ **Physical methods:** a hug, a touch of the hand or a squeeze of the shoulder.
■ **Token methods:** a reward such as a cup of tea or a bar of chocolate.
■ **Tangible rewards:** such as a negotiated visit or trip.

Environment/safety

Consider the environment in which the activity is to take place. The choices available may include the therapy department, the client's home, or a community setting. Consider the facilities, the size, shape, lighting, temperature of the room, the noise, the attitudes of others present. Space is a relevant issue. Clients need to be provided with sufficient personal and work space.

Aim to provide an environment which is free of distractions and where the client feels safe. This environment includes yourself. You must portray a confident and reliable image. Part of feeling safe is knowing the limits. Be clear about what is expected and plan tasks that are within the capabilities of the client and the resources available. It is up to you to set up appropriate conditions with whatever facilities are available.

Activity analysis

If you are to assist an individual to overcome or manage impairment you need to know:

■ The demands the activity will place on the individual.
■ The skills required to perform the activity.
■ How the activity can be adapted to change the demands and skills.

Activity analysis is the process of breaking an activity down into stages. Each stage is analysed to determine the motor, sensory, cognitive and social skills and demands the activity will make on the client.

Activity analysis may be carried out in order to:

■ Carry out a precise assessment of the individual's abilities.
■ Select an appropriate teaching method.
■ Select an appropriate activity to meet a therapeutic aim.
■ Adapt an activity to meet individual needs.
■ Identify the precise part of an activity the individual is having difficulty performing.

> **Box 2** Activity analysis: threading a needle
>
> For a right-handed person the task sequence should look something like this:
>
> (1) Cut the required length of thread.
> (2) Moisten the end of the thread which is to pass through the eye of the needle.
> (3) Take the needle in the left hand with the eye of the needle uppermost.
> (4) Hold the needle at eye level with the eye of the needle facing you.
> (5) Hold the moistened end of the thread in the right hand.
> (6) With the thread at right angles to the needle move the thread forward until it passes through the eye of the needle.
> (7) Remove the right hand from the length of thread and take hold of the moistened end which now protrudes through the eye of the needle.
> (8) Gently pull the thread through the eye of the needle.
>
> A variety of skills are needed to carry out this task, including:
>
> ■ The motor skills of cutting, holding and pulling.
> ■ The cognitive skills such as problem-solving if the thread begins to separate.
> ■ The perceptual skills of spatial awareness and relationship of parts to each other.

Occupational therapists are skilled in undertaking detailed and complex activity analysis. Find a locally based occupational therapist and ask them if you can observe or help with an activity analysis.

As a rehabilitation worker, you will need to identify the skills involved in the tasks that you teach so that you are able to spot any that are causing problems for the client. This analysis needs to take place at the planning stage of a rehabilitation programme and the easiest way to do this is to:

- Perform the task yourself.
- Identify every stage.
- Note any skills that may cause a problem for your client.

Stop and think

Try carrying out an activity analysis on one of the tasks that you frequently teach. Choose something simple. You will be amazed at the number of skills involved.

You need to know the sequence and demands of an activity in order to teach it effectively. The following approaches to teaching may be considered:

- Show the client an example of the finished article, for example in work rehabilitation, before teaching the various stages involved.
- Model or demonstrate the whole sequence of the activity, such as the use of a walking aid, before teaching it step by step.

■ Work beside the client so that each step of the activity is performed first by the rehabilitation worker and then by the client.

Box 3 Checklist for planning

Ask yourself some important questions:

- ■ What is the purpose of this rehabilitation programme?
- ■ What are the client's needs?
- ■ How will you gauge whether the client's needs have been met?

■ Teaching methods

The choice of methods used to implement the rehabilitation programme will be directed by the objectives. As each person learns in their own individual way, the programme's method must reflect the client capabilities, habits and experiences.

Practise

It is essential to provide a means of making opportunities to practise newly learned skills. You need to plan for plenty of practise time. It is important to facilitate secure situations where the client can gain the experience needed. The complete task needs to be practised, as well as the individual components.

Careful observation and monitoring is required to ensure that, where necessary, each skill is being performed correctly, because practise leads to habit and it would be wrong to allow someone to learn a task incorrectly and then have to re-learn it. Usually, short practise sessions will lead more quickly to mastery of a skill; long periods can be tiring and counterproductive but this does depend on the individual person and the objectives of the session.

Feedback

It is important that you give the client regular feedback on their progress, as constructive feedback can support and encourage progress. The way you provide this feedback is crucial in developing a trusting relationship as it conveys to the client how they are progressing and how they are being monitored. Praise for achievement or effort is usually expected and accepted. However, praise for a mediocre attempt may be patronising.

Feedback should be positive and constructive, and as immediate as possible. Begin by asking the client to tell you what he or she feels confident in having done well and what he or she would like to improve (see Figure 3). Your feedback should be based on observation. It should contain enough specific detail and advice to enable the client to reflect and enhance their performance and it should be positive and supportive in tone. The best way to learn how to give effective feedback is to practise.

Case study   Jacques

Jacques is a 25-year-old man who has sustained a closed head injury nine months prior to his referral into the community rehabilitation team. Jacques is fully mobile, with only minimal coordination problems in his right, dominant hand. He has some difficulties with verbal comprehension but is able to engage in conversation. Cognitively, he has difficulties with attention, organisation, sequencing and memory. Jacques lives with his mother. He is not employed and is not able to drive. Before his injury, Jacques worked as a cook but he is no longer able to initiate kitchen activities without being prompted about what to do.

Together with the rehabilitation team, Jacques and his mother identified his first goal as being able to make a hot drink of instant coffee. The rehabilitation worker was introduced to Jacques and his mother, and a regular time was allocated to visit Jacques in his own home to practise making this hot drink. Jacques needed to practise the instant coffee task the same way each time; any change in task presentation negatively affected his performance. The rehabilitation worker recorded his speed, accuracy and approach to the task at each session, as well as the amount of assistance and verbal cueing that was needed. This record was discussed with Jacques at the end of each session to provide him with feedback about his performance. Initially, Jacques needed specific verbal cues to initiate each step, such as 'First you need to find the coffee in the cupboard.' After several repetitions of the task, however, he needed only general cues like 'What do you do first?' or 'What's next?', to help him to remember the steps.

A review of Jacques' records clearly showed that over the course of his sessions he needed progressively fewer specific cues and became much quicker and more organised. Jacques was always pleased to hear the feedback from the rehabilitation worker.

Ongoing review of the records told the rehabilitation worker when Jacques was ready to progress to a different activity, but, before progressing on, the rehabilitation worker introduced variations into the coffee-making activity so that Jacques could learn and practise problem solving and planning strategies. By the end of the fifth week of the rehabilitation programme, Jacques could independently initiate and execute making a cup of hot instant coffee.

Demonstration/modelling

This teaching method refers to the performance, plus an explanation, by the rehabilitation worker of the task to be learned. It is a technique that

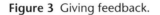

Figure 3 Giving feedback.

is well suited to the teaching of a psychomotor skill but may also integrate cognitive and affective elements. To be successful you need to be a skilled performer of the task and have analysed each component of the task so that each skill or movement can be shown and explained. A demonstration provides the opportunity of seeing a skilled performance but it must be followed by practise, preferably immediately, whilst the demonstration is still fresh in the mind.

Some clients will be capable of observing a lengthy demonstration before practising, whilst others need a task broken down into each stage. Preparing a demonstration requires as much thought and preparation as any other form of teaching. For a demonstration to be clear and interpreted, all necessary items of equipment or materials should be on hand, and in good working order. Think about the speed of the demonstration. Whilst it can be argued that a demonstration at normal speed is useful in showing the eventual goal, the ideal speed for teaching and learning is normally considerably slower.

Commonly, rehabilitation programmes consist of a narrated demonstration, then practice under supervision, followed by feedback. Time for discussion and feedback is essential. The need for repetition of the demonstration should be assessed. The whole, or parts, of a demonstration may have to be repeated. People learn differently and you need to be alert to signs that indicate understanding or lack of it.

Box 4 Guidelines for demonstration/modelling

Set a clear goal or image of the desired outcome by limiting distractions and giving a timely and skilled demonstration.
Provide relevant knowledge and information, either before or after the demonstration, as it may prove distracting if done during the demonstration.
Provide guided practice with constructive, corrective feedback.
Give the clients the opportunity to reflect on their own learning performance.

The following example illustrates a demonstration of a sliding board transfer from a wheelchair to a chair as an example.

■ What is the purpose of this demonstration?
Zaid is a new wheelchair user and needs to be able to transfer independently. The purpose of the demonstration is to teach him to move himself. The utilisation of a sliding board is useful where the heights of surfaces vary or where there is a gap.
■ Preparation of the environment.
As Zaid is sitting in his wheelchair, the demonstration uses two chairs, which are placed side by side. If a wheelchair is used the arm between the two chairs is removed. The floor should be free from clutter.
■ What questions might Zaid ask?
What is the sliding board made of?
Will it hold my weight?
How will I stop the board from tipping or slipping?
How will I carry the board around with me?

Stop and think

Prepare a demonstration to teach someone how to use a walking aid.

■ What would be the purpose of this demonstration?
■ How will you prepare the environment?
■ What questions might you be asked?

Write out the steps for demonstrating how to use the walking aid.
Remember: each individual has their own capacity to learn, and this may be related to their diagnosis, condition or motivation.

Chaining

Chaining is a method of teaching skills in a step-by-step process. There are two types of chaining: forward and backward.

Forward chaining involves learning each aspect of an activity from the beginning to the end.

Backward chaining is mastering the last step first.

Box 5 Example of forward chaining and backward chaining

Task Having a drink of milk

Step	Forward chaining	Backward chaining
(1)	Opening fridge door	Drink milk
(2)	Selecting milk	Pour milk
(3)	Opening milk container	Select drinking utensil
(4)	Select drinking utensil	Open milk container
(5)	Pour milk	Select milk
(6)	Drink	Open fridge door

Chaining enables the rehabilitation worker to monitor very small achievements rather than the whole task. These small but important achievements motivate and encourage the individual to persevere when the rehabilitation programme is slow stream or long term.

Groupwork

As a rehabilitation worker, you may be involved in groupwork in a number of different ways:

■ You may run an activity group which aims to teach task skills and encourage social interaction.

■ You may facilitate or be part of a support group where members share and explore their experiences.

■ Or you may be asked to facilitate a workshop for information or teaching purposes.

Groupwork will be appropriate if the client involved:

■ Has the skills and awareness to interact and share with others in a group.

■ Feels isolated and is without others to offer support or constructive advice.

Grouping people together does not automatically lead to groupwork. Effective groupwork requires several people to work and learn together and helps the individual to consider and respond to the feelings, ideas and opinions of others. Groupwork promotes recognition of similarities and differences. A gathering of people becomes a group when they have the same goals or ideals and when they know they depend on each other to achieve those goals or meet their needs.

If you are running a group you will need to consider the individual needs of the clients, the dynamics of the group, how the members interact and behave

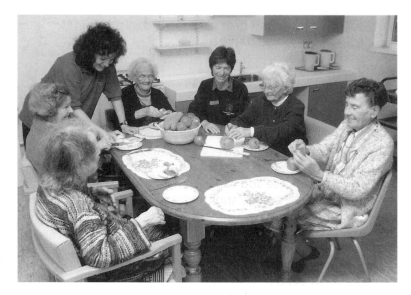

Figure 4 Groupwork.

towards one another, and your own behaviour. Your responsibility is to listen and to respond to the whole group. Listening becomes a problem when the group members regard you as the expert or when you engage with one or two of the more vocal members rather than the whole group.

Box 6 Techniques for the effective facilitation of groupwork

Ensure that group members have an agreed set of ground rules.
Ensure that group members are clear about why they are there.
Look around the room, both when you are speaking and when a group member is speaking. That way the group members will quickly recognise that they are addressing the whole group rather than just you. It will allow you to pick up cues from those who want to speak but are either too slow or are shy.

Preparing for groupwork

Background. If the group is a new one, people will have to get to know each other and find ways of working together. Expectations will be influenced by the advance information given to the members.

Size. The ideal size for a group depends on its purpose. In a small group there is a better chance of gaining participation by all members.

Environment. Groups generally benefit from feeling that they have a defined place in which to meet. The members may arrange the environment to suit themselves. However, for the first meeting it may help to arrange chairs so people can see and hear each other and to minimise distractions such as noise or extreme room temperatures.

Role-play

A role-play is a hands-on opportunity to simulate real life and to practise skills. Role-playing makes use of drama techniques with learners acting assigned parts. Enacting a simulation gives learners a chance to examine their behaviour without the risks that may be inherent in a real-life experience. It allows them the opportunity to practise and experiment with new skills and behaviours, to emphasise different view points, and to receive feedback on behaviour. As role-play draws upon the learners' experiences and knowledge, the subsequent analysis of the interaction is an essential part of role-play. Role-play is particularly useful in social skills training. For instance, in learning how to use communication techniques, a person with poor social skills can be asked to enact initiating conversation in a social situation.

Such issues are often difficult and emotive. Couple this with many people's anxiety and unfamiliarity with role-playing and you can begin to anticipate some resistance to using this technique. For this reason, it is essential to give clear guidelines and safety rules.

> **Box 7   Safety rules for role-play**
>
> All scenarios should be based on learners' needs and their current situation.
> Time out can be called at any time.
> Always conduct a feedback session that reviews and analyses what happened in the role-play.
> Emphasis will be on positive feedback. Constructive suggestions for improvement will be made, rather than negative criticism.
> Never rush processing the role-play. Allow at least as much time for processing the experiences as it takes to enact.

▪ Teaching materials

Audio-visual assisted learning

The use of audio-visual aids can help to stimulate interest and motivate participants to try new behaviours. The content can provide information, and illustrate and model the ideas and skills you are working on during the rehabilitation programme.

Short videos or films can be used in two ways:

(1) Viewing a film.
(2) Filming, then viewing the person carrying out an activity.

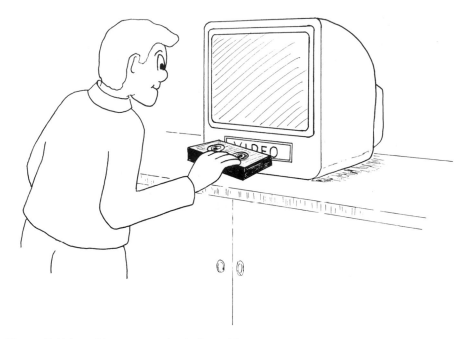

Figure 5 Using video as a method of teaching.

Viewing a film

Since people are passive as they view a video/film, this method should be combined with a discussion, so that there is active participation.

You may watch the film with the individual, or leave it with them to watch at another time. Either way you need to follow these steps for using video/film watching in rehabilitation programmes:

(1) Prepare for showing.
(2) Check that the equipment and resources are compatible.
(3) Preview and identify the important points you want the person to get from viewing the film.
(4) Check the equipment works.
(5) Provide instructions.
(6) Tell the individual(s) what they will see and why.
(7) After the viewing, discuss and summarise the major points.

Stop and think

Select a film/video that you may use during a rehabilitation programme. Preview it and answer these questions:

How could I introduce this video into the rehabilitation programme?
What would be the advantages/disadvantages of doing so?

Filming the client

This is an excellent way of capturing pre- and post-learning, and also for the individual to view themselves and identify the difficulties they have. Consent will need to obtained from the individual, and consent forms need to be filled in if the film is to be used for any purpose other than feedback to the individual.

Computer assisted learning

There are a vast number of computer packages that aid learning, from simple touch screens, which rely on reinforcement, to complex problem-solving games. Technology often appeals to technically minded individuals and can work well in some cases. See also 'E-Learning', p. 304.

Information sheets

Written materials are one of the most important teaching tools available. They can be used for direct learning and can be left with the individuals to reinforce any messages given.

Box 8 Preparing information sheets

The sheet should be easy to understand and learn from.
Use simple language and avoid overlong sentences or statements.
Diagrams can help to clarify a complex message.
Aim to have a consistent style throughout.
Ensure any sheets are produced to a high quality.
Frequently photocopied pages look scrappy and may be difficult to read.

There are a number of computer packages that can help with both the format and content of these sheets.

▪ Evaluation

Just as it is important to evaluate the whole rehabilitation programme, you also need to continually evaluate the particular teaching techniques you have used. The purpose of evaluation is to gather and interpret data to determine the extent to which your teaching techniques have been successful. There are three reasons for this:

(1) To provide guidance on how to improve further rehabilitation programmes.
(2) To contribute to the assessment of an individual's need for further rehabilitation sessions.

Teaching for rehabilitation

OUTCOME

- What changes occurred in the client's knowledge or behaviour?
- Did the client consider he/she had benefited?
- Were the client's objectives (goals) achieved?
- Is there evidence of transferable skills?

EVALUATION

STRUCTURE

- Were the facilities and resources adequate?
- Was there sufficient time?
- Was the environment conducive to learning?
- Was the programme logically ordered?

PROCESS

- How did the client participate?
- Was feedback given and received?
- Did the teaching methods build on existing experiences and abilities?

Figure 6 Evaluation chart.

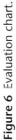

(3) Feedback for the rehabilitation worker, which will indicate strengths and weaknesses, allowing for improvements in providing services and for job satisfaction.

The evaluation can examine the structure, process and outcome of a programme or educational package. The evaluation chart (Figure 6) suggests some questions and areas to guide the evaluation process.

■ Conclusion

This chapter has shown that teaching is a vital part of the role of the rehabilitation worker. Much of rehabilitation is directed at assisting the individual to adapt to new circumstances or environments. Since learning is an essential part of adaptation, it can be argued that all rehabilitation is teaching. Teaching is challenging, satisfying and sometimes frustrating. It should be recognised and carried out as a purposeful activity, with time spent planning and evaluating teaching strategies. Teaching and learning are interactive processes. The individual learner should be involved in planning and evaluating their own personal learning wherever possible.

■ Further reading

Doak, C.C., Doak, L.G. & Root, J.H. (1996) *Teaching Patients with Low Literacy*. Philadelphia, J.P. Lippincott. *This book offers practical advice for developing and evaluating written client education material.*

Finlay, L. (1993) *Groupwork in Occupational Therapy*. Cheltenham, Nelson Thornes Ltd.

Kiger, A.M. (2004) *Teaching for Health* (3rd edition). London, Churchill Livingstone. *This book offers a comprehensive coverage of the basic elements of teaching. Its focus is health promotion rather than rehabilitation, but Chapter 5, on teaching techniques and aids, provides a useful overview.*

Knowles, M.S. (1970) *The Modern Practice of Adult Education: Androgogy versus Pedagogy*. New York, Association Press.

Section 2
Enhancing function

Enhancing function

Susan Nancarrow, Hazel Mackey, Kelly McPhee, Sue Ball, Martin Ridgeway, Beverly Palin & Anna Moran

INTRODUCTION

As a rehabilitation worker, it is likely that one of your major tasks will be to help clients become as independent as possible in their activities of daily living. The client's ability to perform many activities that most of us take for granted: getting in and out of bed and being able to go to the toilet, wash and get dressed in the morning, can make the difference between being able to live alone or needing intensive daily support. This section of the book is dedicated to helping you work with the client to optimise their function during their day-to-day activities, or commonly performed tasks.

Deficits in the client's activities of daily living are normally assessed by a rehabilitation team. Similarly, the input of an interdisciplinary team is normally required to develop a programme to help regain independence. It is valuable to monitor the client's ability to undertake their daily activities in their normal environment. A client may manage perfectly well in a therapy kitchen in a residential rehabilitation setting, then return to their own home which may have uneven flooring, cupboards they can't reach and broken drawer handles, making it difficult to function. It is also useful to see the client's normal routine and patterns, so the rehabilitation programme can be tailored to be as achievable as possible for the client. However, this does not mean that clients cannot learn valuable skills in a dedicated rehabilitation setting before they return home.

Additionally, every client will have different habits and different living arrangements. Some clients live with very able-bodied, supportive family members, whilst others live alone. A client with hemiplegia living in a single-storey bungalow will have quite different support needs to the same person living in a house with lots of stairs. Some clients might be very tidy and highly organised, whereas others could be extremely untidy and disorganised, which could create difficulties moving around the house, or finding appropriate clothing, for instance. In some cases, the client's home environment might be a safety risk to both them and you. Alternatively, you might identify a client who has memory loss or cognitive impairment. It is important to take into account the skills and limitations of the client. Section 1: Teaching for rehabilitation highlights some of the issues you need to consider when you are developing a programme for a client.

In your role as a rehabilitation worker, you are ideally placed to monitor changes in the client's abilities or identify particular difficulties they might have and notify the relevant member of your team to have the issues addressed.

Levels of independence

Activities of daily living can be divided into two categories:

(1) Basic activities of daily living (BADL).
(2) Instrumental activities of daily living (IADL).

BADL are those activities that enable the client to maintain themselves in their home living environment. They include personal hygiene, bathing, dressing, feeding and functional mobility. IADL allow the client to function more fully within their local community or society and require more advanced skills such as problem solving and social interaction. Examples of IADL include home management, such as meal preparation and shopping, catching public transport and managing medication. This section will not cover the full range of IADL, but will cover some of the most common areas likely to be required by rehabilitation workers when working with clients.

To monitor change, and have a way of communicating levels of dependence or independence with other team members, it is useful to be able to rate different levels of independence. Two common tools used to describe levels of independence on ADL are the Barthel Index and Functional Independence Measure (FIM). These tools enable the assessor to rate the client's level of independence on a scale that ranges from complete dependence to full independence.

Box 1 provides a way of describing levels of independence.

A client is only deemed to be independent when they can perform an activity without any assistance or assistive devices, and within a reasonable length of time. You can include a note of the client's level of independence in performing a particular activity in the progress notes (see Section 1: Agreeing and reaching goals, for more detail).

Box 1 Describing levels of independence

Dependent	Client requires total assistance, or more than 75% support to complete a given activity.
Maximal assistance	Requires between 50% and 75% physical assistance to complete an activity.
Moderate assistance	Requires between 25% and 50% physical assistance to complete an activity. The client may require some cues or assistive devices to help them with the activity.
Minimal assistance	Less than 25% physical assistance required to complete the task as well as some supervision and cues.
Supervision	The client can complete the task themselves, but requires supervision.
Independent	The client can perform the activity without any assistance, physical or verbal support and without the use of assistive devices.

(*Source*: Hamilton, B.B., Granger, C.V., Sherwin, E.S., Zielezny, M. & Tashman, J.S. (1987) A uniform national data system for medical rehabilitation. In: M.J. Fuhrer (ed.), *Rehabilitation Outcomes: Analysis and Measurement* (pp. 115–150), Baltimore, Md., Brookes.)

■ Being prepared to help support function

Before you can help the client develop skills in a particular activity of daily living, you need to become familiar with the task yourself. This means familiarising yourself with any equipment you might need to use and being able to demonstrate activities and the use of equipment. Section 1: Teaching for rehabilitation provides more information about the range of different teaching approaches you may need to use to teach a particular skill or activity. Don't forget that you will not just be teaching the new skill or activity to the client. In many cases, you need to work closely with carers or other family members to teach them how to support the client around particular activities.

The other important skill you need is a good ability to observe and listen. *Watch* the client performing a particular activity and consider the factors that are helping them, and those that are causing them difficulty. *Listen* to the client, ask them questions about their progress. Ensure that you use these important cues to inform your decision making about the appropriateness of the intervention, and the client's progress against their goals. The intrinsic–extrinsic framework below can form a valuable basis for your observations. You should provide feedback to the team about your observations.

■ ■ CASE STUDIES

Eight case studies are outlined below. They are based on real clinical experiences and provide an indication of the variety of individuals you will meet, and the different types of interventions you might deliver during the rehabilitation process. Space does not permit an in-depth exploration of the complexities of each case. Nevertheless, they are referred to throughout the rest of this section, to emphasise the practical application of rehabilitation interventions. Each client's preferred name or title is written in brackets beside their name, and this is the name that is used throughout the text.

Case study 1 Ms Vinita Gupta (Vinita)

Vinita is a 45-year-old mother of two school-aged daughters. She was diagnosed with rheumatoid arthritis six months ago. She and her husband moved to England from India 20 years ago, and whilst she has good community support, all of her extended family still live in India. They live in a three-storey house and she has some difficulties getting up and down the stairs, particularly during acute phases of her arthritis. She often feels fatigued, and has aches and pains in her hands and feet most days. However, she is able to carry out her normal daily activities despite some discomfort and limited movement in some joints. Every morning, Vinita wakes with pain and stiffness in her wrists. Her ability to reach and manipulate objects is reduced, as is her ability to lift and carry. She has regular 'flare-ups' of her arthritis when her joints are very painful and swollen and her movements severely limited. At these times her activities are limited to self-care only.

Case study 2 Mrs Phyllis Heath (Mrs Heath)

Mrs Heath is 85 years old and lives with her husband, Jack, who is 87. They have no children. Mrs Heath is very bright and alert. She is well educated and teaches piano to students who come to her home. Up until five years ago she also worked as a volunteer, delivering meals to housebound and disabled people. She is a regular church attender, and has a good network of friends. Recently, she tripped and fractured her left hip. She was admitted to hospital and underwent surgery for a total hip replacement. She also suffers from urinary incontinence which has become worse since her hospitalisation.

Case study 3   Mr Giuseppe Rossi (Mr Rossi)

Mr Giuseppe Rossi is 63 years old. He was diagnosed with Parkinson's disease ten years ago. His condition has deteriorated steadily and two years ago he retired from his job as a bank manager. Mr Rossi's mobility has deteriorated recently, resulting in four falls in one month. Mr Rossi has a fixed posture when he walks, his neck is held flexed, his spine is rigid and he cannot swing his arms. He has difficulty initiating movement and walks with short shuffling steps. He finds turning and walking through doorways difficult. He has difficulty being understood as he cannot raise his voice, and finds eating and drinking difficult.

Case study 4   Mr Mick Black (Mick)

Mick is a former miner who stopped working when the local pit closed in the early 1990s. He was a heavy smoker but stopped smoking two years ago. He is 55 years old and has chronic emphysema. He lives in a three-storey terraced house which is at the top of a steep hill. He has difficulty getting a loud enough voice to talk to people. His wife, Esther, gives good support but she worries about his wheezing and inability to sleep at night. She is also concerned about his frequent coughing or choking during eating and drinking. Mick feels tired all the time. He becomes breathless on exertion. He no longer socialises with his friends as he has difficulty talking and getting out of the house. Recently Mick has been neglecting his personal hygiene and he rarely washes or showers.

Case study 5   Ms Maryanne Yin (Maryanne)

Maryanne is a petite, attractive, 59-year-old, divorced business woman who owns a number of well-known and successful beauty salons. She prides herself on always looking smart and well presented. She has a wide circle of friends and enjoys social gatherings such as eating at the best restaurants, attending galas and balls and going to the theatre. At work she wears tailored suits with heeled shoes, and during her leisure time she wears coordinated smart casual wear. She has a wide selection of earrings, necklaces and bracelets, and friends often tell her that they can judge her mood according to the jewellery that she is wearing. One afternoon, whilst at work, Maryanne had a right CVA (stroke) which resulted in a left-sided hemiplegia. English is her second language.

Enhancing function

Case study 6 Mrs Frances Yves (Frances)

Frances is a 68-year-old woman who was widowed six months ago when her husband of 45 years died suddenly. Following her husband's death she has suffered depression which is being treated with antidepressants. Frances has been an insulin-dependent diabetic since she was a teenager. Over the past ten years she has developed severe peripheral neuropathy and peripheral vascular disease which causes coldness and numbness to her feet. Her eyesight has begun to fade due to diabetic retinopathy.

Case study 7 Mr Bob Wright (Bob)

Bob is a 28-year-old single man with Down's syndrome. He has significant difficulties with reading and writing, and people find his speech difficult to understand. He lives with his elderly grandmother. Bob is independent in eating, dressing, bathing and simple food preparation. He would like to get a job but he lacks confidence in going out alone. He easily becomes flustered when things don't go to plan and is anxious when he is required to interact with people he doesn't know. Bob's grandmother has asked for help to prepare Bob to live alone when she dies.

Case study 8 Mrs Elena Kalnina (Mrs Kalnina)

Mrs Kalnina is a 52-year-old widow who has a history of depressive illness over a 20-year period. Three years ago, she completed a degree in history after studying at her local university on a part-time basis. Since then she has had a number of short-term jobs such as clerical assistant, tour guide and assistant librarian. However, she has been unable to maintain full-time, permanent employment due to relapses of her anxiety and depressive illness.

Mrs Kalnina lives alone. She has difficulty sleeping and wakes each morning feeling depressed. She spends a great deal of time alone. Her leisure interests are reading, watching documentaries on the television and needlepoint. She is able to complete all her personal care and household tasks but does so with little energy or enthusiasm. Recently, Mrs Kalnina has lost confidence in going out alone. She would like to return to work in order to supplement her income, to gain new social networks and to have more structure to her day.

■ Identifying solutions

Helping a client become independent in their activities of daily living involves two main approaches:

(1) Restoring impaired skills through retraining.
(2) Adapting the disability through environmental adaptations.

Breaking these two approaches down further, it is useful to consider those factors that impact on the client that are intrinsic, or internal to the client, and extrinsic. **Intrinsic** factors include the following:

- **Physical factors:** such as the mobility of the client, their level of fitness, integrity of their joints and skin.
- **Medical factors:** such as the underlying disease, diagnosis or pathology.
- **Emotional and psychological factors:** including motivation, spirituality, self-esteem and depression.

Extrinsic factors include:

- The **physical environment:** this is the setting in which any of the client's activities take place, including home, work and social activities.
- The client's **financial** situation: can the client afford the intervention that you are considering?
- **Social** factors: such as cultural and religious considerations, employment and interactions with friends and family.

It is useful to consider the intrinsic and extrinsic factors surrounding all of the activities of re-enablement, and in the context of the goals of the client. Generally, the client assessment will identify these issues, but as a rehabilitation worker, you are ideally placed to consider these issues as they arise to help you identify some of the problems, and consider the solutions.

For most 'problems' of rehabilitation, there are a number of possible solutions that will depend on the client's situation and desires. You can use the intrinsic/extrinsic framework above to identify the problems, and to consider a wide range of different solutions. You will need to discuss these with the client and with your team to determine the most appropriate approach to address the problems.

Review the case study of Mrs Heath (case study 2) to consider the factors that may place her at risk of falling again. You work with Mrs Heath for two mornings, and make the following observations about her intrinsic and extrinsic risk factors for falling:

Intrinsic risk factors

- Poor eyesight
- Muscle weakness
- Painful joints
- Sore feet
- Lack of confidence

Enhancing function

Enhancing function

- Incontinence and urgent need to get to the bathroom
- Reduced mobility following hip replacement

Extrinsic risk factors

- Steep stairs to get to the bathroom
- Loose rugs on the floor
- Poor lighting in the house
- Poorly fitting shoes

There are likely to be many more intrinsic and extrinsic risk factors for clients at risk of falling. You may think of some yourself, or refer to Section 3: Falls, for more ideas.

Now think about some of the ways that you might go about addressing some of these risk factors for falling. Some of the risk factors are more easily modifiable than others. For instance, poor eyesight can be difficult to correct, although you may want to consider whether Mrs Heath has the right glasses to treat her condition. Similarly, steep stairs could be very expensive to alter, and most of the alternative solutions, such as a stairlift, or putting an additional toilet on another floor of the house, are expensive. You may identify ways to address Mrs Heath's muscle weakness, painful joints and sore feet, and to improve her mobility. Can you think of any other solutions?

Each of these options needs to be considered within the team, and in consultation with Mrs Heath to identify the most appropriate treatment option to address her needs and circumstances.

Stop and think

Review the case studies of Bob (case study 7) and Mrs Kalnina (case study 8) and think about some of the intrinsic and extrinsic factors that may impact on their ability to achieve their goals.

The remainder of this section considers these two main approaches to enabling independence in a range of activities of daily living. The activities included in this section are:

- Mobility and transfers
- Washing and hygiene
- Dressing
- Toileting and toilet management
- Food preparation, handling and eating
- Swallowing difficulties
- Managing medication
- Going out

■ ■ MOBILITY AND TRANSFERS

Mobility is fundamental to enabling independence. Supporting mobility in the home and community is a key goal of rehabilitation. For individuals to be able to participate in the activities and tasks of their life roles, they must be able to move around their surroundings. This may entail moving around in bed, dressing or toileting, moving around the house to cook or clean, or moving about the community to a workplace, shop, theatre, or church. Rehabilitation workers are concerned with a person's mobility with regards to positioning and posture, therapeutic exercise, transfers, walking, and the use of assistive devices or adaptive equipment.

Stop and think

Think of some people you have worked with in the past, or people you know whose mobility is restricted.
How did their mobility difficulties affect their participation in everyday activities?
How did their family and friends react?
What equipment or adaptations were required?
What was the psychological effect of their loss of mobility?

■ Barriers to mobility and transfers

Many intrinsic and extrinsic factors impact on mobility and transfer difficulties, including the underlying pathology, the individual and their environment. Mobility and transfer difficulties can arise from either neurological or mechanical (musculoskeletal) origins, or a mixture of both. Cardiorespiratory diseases can also impact on mobility because they cause breathlessness and a lack of energy.

Neurological impairments

Neurological impairments result from damage to the central nervous system (the brain or spinal cord) from conditions such as multiple sclerosis, motor neurone disease and cerebrovascular accidents, or from direct trauma/lesion through head or spinal injury. Mr Rossi (case study 3) has Parkinson's disease, which is a neurological impairment.

The effects of neurological impairments may include:

■ Abnormal muscle tone.
■ Loss of the ability of muscles to work together.
■ Loss of sensory feedback and perceptual cues that are vital for judging distance and depth to accomplish desired movement.

■ The loss of postural reflexes needed to provide stability and balance when moving.

The approach to rehabilitation will vary, depending upon the extent and location of the damage to the central nervous system. Cerebellum (brain) damage affects muscle tone and coordination, whilst spinal cord injury impacts upon muscle use and sensation below the level of the lesion. Often the treatment and techniques used will focus on maintaining function and reducing the effects of the disability. The central nervous system cannot regenerate, unlike peripheral nerves, so the intervention must include effective problem solving that enables the client to work out new ways of managing their activities of daily living. Damage to peripheral nerves is common and may result from direct injury from crushing or cutting, or from the effects of infection and disease such as meningitis or diabetes mellitus. Frances' peripheral neuropathy is caused by her diabetes. Sensation and muscle use will be reduced but it is sometimes possible for the nerves to repair, thus enhancing the potential for rehabilitation.

Musculo skeletal impairments

Any change to the body's musculoskeletal system resulting from trauma, disease or growth problems can affect movement. The causes of these changes include bone trauma and fractures, joint injuries, muscle damage, and soft tissue injuries to ligaments and tendons. Some conditions may cause skeletal abnormalities such as scoliosis; whilst other diseases like osteoporosis, osteoarthritis and rheumatoid arthritis impact on bone strength, joint movement and joint stability. Some of the effects of musculoskeletal damage can include muscle imbalance and weakness, pain, restricted range of movement or the skeleton being unable to bear the body's weight. Mrs Heath's mobility problems are of musculoskeletal origin.

Careful consideration should be given to the client's medical stability before starting rehabilitation. It is crucial to liaise with other members of the team involved in the individual's care before implementing an intervention. A thorough risk assessment may be necessary to avoid further damage to the musculoskeletal system. For example, clients with balance problems or bone/muscle weakness may be at risk of further fractures due to a high risk of falls. Conditions such as rheumatoid arthritis leave joints susceptible to further damage and deformity if too much strain is placed upon them when the disease is in its acute or active phase.

Psychological and social impact of mobility and transfer problems

In addition to the physical impact, it is important to consider the psychological and social impact of reduced mobility on the client and their family or carer. Many factors will be involved, including age, cause of disability, responsibilities and roles, lifestyle, relationships, environment, motivation, general health, confidence, self-esteem, support networks and employment status. The way

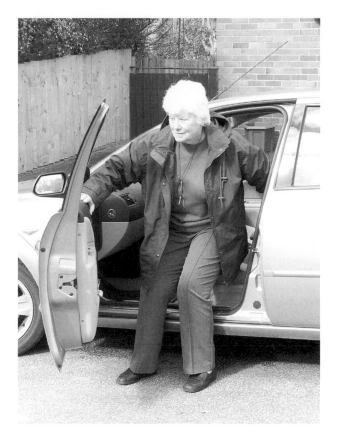

Figure 1 Imagine if you lost your ability to move around as freely as you currently do.

these factors impact upon a situation will ultimately depend upon the individual's circumstances, the personalities involved, and this can only be ascertained by thorough assessment. You should not make assumptions, and all cases should be considered on an individual basis.

Stop and think

Imagine if you lost your ability to walk, drive, or to move around as freely as you can now. What activities would you no longer be able to do? How would you shop, cook, clean, go to work or look after children? What impact would your loss of mobility have on your social life? Now consider how these changes would affect your self-esteem and confidence.

Reflect on the impact that a loss of mobility must have on your clients, whether it is sudden or gradual.

For example, consider the effects of Mr Rossi's Parkinsonism and Mrs Heath's hip fracture. Both individuals may experience emotions such as depression,

Enhancing function

a sense of loss, grief, frustration, embarrassment, anxiety, bitterness, anger or shame. They may have problems accepting assistive equipment, home adaptations or reliance upon someone else to help them with some personal or domestic activities of daily living. Equally, both individuals may share a strong desire to accept their disabilities and be motivated to work hard and become as independent as possible.

Consideration of how disability impacts upon the psychological and social issues is paramount if the wishes and aspirations of the individual are to be identified and addressed by the rehabilitation team. Section 3: Psychological aspects of rehabilitation provides more information about how to provide or access psychological support for your client.

■ Walking

It is useful to consider and observe what constitutes normal movement patterns associated with mobility and transfers. When humans stand upright, our centre of gravity lies slightly to the front of the middle of the pelvic region. The normal walking pattern consists of two phases: the support phase and the swing phase.

- **Support phase:** this begins when the heel of the leading leg strikes the ground and the body's weight shifts to this side as the foot is placed flat on the ground. The body is now supported to allow the trailing leg to commence the swing phase.
- **Swing phase:** this begins when the toes of the trailing leg leave the ground and commence the swing forward through to heel strike.

It is helpful to observe someone from the front and side to highlight the degree of flexion and extension required at the hip, knee and ankle joints to accomplish a normal walking gait. Also, notice how the head and trunk move to accommodate the changing centre of gravity, therefore maintaining the necessary balance through each phase.

These phases involve readjustment of the pelvis to ensure the body's centre of gravity is over the supporting foot to produce balanced upright movement. An individual unable to move their pelvis in this way will have difficulty walking.

An abnormal walking gait will occur if a mechanical or neurological impairment is present that affects the body's ability to achieve the two phases of walking described above. Types of abnormal walking gait include:

- **Shuffling gait:** commonly affecting people with Parkinson's disease, whereby the pelvis and knees become quite rigid resulting in short, shuffling type steps.
- **High stepping:** due to lack of sensory feedback from the sole of the foot, leading to the foot being lifted high off the ground in the swing phase.
- **Spastic and hemiplegic gait:** whereby high or low tone, due to neurological damage of the central nervous system, affects the swing phase and results in problems achieving correct heel strike, coordination and balance.

■ **Waddling gait:** caused by muscle weakness and lack of pelvic support, leading to pelvic tilt and exaggerated side-to-side movement of the trunk.

Gait abnormalities make walking less efficient and mobility more difficult, which means that the client will use more energy to move around. Normally, another part of the body will need to compensate for the abnormal gait. This might occur at the knee, hip or lower back and could result in pain, or muscle or joint strain.

A further risk of gait abnormalities is that it affects the normal interaction between the muscles and bones of the leg that take place during walking to ensure normal circulation. Our bodies use gravity to allow blood to flow down to our legs and feet and we have a complex system of built-in pumps in our calf muscles that move the blood from our feet back up to the heart. If someone is immobile for a long time, or is unable to walk properly, the 'calf muscle pump' will not work effectively, which increases their risk of developing circulatory problems in their legs and feet. This is one reason that people are mobilised fairly quickly following hospitalisation for conditions like a hip fracture.

To help Mr Rossi walk, the rehabilitation worker reinforces the walking techniques taught by the physiotherapist. During walking practice, the rehabilitation worker emphasises the heel–toe gait, arm swing and upright posture. Mr Rossi sometimes 'freezes' and is unable to initiate any movement. As well as being frustrating, this can increase his risk of falling. In these circumstances, the rehabilitation worker uses auditory and verbal cues, for instance encouraging Mr Rossi to deliberately shift his body weight onto one foot. Mr Rossi has been advised to remove the loose rugs within his home as these are potential hazards for slips and trips, and to wear non-slip footwear.

■ Posture and positioning

Rehabilitation workers both practise and teach the principles of proper body mechanics. These are used not only for lifting and carrying, but for nearly every movement undertaken. The principles of body mechanics are:

■ Ensure good posture by maintaining the natural curves of the spine, knees slightly bent and weight over the centre of the body.
■ Maintain a stable base of support, feet usually shoulder width apart, using both sides of the body equally.
■ Bend from the hips and the knees and do not use the back muscles to perform work.
■ Do not twist the body when lifting, pivot or shift the feet to turn.

Correct positioning is essential for preventing the complications associated with restricted mobility. Mr Rossi has the characteristic stooped posture associated with Parkinson's disease (see Figure 2). This affects his mobility and ability

Enhancing function

to transfer. Mr Rossi was advised to concentrate on his standing posture and to carry out exercises to prevent further deterioration (see Figure 3).

Stop and think

Consider the ways that problems with posture can affect self-care and participation in wider community activities.

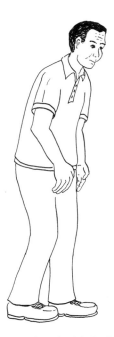

Figure 2 The characteristic stoop associated with Parkinson's disease.

Choosing a chair

Sitting posture is important, especially as people with restricted mobility spend a lot of time in chairs. Feet should be flat on the floor and the hips well back in the seat, with weight distributed evenly over the hips. It is easier to get out of a high chair than a low one. There are many different styles and shapes of chair. As a rehabilitation worker you may be asked to advise on the purchase of a new chair. Always advise the individual to try out the chair before purchasing as the size, shape, weight and physical condition of the individual affects the suitability of the chair even if it is specially designed for those with restricted mobility. Don't forget to consider the cost and the environment in which the chair will be used to ensure that they are appropriate for the needs of the client.

Enhancing function

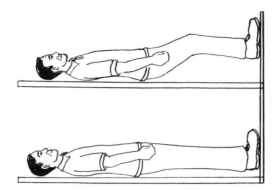

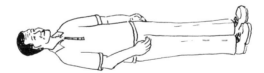

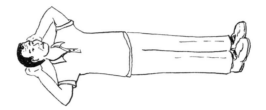

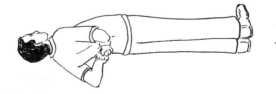

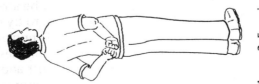

Figure 3 Exercises to improve posture.

Box 2   General guidelines on choosing a chair

- Choose the highest chair that allows the client's feet to be flat on the floor.
- Armrests are important to aid rising from a chair. Look for a good hand grip which allows the fingers to be wrapped around the end. The height of the armrests is important for support and comfort. Armrests that are too high cause the shoulders to hunch, but if they are too low the elbows will not be supported.
- It is easier to get out of a chair if the client's feet can be tucked back slightly underneath the seat of the chair. This allows them to move their weight over their feet more quickly. Therefore, avoid chairs that have no space between the seat and the floor.
- The seat of the chair should offer support, comfort and a firm base to push up from.
- Avoid sagging seats.
- The chair should be wide enough to allow changes in position.
- The seat should be just deep enough to give full support to the thighs.

Box 3   Alerts when mobilising a client following hip replacement

Precautions need to be taken following a hip replacement to:

- Prevent dislocation of the new joint.
- Prevent infection.

This will be achieved by:

- Avoiding forcing the range of movement of the joint.
- Avoiding aggressive exercise initially.
- Maintaining good posture.
- Initially, avoiding hip flexion beyond 90°, as well as internal rotation and adduction.

In addition to her arm chair, what other items in Mrs Heath's home may need raising? What advice would you offer Mrs Heath about bathing and dressing?

Consider the impact of Mrs Heath's hip replacement on her sitting posture and seating needs. Initially, she will need to take precautions to prevent dislocation of her new hip. This includes maintaining a good sitting posture that does not flex the hip beyond 90°. At home, Mrs Heath's chair is low. She is advised against using an extra cushion because although this raises the seat height, arm support is reduced. Instead, the rehabilitation worker firmly applies chair raisers to the legs of the chair.

■ Transfers

Transfers are the process of moving from one surface to another, such as from a bed to a wheelchair, from a wheelchair to a toilet, or from a wheelchair to a car. The complexity of the transfer will depend on the surfaces that the client is transferring between, and the physical ability of the client.

Understanding a normal sit to stand movement (see Figure 4) is useful to help you identify dysfunctional techniques:

- Before attempting to stand, move forward to the edge of the seat.
- Lean the trunk forward to allow the centre of gravity to be positioned over the feet.
- A solid base of support is established by placing the feet slightly apart with the preferred foot forward.
- By keeping the head up and pushing up with the hands and feet standing is easily achieved.

Stop and think

Try to stand without shifting your centre of gravity forward. How much more effort do you use to stand this way, compared to the recommended technique?

Think about the impact of poor standing technique on someone with a physical impairment or who is fatigued.

Techniques to assist moving and walking

There are various techniques and methods for performing a transfer. The most appropriate approach will depend on the individual, the help available and the layout of the environment. A thorough assessment of the intrinsic and extrinsic risk factors is necessary before encouraging or assisting the individual to stand or walk.

The upper body contains 60% of our total body weight. Therefore, in order to mobilise or transfer it is important to consider strength, joint mobility and balance of the upper body trunk and arms as well as the spine and lower limbs.

Besides balance, a range of other factors also need careful consideration, including muscle power and stamina, ability to weight-bear through both legs, the range of movement of participating joints, coordination, sensation and cognitive status. The need for adequate footwear, splints or orthoses, and consideration of whether pain is a problem are also important factors.

Before considering transfer techniques and approaches, it is important to consider sitting balance. If the client is able to sit on the edge of a bed or chair and maintain this position for a few minutes then they are said to have 'sitting balance'. Many people who have suffered a stroke have poor sitting balance

Enhancing function

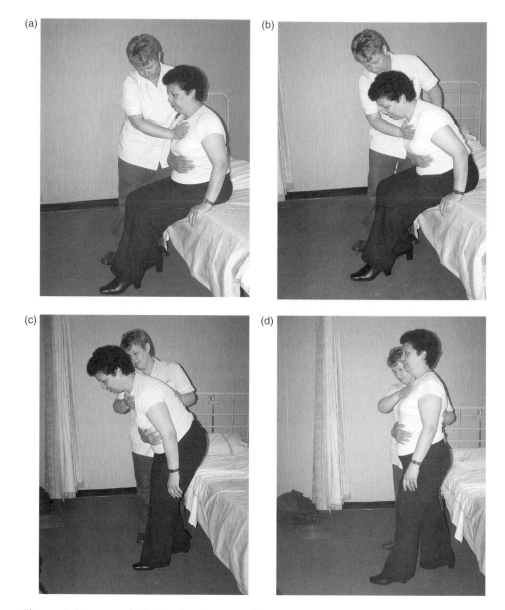

Figure 4 Sequenced photo of a client standing.

initially and have to re-learn good sitting balance to be safer when they sit, transfer or mobilise. Clients who are unable to maintain adequate sitting balance are likely to have difficulties achieving and maintaining safe standing.

Whichever transfer the client is undertaking, they need the ability to bring the weight forward and away from the buttocks. This can be done either independently or with assistance.

Family members can be trained to perform each step of the transfer as part of the rehabilitation programme. The family member should practise with the appropriate team member and the client in a protected, supervised environment. It is important to practise proper body mechanics throughout any transfers to protect the helper as well as the person being transferred.

There are three levels of transfer:

■ **Assisted transfer:** client requires assistance of one or more persons.
■ **Sliding board transfer:** client uses a sliding board to bridge the gap between two surfaces.
■ **Independent transfer:** client can perform all steps of a transfer with no assistance from another person, although an assistive device may be used.

A graded training programme, moving through the levels of transfers, may be necessary as the client progresses through rehabilitation.

Assisted transfers

Assisted transfers (see Figure 5) may be necessary for people with impairments that do not allow them to move independently, or until the client can begin to learn independent transfers. When you are working with the client to provide assisted transfers, both you and the client must have confidence in one another. This confidence comes from knowing each other's moves, and being clear about your own role in the procedure. Regardless of the transfer method the following guidelines should be used:

■ Discuss with the client the type and amount of help they require. Often the client will be able to tell you which transfer method they normally use.
■ Use correct body mechanics. You should ensure that before and during the manoeuvre your own hips and knees are flexed, your spine is straight, your head is erect, your feet are well spaced to give a firm base, and that you maintain balance throughout.
■ Prepare the environment before you undertake any manoeuvre. Ensure that you create an obstacle free passage from start to finish.
■ You should be suitably dressed, with shoes that provide firm support and clothes that allow adequate movement without creating any hazards.
■ Sometimes the client's condition can deteriorate and their normal transfer technique will be unsafe. You should never do a transfer with someone who you think may be unable to transfer, who is unsafe or who you are not confident about. If in doubt, check with the appropriate team member to reassess the client or consult your manual handling adviser.

Sliding board transfers

If someone is unable to stand to transfer, they may use a transfer board to bridge the gap between two surfaces and then slide their buttocks across the board to the new surface. The client must be able to put their legs in place after the transfer, or have assistance at hand.

Enhancing function

Enhancing function

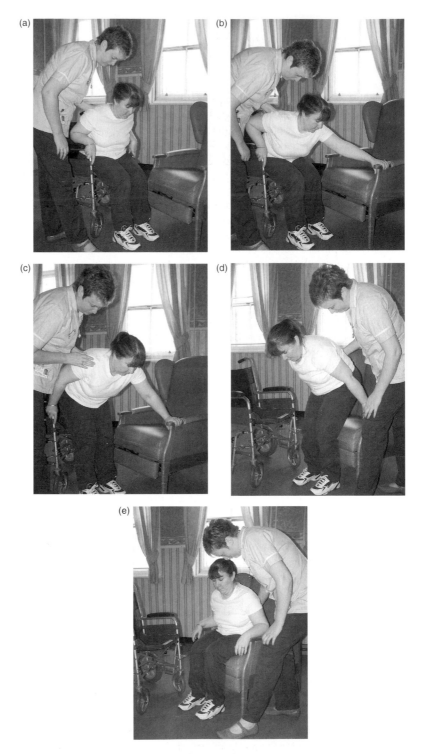

Figure 5 Assisted transfer from wheelchair to chair.

> **Box 4** Sliding transfers for people in a wheelchair
>
> ▪ Wheelchair or chair placement is usually at a 45° angle, although straight sideways and backwards transfers are also possible.
> ▪ Lock brakes and castors and remove any armrests.
> ▪ Level surfaces greatly aid the transfer, although gravity can be used to assist when sliding to a lower surface.
> ▪ Place transfer board to bridge the two surfaces. The individual leans to position a portion of the board under the buttocks and then sits and regains balance.
> ▪ The client performs shoulder depression with the elbows extended and locked to perform a series of little push ups along the surface of the board. Although the term 'slide' is used, the client does a lift and bounce movement rather than a slide as this could damage the skin.
> ▪ At destination, the client tilts the trunk and removes the board.

There are a variety of shapes, lengths, weights and styles of transfer board. A transfer board may be used to facilitate movement between different types of seating areas. This type of transfer may be particularly useful to support transfers in and out of a car.

Independent transfers

Clients with adequate strength to push up and move their trunk and lower limbs can transfer independently, although risk assessments still need to be carried out.

▪ The surfaces for transfers should be stable and as equal in height as possible.
▪ Brakes should be applied to any wheeled chair before the transfer is attempted, and any environmental hazards such as footrests should be removed.

Following her hip operation, Mrs Heath needed to learn how to stand from sitting whilst using a walking aid. One of the temptations of using a free-standing walking aid is to pull up on the aid to assist with standing. This is unsafe because the walking aid can tip and move as the person's weight moves. Mrs Heath was shown how to bring her body forward and to push up using the arms of the chair before reaching for the walking aid (see Figure 6).

Without adequate instruction and advice, walking aids can be hazardous when transferring as they can get tangled in the individual's feet, or tip over if the individual puts too much weight though them.

Enhancing function

Enhancing function

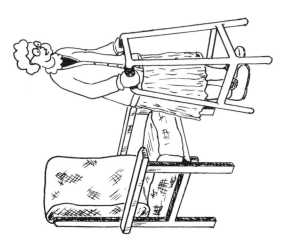

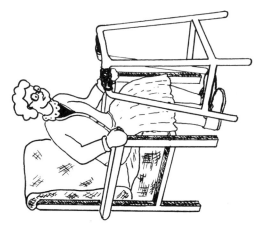

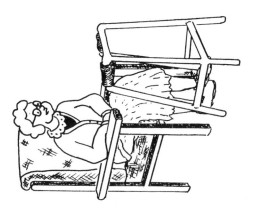

Figure 6 Standing using a walking frame.

■ Assistive equipment

There is enormous variety in the different types of equipment available to promote mobility and simplify client moving and handling. This section will not attempt to cover the full range, but will highlight some of the most common types of assistive equipment and give a brief description of their use. Links to more information about assistive equipment can be found at the end of this chapter.

Wheelchairs

Wheelchairs provide mobility for people who cannot walk or have limited walking ability. There are many different types of wheelchairs catering for a wide range of client needs. For example, self-propelling wheelchairs are appropriate for clients with the ability to drive the wheelchair using their arms or legs.

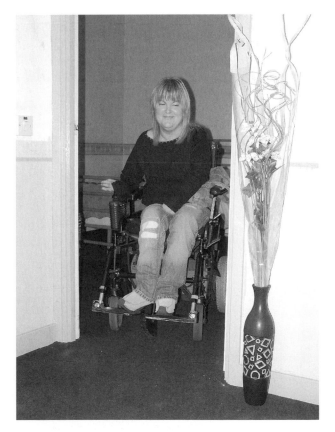

Figure 7 Client negotiating a doorframe in a wheelchair.

Enhancing function

Powered wheelchairs are useful for people who lack the ability to propel, or for people with low endurance levels who are cognitively aware and able to manage the controls. Attendant-propelled wheelchairs require a helper to walk behind and push them. The accurate prescription of a wheelchair is essential to the client's comfort and function.

Box 5   Considerations when selecting a wheelchair

- How often will the chair be used?
- Where will the chair be used? Indoors, outdoors or both?
- What are the environmental factors which need to be considered?
- How does the individual transfer?
- How will the wheelchair be transported?
- Has the individual any specific needs, for example continence issues, pressure areas?

The height and width of the wheelchair is based on the individual's physical requirements. The back and sides of a wheelchair can be modified to alter the amount of support provided.

It is important to consider how the wheelchair will be transported. Folding wheelchairs with detachable arms and footrests are transported easily. People

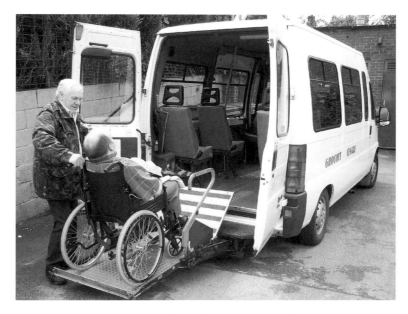

Figure 8 Community transport moving a client in a wheelchair.

with upper body strength often learn how to load their own wheelchair into a car. Alternatively, a selection of hoists and lifts are available.

Wheelchair users are often hindered by poor access to buildings, transport and public spaces. Narrow doorways, steps and insufficient turning spaces may restrict a person's ability to participate in community activities or reduce their independence. Accessibility and the physical space available are important considerations when planning any outing for a person with reduced mobility.

You may be involved in indoor and outdoor mobility training to help familiarise the client with their new wheelchair. The rehabilitation programme will include learning to handle and manoeuvre the wheelchair in many circumstances. The first phase of training involves propelling the wheelchair on a smooth, uncluttered surface, and transferring in and out of the wheelchair. The second phase involves learning to use the wheelchair outdoors, including using ramps, going up and down kerbs, and pushing a shopping trolley.

Stop and think

List the potential problems a wheelchair user faces when visiting the local supermarket for their weekly household shop. Consider the restrictions you have identified and suggest possible solutions.

Walking aids

A vast array of walking aids exist including:

- Walking sticks of various designs, including tripods and quadruped sticks.
- Elbow crutches.
- Walking frames.
- Wheeled frames.

All have their merits, but a thorough assessment by the physiotherapist is advised to ensure the most appropriate equipment is identified to meet the particular needs of the client. Ensure that you familiarise yourself with the equipment and its correct use.

Mechanised equipment

Mechanised equipment should be considered for those clients who regularly require assistance with transfers. The range is vast and includes:

- Devices attached to beds to raise and lower mattresses
- Leg lifters

Enhancing function

■ Profile beds
■ Lift and recline chairs
■ Lifting cushions
■ Powered toilet risers
■ Hoists

Hoists

The most common types of hoists used are mobile hoists and ceiling track hoists. Mobile hoists are often issued in crisis situations when a person's mobility has deteriorated to such an extent that they require lifting (see Figure 10). They take up a lot of room and long term they can present problems due to storage difficulties, incompatibility with the client's environment and furniture, limited lifting height and manoeuverability problems. Ceiling track hoists may be installed for long-term problems and are often fitted in hospitals, nursing and residential homes, and day centres. They are becoming more common in people's homes as they are less intrusive and easier to use than mobile hoists.

Both types of hoist require slings in order to lift the client safely. Many types of sling are available and they can be made to suit a client's individual needs, although they must be compatible with the equipment. Thorough assessment will identify the correct sling for the task and ensure the comfort and dignity of the client.

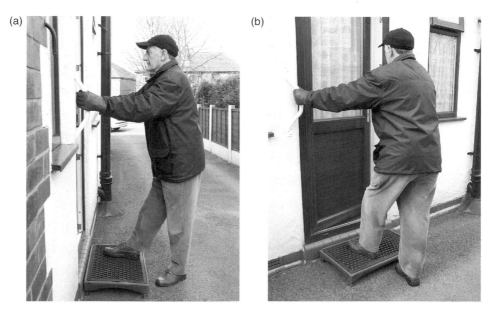

(a) (b)

Figure 9 Using a grab-rail and half step to improve access to a client's house.

Box 6 Other types of aids that can be used to assist transfers and mobility

Rails	Many types of grab-rails are available for various situations, and enable individuals to support themselves whilst transferring. These are often a first consideration as they are simple to install, reduce risk and promote independence (see Figure 9).
Chair, bed and toilet raisers	Again, many types and sizes exist to suit the individual needs of the client as well as the individual nature of the furniture and toilets encountered. They increase the height of the chair, bed or toilet to promote an easier and usually independent transfer.
Transfer boards	These bridge the gap between two points. Many types exist, consisting of polished wood or plastic construction. Selecting the appropriate design will depend on the client's particular needs identified at assessment.
Handling slings	These enable carers to assist with standing transfers and moving on a bed. In addition, they are effective for moving legs on and off beds or stools. It enables a safe working posture for carers.
Handling belts	The individual wears this securely around the waist to enable one or two carers to assist with transfers and mobility. A series of hand holds on the belt allow maintenance of good grip whilst promoting the carers safe working posture.
Low friction slide sheets	These are very versatile items of equipment which allow the easy movement of people in bed, on chairs or even some floor surfaces without the need for lifting. They reduce the effects of friction upon the individual's skin and protect carers from the risks associated with manual handling.
Turntables	These are used to rotate the client whilst sitting or standing and enable the carer to control the turn with minimal effort. They are used for standing and seated transfers, for example from bed to chair, or car transfers.
Client standing aids	These are designed for clients who have a reasonable degree of strength in their arms and legs. The client uses the equipment to pull on from a seated to standing position. The equipment can then be rotated to the desired position by the carer, allowing the client to lower themselves to sitting once again.

Enhancing function

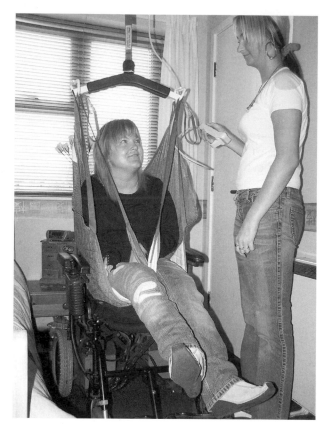

Figure 10 Hoist.

■ Therapeutic exercise

Regular exercise is essential to help people maintain function and prevent further problems. Exercise helps prevent contractures and maintain muscle tone, improve strength and function and enhance balance and coordination. There are a variety of different types of exercises:

■ **Range of movement exercises**
Range of movement exercises involve a precise set of actions to move the joints through their range to help reduce stiffness in muscles and joints. Few joints are put through their full range of movement during normal daily activity. This is not a problem in a healthy joint but in a diseased joint, progressive loss of joint range of movement will occur. Exercises may be passive (performed for the person), active (performed by the person independently), or active with assistance. The exercise programme must be performed correctly to be effective and safe. The client's everyday activities offer opportunities to integrate exercises into daily living. Joint instability is common in diseased joints. Damage to the joints, pain and other problems may result from improperly administered exercises. You

have a responsibility to ensure that exercises are performed properly, safely and at regular intervals.

■ **Muscle strengthening exercises**

Muscle strengthening exercises require moving the muscles against some sort of resistance. The two main types of muscle strengthening exercise are isotonic and isometric. Isotonic exercises involve contracting the muscle to move the joint, for example weight training with dumb-bells. A client with very weak muscles may find that simply moving their limb against gravity provides sufficient resistance to help gradually build up strength. Isometric exercises involve contracting muscles without moving the joint. An example is pushing against a wall, where there is no movement of the joint, but tension builds up in the muscles. Isometric exercises require the participation of the client. The most common isometric exercises involve the abdominal, the thigh and buttock muscles. These exercises may be performed in bed, for instance following hip or knee surgery. Isometric exercises can be helpful to people with joint disease, such as Vinita with rheumatoid arthritis, to help build up muscle strength without putting strain on diseased joints. However, it is important that any exercise programme is carefully monitored by an appropriate professional.

■ **Aerobic exercise**

Walking, cycling and swimming are examples of aerobic exercise. A wide range of exercise equipment is available to support therapeutic exercise designed to maintain overall fitness. A good deal of success with exercise begins by incorporating it into everyday activities. The programme needs to be tailored to meet the client's fitness ability, rehabilitation needs and access to appropriate facilities and equipment.

Hydrotherapy or aqua-aerobics can be beneficial for people with joint problems.

■ ■ WASHING AND HYGIENE

Washing and personal grooming are an important part of everyone's daily routine. Not only are they necessary for the maintenance of good hygiene and prevention of infection but they also affect our feelings of general well-being, morale and confidence in social interactions. Habits vary from person to person.

Stop and think

List the possible reasons for Mick's (case study 4) self-neglect. Make sure you consider the intrinsic and extrinsic factors.

Enhancing function

■ Washing

Washing is an area of self-care in which the majority of people have a great desire to be independent. Everyone has their own routine for washing and bathing. It is important that these routines continue and that the client's own preferences are catered for.

Stop and think

Methods of washing may be determined by religious practices and cultural norms, or by family habits. How could you find out about any special rules, customs or rituals the individual may use in self-care activities?

Maintaining personal dignity

The client may be embarrassed by the presence of someone else whilst washing and bathing. Rehabilitation workers need to show sensitivity and tact, and to respect the privacy and dignity of the client. Try to make the experience as pleasant and relaxed as possible. Ensure that all essential items are ready at hand before starting, and that interruptions are unlikely. Wherever possible, the client's own choice of toiletries should be used.

Let the person do as much as they can by themselves, but remember safety. Most people can manage to wash their own hands and face provided they have access to hot water, soap, washcloth and towel. It is not always necessary for the person to go to the washbasin. Instead, a bowl of warm water can be taken to a more accessible but private place.

Stop and think

It is worth taking a little time to consider the following questions:

- Where does the client prefer to get undressed?
- Do they prefer a wash/bath/shower?
- What toiletries do they need?

On assessment, it was found that Mick was struggling to wash himself due to decreased strength and endurance. Because of his disturbed sleep patterns, he had very little energy in the morning. Fatigue and breathlessness made climbing the stairs very difficult, so Mick prioritised using his energy for the stairs rather than washing. He insisted that he did not want anyone to help him with washing but he was embarrassed about his uncleanliness.

Mick's main bathroom was upstairs; however, there was a toilet with washbasin, downstairs. Although it was a change to his lifetime routine, Mick agreed to move his toiletries to the downstairs toilet. He can now descend the stairs, rest a while, then wash. Standing to wash is still not possible, so Mick minimises his breathlessness on exertion by sitting to wash. There is insufficient space for a perching stool, but Mick can sit on the toilet and reach the washbasin. His wife makes sure that everything is within easy reach and Mick manages to wash independently.

■ Bathing/showering

Bathing or showering are energetic activities requiring a high degree of strength, balance, coordination and tolerance to temperature change.

> ### Box 7   Safety in the bathroom
>
> - Bathrooms and toilets should be well-lit, either by daylight or artificial lighting.
> - The use of bath oils should be discouraged to reduce the risk of slipping.
> - Check that the floor is not slippery.
> - Check that the water temperature of the bath or shower is not too hot or cold.
> - Make sure the room is warm before the person undresses.
> - Leave doors unlocked, or replace locks with those that can be opened from outside as well as inside.
> - Narrow bathroom doors can be removed and replaced with curtains or made into sliding doors, for greater access.
> - Non-slip mats in baths or showers are essential.
> - Insulate or cover hot water pipes.
> - Eliminate clutter and loose towels, clothing or rugs.
> - Install grab-rails and discourage the use of taps, soap dishes etc. as items to pull up on.
> - Angle showerhead away from head and face.

■ The bathroom environment

Bathrooms are often small, with awkward access and potentially slippery surfaces (see Figure 11). Yet most of the activities that take place in the bathroom: showering, toileting, washing and bathing, require a great deal of physical mobility. The person may be wet, soapy and loosely dressed.

Enhancing function

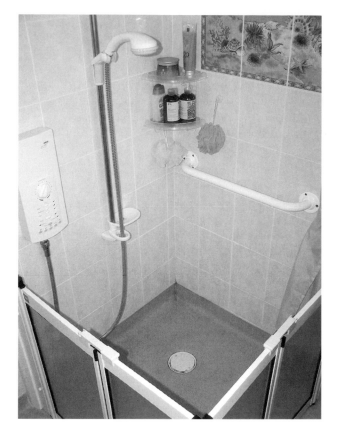

Figure 11 Showers are often in a confined space.

▪ Assistive equipment

Assistive equipment can play an important role in energy conservation and safety. An occupational therapist will be able to advise on the fitting and correct usage of assistive equipment. Items which may assist those with limited range of movement and strength include long-handled sponges or lightweight lambs-wool pads which may help with washing and drying the feet and back, or a mitten flannel which will stay on the hand without being gripped. Soap on a rope might make it easier to keep control of a slippery item.

Grab-rails

Grab-rails are fitted to help people with weak muscles, painful joints or poor balance to get around. They have four basic functions:

▪ Pushing up.
▪ Pulling up.

- Steadying when lowering.
- Security when transferring.

Horizontal grab-rails mainly help in pushing up, whereas vertical rails assist in pulling up to stand. In bathrooms, plastic grab-rails are required, and those with ridged or anti-slip surfaces give the best grip when wet. For a person with painful hands, the rail must be shaped for comfort. Grab-rails are available in various designs, materials and finishes. They may be fixed, hinged, straight or curved. Rail systems allow the rails to be built up in various configurations for different applications.

Taps and tap turners

Stiff taps can often be improved by servicing. Replacing perished washers will make them easier to turn on and off. Lever taps take much less effort to turn on and off. They are more comfortable to use for people with limited strength or grip, as the lever requires only a 90° turn and can be pushed with any part of the body. Most types of tap head can be replaced with a lever tap by a plumber or someone with appropriate skills. An alternative solution is to use a tap turner. These are detachable levers which can be used on standard tap heads.

Tap turners are difficult to use if there is not enough space between and behind the taps. Mixer taps are useful because they only require one hand to adjust the temperature. It can be beneficial to set a thermostat to ensure that the water in the bath or shower cannot exceed a safe level. This is especially important for people with impaired sensation or those that cannot move away quickly, for instance people with reduced mobility, or those with epilepsy who are at risk of having a fit in the shower.

Bath boards and seats

Bath boards provide a stable platform to help people get in and out of the bath. They are particularly useful for people who have difficulty getting over the side of the bath because of stiff joints, poor balance, lack of coordination or weakness.

A bath seat can help someone who is unable to get directly on and off the bottom of the bath because of poor balance or limited movements or weakness in their lower trunk and legs. The client will need strong arms to lower themselves onto the seat. They may choose to remain on the seat to bathe, or may lower themselves onto the bottom of the bath. A bath board can be used with a bath seat.

A bath board can also be used to sit on for washing, showering or drying. Drainage holes aid drying and lessen the chances of slipping. There are a wide variety of bath boards and seats available. The bath board or seat chosen should be suitable for the bath and fitted safely (see Figure 12).

Enhancing function

Enhancing function

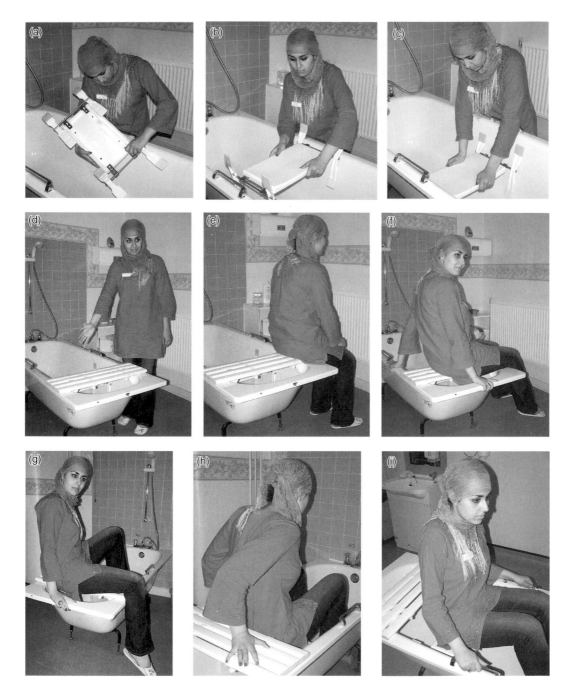

Figure 12 Installing and using a bath board and bath seat.

> **Box 8**   Using a bath board
>
> (1) Check that equipment is fitted securely.
> (2) Sit on the board with feet outside the bath.
> (3) Slide backwards on the board.
> (4) Turn to swing the legs over into the bath.
> (5) Slide to the middle of the board.
> (6) Lower to the bath seat or the base of the bath.

Bath boards are fitted to the bath with adjustable brackets which brace against the sides of the bath. The brackets must wedge firmly against the sides of the bath and should not slip or slide. It should be checked regularly to ensure the fittings are tight. Most baths will take bath boards and seats. However, some plastic and fibreglass baths are not robust enough to take wedge-in bath seats. In these cases, a bath seat may be suspended from the rim of the bath or stood in the bottom of the bath. It is difficult to fit bath boards to some baths with shaped or uneven top surfaces. Check the manufacturer's recommended maximum weight limit. It is important to ensure that the bath board is the correct length. The board should not overlap the edge of the bath or it could tip while it is being used. Stronger bath boards and seats are available for heavier people.

Enhancing function

Bath step

A bath step is a raised platform which is placed beside the bath to make it easier for a person with painful or limited hip or knee movement to step into the bath. The step must be stable in use and the surface needs to be non-slip when wet.

Bath lifts

A bath lift is a type of dedicated hoist that helps the client get in and out of the bath. There are a variety of powered or manual bath lifts available. Some can be operated independently by the user, others are operated by a helper.

Shower seats

Shower seats are water-resistant seats that allow the client to sit while showering. They can be wall-fixed seats, hinged seats, free-standing stools or chairs for ambulant users, or mobile shower chairs which can be used by people who are less mobile. Sanichairs can be used in the shower, as commodes or over the toilet, therefore reducing the need for transfers.

Shower seats should be stable, drain well and have a cut-away section to make washing the genital area easier. Seats vary in size, shape and contour, and need to be matched against the needs and abilities of the user. It is important to consider the space available and the method of transfer when choosing a shower seat.

Mick was supplied with a free-standing shower stool. Using a long-handled sponge, with shower gel applied whilst he was seated, meant that he could clean his feet.

Other tips for bathroom mobility

- Mobile hoists need access beneath the bath to ensure correct positioning for stability. Side or end bath panels may have to be removed.
- Wheelchair users require the bath to be a similar height to the wheelchair seat if independent transfers are to be facilitated.
- If a helper is needed, the bath may need to be higher than usual to facilitate moving and handling, and to prevent back strain.
- Washbasins, work surfaces and mirrors may need to be lowered, and a space under the washbasin allows the client to sit in a chair to wash.
- For many people a well-designed and positioned shower provides a safer and more suitable method of washing than a bath. A shower that has level access allows the use of wheeled shower chairs so the client can easily be moved into the shower area.

◼ Drying

Drying the body requires grip, coordination, flexibility and strength. In cooler climates, a warm room and a heater to warm a towel or bathrobe are also useful. It is important that the person is thoroughly dried, especially in the skin folds, as it is easy for skin to become chafed and sore. Hot air drying facilities are available.

A large bath-sheet in which the person can wrap themselves will aid drying with a minimum of effort. Tapes or loops placed on each end of the towel will help with drying the back and legs. Thick soft towelling mittens may be used by those with impaired grip.

Mick found that by putting on a large bathrobe and resting after showering, he could keep warm, rest and dry himself with little assistance (see Figure 13).

◼ Grooming

Daily grooming activities include the ability to obtain and use the necessary supplies, remove unwanted facial and body hair, apply and remove cosmetics; washing, drying, styling and brushing hair; caring for finger and toe nails; skin care and applying deodorant.

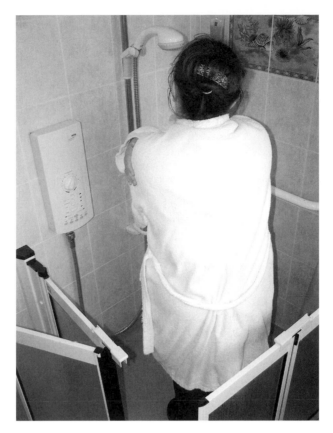

Figure 13 Drying in the shower with the aid of a bathrobe.

Hair care

Keeping hair washed and well brushed can be difficult for clients who cannot lean over, raise their hands above their head, move their hands, or have difficulty balancing.

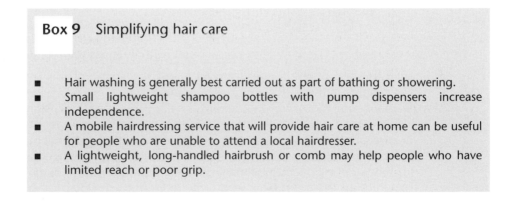

Box 9 Simplifying hair care

- Hair washing is generally best carried out as part of bathing or showering.
- Small lightweight shampoo bottles with pump dispensers increase independence.
- A mobile hairdressing service that will provide hair care at home can be useful for people who are unable to attend a local hairdresser.
- A lightweight, long-handled hairbrush or comb may help people who have limited reach or poor grip.

Enhancing function

- Built-up handles offer a better grip, whereas long and curved handles help with reach.
- A brush with an angled head will help with reach, and a thick, grooved handle will help with grip.
- A wide-toothed comb or hard nylon-bristled hairbrush is easier to use than a narrow toothed comb or soft brush.
- Loops strapped to the rear of a brush head enable a person with limited hand movements, to slide the whole hand through the space and facilitate use.
- An adjustable mirror, or two wall-mounted mirrors angled so as to be able to see both front and back may be useful, and can act as reminders for those with partial body neglect.

Nail care

Proper care of finger and toe nails is essential for hygiene, appearance and mobility. Nails tend to become thickened and brittle with age and as a result of some illnesses like psoriasis. Nail care may be difficult for a person who cannot manage implements, or who has problems with bending or balancing.

Box 10   Nail care

- A nailbrush with a curved handle can be helpful for people with a weak grip.
- Suction pads can be used to attach the nailbrush to the side of the basin for those who are only able to use one hand.
- Nail clippers are easier to use than scissors for thick nails. Nail clippers fixed to a small base can be placed on a table and operated with the palm of the hand to help people with weak or painful grip, or unsteady hands.
- Self-opening lightweight nail scissors are useful for people with weak or painful hands.
- People with impaired vision may benefit from a magnifying glass that can be stabilised or worn around their neck.

Toe nails should be trimmed neatly and evenly, so that they are slightly shorter than the end of the toe and should follow the shape of the end of the toe. Examine all of the nails for ingrown toe nails, which are most common on the big toes, but can occur on any of the nails. They may show signs of redness, inflammation, pus or bleeding around the nail. If the nails are extremely long, or in a poor state of repair, ask the client how they get their nails trimmed. If they are struggling to care for their nails themselves, alternative arrangements for foot care will need to be made. A family member could undertake the basic foot care, or the client may need to be referred to a podiatrist. Any client with diabetes or poor circulation should be referred to a podiatrist for a thorough foot assessment and advice on ongoing foot care.

Oral hygiene

Dental care is important for everyone, but it is particularly vital for people who take regular medication. Absent teeth or ill-fitting dentures can make communicating and eating difficult and contribute to poor nutrition. A build-up of bacteria in the mouth and saliva can lead to chest-related illnesses. Ensure that the client has access to the appropriate supplies to clean their mouth (for example toothbrush and toothpaste), and can clean their teeth or dental prosthetics.

> ### Box 11   Oral hygiene
>
> - Toothbrush handles can be enlarged to assist people with weak grip.
> - A toothbrush with a long handle may be needed by someone with limited reach.
> - A wall-mounted holder for toothpaste or a pump action dispenser may make dispensing toothpaste easier. In some cases it may be easier to apply toothpaste directly to the teeth.
> - An electric toothbrush may be useful, provided the brush is not too heavy and the controls are easy to use.
> - Medicated mouthwash can reduce bacteria in the mouth.

Shaving, skin care and applying make-up

> ### Box 12   Shaving/make-up and skin care
>
> - Adequate lighting and a suitably placed mirror will greatly help with these tasks.
> - Extended handles can assist people with limited reach.
> - Women may be able to use depilatory creams or foam to remove underarm or leg hair.
> - Men may find an electric razor less hazardous than wet shaving, but it is usually heavier.
> - For men with diminished facial sensation, it is best to encourage the use of an electric shaver.
> - Cosmetic jars can be opened with one hand when the base of the container is stabilised to a table using a suction cup.
> - Moisturisers, creams and soaps may be more accessible from a pump dispenser than screw top containers.
> - Being able to sit whilst performing tasks may reduce fatigue.

Enhancing function

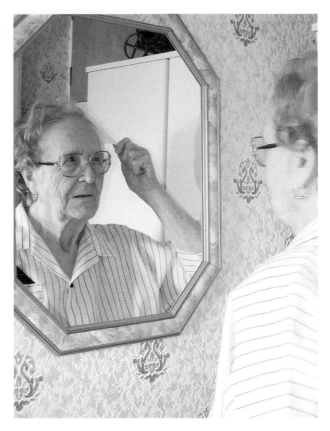

Figure 14 Adequate lighting and a well-placed mirror make grooming easier.

Stop and think

A knowledge of sexual needs, sexual expression and sexual identity is an important part of rehabilitation of the 'whole' person. Mood disorders, physical illness, acquired disability and medication, can all affect sexual functioning. The person may be reluctant to raise their intimate concerns immediately, but may begin to mention them as certain tasks within the rehabilitation programme develop. You should be able to discuss these issues with the person and their family and refer on to the most knowledgeable team member.

▪ ▪ TOILETING AND TOILET MANAGEMENT

Independence in toileting can be one of the most crucial aspects of a rehabilitation programme, for both convenience and psychological reasons. Clothing management needs to be assessed as part of toileting, as alterations to the client's clothing, especially their underwear may be required. The toilet is usually the smallest room in the house. Generally, the more disabled a person, the more space they will require to manoeuvre. Even when it is combined with the bathroom there is not always suitable space. Major structural alterations may be required, particularly for wheelchair users.

Assistive devices for toileting

There are a number of assistive devices to help with toileting.

Toilet seats

If a person has difficulty getting on and off a standard height toilet a raised toilet seat and rails may be useful. A raised toilet seat attaches to a standard toilet bowl, with the existing toilet seat being lifted up, or removed. This can be a temporary measure, to help someone after injury or surgery, or be a more permanent fixture. A variety of heights and styles are available. A raised toilet seat, used on top of a standard seat, may be moved to another toilet or removed when another person wishes to use the toilet.

Combined toilet seats and frames are available. The height of the frame may be fixed or adjustable. The frame may be free-standing (see Figure 15) or fixed to the floor. Free-standing frames are not stable enough for anyone who pushes on only one side of the frame when getting up or down. In this case, a floor-fixed version will be required.

The type of seat required is determined by comfort and the ability of the person. A horseshoe shape, which is open at the front, makes cleansing easier for some people. Inclined seats can be used by those with stiff hip and knee joints. A raising toilet seat may help someone who is very stiff, with weak or very limited movement. They are likely to suit people who find a spring chair seat raiser useful. Some transfer of weight forwards and upwards is needed to initiate standing. See Box 13 for other options to assist toileting, and Box 14 for advice for toileting wheelchair users.

■ ■ DRESSING

For many of us, the clothes we choose to wear and the way we wear them are a means of asserting our personal and sexual identity. Whether we spend hours selecting the perfect outfit for an occasion, or throw on the nearest garments at hand, we are expressing something about ourselves, our priorities and our way of life. The clients we work with are no different. Do not make assumptions about appropriate techniques and outfits based on your own values and habits. Wherever possible the client should choose what they would like to wear and the method of dressing. When planning a dressing programme, consideration should be given to the person's level of ability, choice and style of dress and any habits.

Enhancing function

Box 13   Other assistive devices to aid toileting

Rails	Rails are useful for people who need help to get on and off the toilet, as it is not safe to rely on putting weight onto washbasins, toilet roll holders, door handles, etc. An individual assessment is often required to ascertain the most suitable size and positioning of rails. Some people can manage with one rail, others need rails at different angles for support when sitting and standing. Toilet support frames are available and may be free-standing or floor-fixed. Some have arms, which are hinged and can be raised for sideways transfers.
Sanichairs	For people who cannot manage to transfer from a wheelchair to the toilet, Sanichairs are available, which can either be self-propelling or attendant propelled and can be positioned over the toilet pedestal.
Bidets	A bidet may be used for personal cleansing after defecation and during menstruation. Lightweight portable bidets are available. Combined toilets and bidets, which wash and dry, can be installed for people who struggle to cleanse themselves independently.
Commodes	If a standard toilet is inaccessible, a commode can be used. Commodes may be static or mobile. A wide range of commode chairs are available. Most commodes have a weight limit.
Bottom wipers	Angled toilet paper holders are available to help a person with limited reach or hand function. They may be used from the front or the rear, depending on the person's range of movement and personal preference.
Bedpans and urinals	If a person is unable to use a toilet or commode, bedpans and urinals can be used.

Box 14   Toileting for wheelchair users

Wheelchair users will need the toilet and wheelchair seat to be at the same height for ease of transfer.

Transfer techniques may need to be adapted with side, forward and backward transfers considered.

Sideways transfers are easier if the toilet pedestal is set further forward from the wall than usual.

Detachable wheelchair armrests, chassis design which permits close approach and folding and removable backrests, should all be considered.

Consider the issues around toilet transfers when you are choosing a wheelchair.

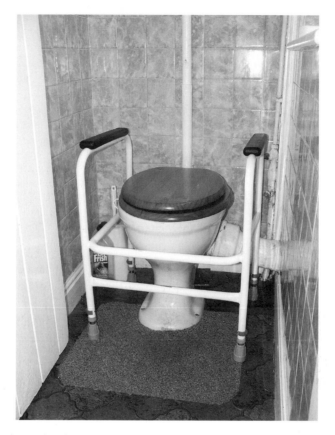

Figure 15 Toilet with adaptations.

Try to keep to the routine the person is used to. For example, a person may prefer to dress their lower half first, or they may prefer to put on all their underwear first. Some people stand to dress, others sit. There may be gender differences. For example, when pulling off a jumper or sweater, men tend to grasp the upper back and pull it over their head, whereas women often pull the garment from the waistband up over the arms and head.

■ Dressing programmes

Think about all of the activities involved in getting dressed. You need to be able to decide what clothes and accessories to wear; find the clothes; and then have the dexterity to pull on pants, trousers or stockings in a logical sequence; fasten zippers and buttons and reach down to put on hosiery and footwear. Some clients will have to manage putting on prostheses or orthoses.

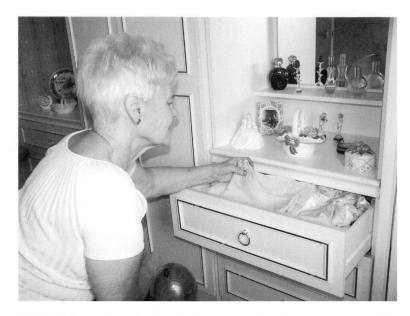

Figure 16 Full independence in dressing includes being able to choose clothing.

Full independence in dressing includes an ability to perform tasks that require mobility and balance, perception and cognition. Critical observation of dressing often pinpoints areas of difficulty that require further interventions. A dressing programme cannot exist in isolation from other parts of the rehabilitation programme. Because of the complexity of dressing, there are a number of intrinsic and extrinsic factors that can impact on a client's ability to dress themselves.

Stop and think

Consider the possible intrinsic and extrinsic factors that might impact on Maryanne's ability to dress herself. How might she overcome these?

A dressing assessment should start by gathering information about the history of the specific problem and reviewing past function. Identify whether any assistive devices have been used in the past. A dressing assessment will examine all of the tasks described above, but it is also a good way to evaluate the client's psychosocial, emotional and cultural issues, as well as carrying out neurological and musculoskeletal assessments.

Generally, undressing is easier than dressing. It is less tiring. It may be appropriate to begin the rehabilitation programme with an undressing programme. Maryanne began her dressing programme by learning how to take off her upper garments, followed by her lower ones, and finally her shoes. For safety reasons it was important that her footwear was left until last so that her feet were supported when standing. Maryanne was encouraged to prepare for the following day's dressing. Clothes to be worn the next day were to be left folded and ordered, ready for putting them on.

Offering Support

Deciding at what stage to intervene is crucial. Consider pain levels, stiffness, slowness and weakness. The level of independence aimed for should take into account the individual's circumstances. Total independence may be unrealistic. Remember that it is sometimes more important to save a person's energy for a more rewarding activity later in the day. Do not allow the person to become too cold or too fatigued. Decide when to step in to maintain an atmosphere of encouragement without frustration. Plan to provide cues, repetition and reinforcement (see Section 1: Teaching for rehabilitation) and keep environmental distractions to a minimum.

Box 15   Key messages

- Be consistent.
- Organise the environment.
- Acknowledge person's preferences/lifestyle.
- Encourage independence with easier tasks first.
- Time a programme to fit in with individual's and family's routine.
- Allow ample time.
- Have a plan of support ready.
- Ensure that the room is private and warm and comfortable.

Clothing

Selecting clothes

Clothing must fit with the person's condition, any sensory impairment, the environment and the weather. Several layers of thin clothing may be more adaptable to changing temperatures, but also take longer to put on, which means more effort. Choose fabrics which are lightweight, warm and allow the skin to breathe. There are several points to remember when selecting garments to wear. Ideally, garments should be simple and loose fitting, with a minimum of fastenings. Elasticised waists are often easier to manage.

Particular attention should be paid to comfort, as the person may have to spend many hours in the same position. Beware that clothing does not cause complications. For example, denim jeans and tight socks can cause skin breakdown if the rigid seams cut into the skin. Pockets are useful as they enable the person to carry small items around, whilst leaving both hands free.

Enhancing function

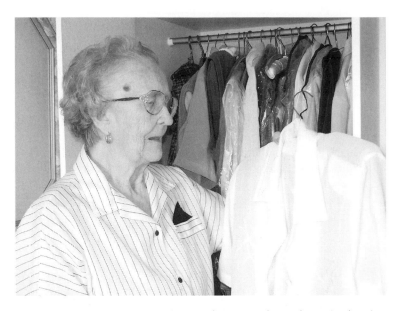

Figure 17 Appropriate storage of clothing enhances independence in dressing.

Storing clothes

People with poor eyesight sometimes have difficulty differentiating between clothes of different colours, or even finding the right garments. The dressing area should be well lit, and it can be helpful to install a light inside the cupboard.

Clothes can be organised in a way that makes them easier to find and select. Similar types of clothes can be hung or arranged together, such as hanging skirts or trousers in one part of the wardrobe and shirts or blouses separately. Alternatively, complete matching outfits could be hung together on the same coat hanger. Clothes of similar colours could be grouped together. It might be useful to 'tag' clothes in a way that helps the client to identify the colours. You might use wire coat hangers for red clothes and plastic coat hangers for green, for instance. Alternatively, you could use a tactile marker on the clothing label, such as safety pins, to denote clothes of a particular colour. Wardrobe planning can be useful in this instance, and it may be beneficial to limit the range of different colours to reduce the need for a great deal of tagging and arranging of different clothes.

Clothing adaptations

Ill-fitting clothing is uncomfortable and distracting. Careful selection and adaptation of clothing can ease the situation. Adaptations have to be considered when difficulties are experienced with ordinary clothes. The most common alterations are:

- Enlarging openings to ease putting on or taking off.
- Moving fastenings (normally to the front) so that they are within easy reach.

- Changing the types of fastenings, for example using Velcro instead of hooks and eyes or buttons.
- Inserting elastic into waistbands.
- Adding loops or extension tabs to zip fastenings.
- Large buttons or hooks.

Stop and think

Consider Maryanne. The tight-fitting, tailored clothes she usually wears are difficult for her to manage independently but she refuses to wear baggy sweatshirts and jogging pants, even though she could manage to dress herself if she wore these.

- Why is it important to Maryanne to wear the clothes she has chosen?
- How could you adapt her clothes to make them easier to put on?
- What advice would you give to Maryanne about buying new clothes?

Footwear

Encourage clients to wear shoes when they are out of bed, to protect their feet. Sometimes older people have very thin, frail and inelastic skin which is particularly vulnerable to damage, and takes some time to heal. Foot and lower leg protection is very important to prevent injury in these cases (see Box 16). Clients with sensory deficits (nerve damage) will not feel pain, such as heat, bumping against a chair leg, or pressure, which can lead to skin breakdown or ulcers. People are at particular risk of suffering from sensory deficits in their feet and legs if they have diabetes or a history of alcohol abuse.

Stop and think

Frances has severe peripheral neuropathy in both feet as a result of her diabetes mellitus. She is unable to detect pressure, pain or different temperatures in her feet, which means that any injury may go undetected. She first noticed her peripheral neuropathy when a pin became embedded in her foot and became infected. She went to her GP who noticed the head of the pin in the middle of the infected lesion and removed it. She was successfully treated with antibiotics. However, her GP highlighted the risk of developing a serious infection which could lead to ulceration or worse, amputation. She now sees a podiatrist regularly for her foot care, and is required to wear protective footwear at all times. She inspects her feet every day as part of her washing and bathing routine to make sure that she detects any damage or injuries to her feet.
What other precautions might Frances take to protect her feet from damage?

People who have poor blood flow to their feet also need to take particular care to protect their feet from injury, because any injury will take longer to heal. People most at risk are those with diabetes and vascular disease, and heavy smokers.

It is important that the client's shoes fit properly, and are comfortable and appropriate for the purpose. You probably know yourself that when you wear tight or uncomfortable shoes, or just have painful feet it impacts on everything else you attempt to do. But even more importantly, painful feet and poorly fitting shoes have been found to significantly increase the risk of falling. In other words, well-cared for feet and appropriate shoes are an important component of client safety, comfort and risk reduction.

Box 16 describes the types of features you should look for in the footwear of someone who has compromised foot health and when their feet require protection (for instance diabetes or peripheral vascular disease).

Encourage the client to wear supportive shoes rather than slippers or 'scuffs'. Slip-on shoes do not provide much protection, and can increase the risk of falling.

■ Dressing techniques

Depending upon the problem, the client may need to be taught new tips and techniques for dressing. In Maryanne's case she has reduced strength and movement in her left arm and leg and minimal functional use of her left hand. In addition to this she has some perceptual and cognitive disturbances resulting in the neglect of her left side and inconsistent concentration.

Because Maryanne has suffered a cerebrovascular accident, it is important that any dressing technique used not only encourages functional independence, but also inhibits patterns of spasticity. In addition to Maryanne's physical difficulties, she has had some perceptual disturbances. The following tips may help when carrying out a dressing programme with people who have perceptual problems. See also Boxes 17 and 18.

Dressing techniques: bra

Women may experience difficulty with putting on and taking off bras. For comfort, and appearance where it has been identified as important to the client, it is preferable to alter techniques or adapt clothing, rather than to advise female clients not to wear a bra.

For those with the use of only one hand a clothes peg may be used to hold the bra to the top of a waistband, acting as the stabilising hand whilst the unaffected hand closes the hooks. Velcro may be used to cover hooks if these are difficult to fasten. If a client can manoeuvre her upper limbs a sports bra or stretch bra can be sewn closed and pulled down into position.

Box 16   Optimal shoe fit

Length	Approximately 1 cm between the big toe and the end of the shoe when the client is weight-bearing in the shoe.
Depth	The shoe should be wide enough and deep enough to prevent rubbing on the toes.
Heel support	The heel (back) of the shoe should be firm. It should not squash easily when it is squeezed sideways or from the top.
Cushioning material	The sole should contain some sort of cushioning material, such as rubber or another cushioned material.
Sole	The sole should be stiff, and only bend under the ball of the foot.
Restraining mechanism	The shoe should have some sort of restraining mechanism such as buckles, laces, straps, Velcro or elastic; otherwise the toes have to 'scrunch up' to hold the shoe in place.
Heel height	Less than 3 cm.
Style	Should protect the toes, enclose the heel, and protect the foot from entry of any foreign objects.
Materials	Should allow ventilation and be pliable enough to prevent injury to the toes or foot.
Shoe shape	The shoe should be the same shape as the foot. To test this, trace around your foot whilst standing barefooted, then put the shoe over the foot tracing. If any part of the foot protrudes, then it is likely that the shoe is the wrong shape.
Injury	The shoe should not cause injury to the foot.

Source: Adapted from Nancarrow, S.A. (1999) Footwear suitability scale: a measure of shoe fit for people with diabetes. *Australasian Journal of Podiatric Medicine*, **33** (2), 59–64.

Enhancing function

Box 17   Dressing

A well-balanced starting position, for example a chair with arms and a wide seat, will offer support when twisting, reaching or leaning.
Another person may find that lying on the bed is best for dressing the lower half, whilst preferring to sit on the side of the bed to dress their top half.

Box 18 Devising a dressing programme with people who have perceptual problems

Encourage the person to feel part of the clothing that will assist in recognising it, for example trace the line of buttons on the front of a shirt.
Use labels to distinguish front/back, outside/inside.
When buttoning a shirt, match the first button, then you may encourage the person to continue with the others.
When teaching people who have disturbances of body scheme, always touch the body part when naming where garment is to be placed.
People with unilateral neglect need to have the neglected side stimulated:

- Place clothes on the person's neglected side, and then teach scanning techniques to enable the person to find their clothes.
- Touch the neglected side when assisting with dressing.
- Use frequent verbal cues to remind the person to consider their affected side.
- Use the same sequence of dressing each time, as this will build up a trigger system to remind the person of their affected side.
- Always approach the person from the affected side.

People with difficulty distinguishing items benefit from having clothes laid out on a plain background that is unlike the colour of the clothing.
Remove clutter and any unwanted clothing.

Dressing aids

Simple dressing aids should be considered if alternative methods or alterations are not adequate.

Box 19 Dressing aids

A dressing stick	For pulling on or pushing off clothing, may be useful for people with severe shoulder limitation.
Long-handled shoehorn	For those who cannot reach their feet to pull the backs of their shoes over their heels.
A button hook	Helpful to those with the use of only one hand.
Long-handled pick up sticks	Used to pick up items beyond a person's reach, but can be equally useful in pulling up pants/trousers.
Stocking aids	Can be used to help put on lightweight socks, stockings, or tights.
Elastic shoelaces	Can be used to convert lace-up shoes to slip-ons, making them easier to get on/off.

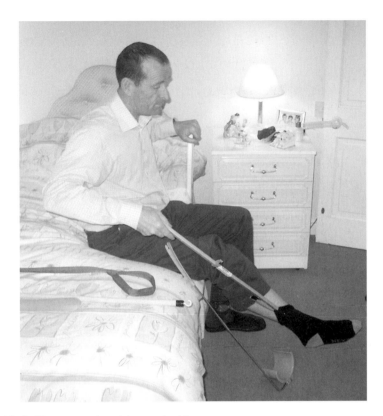

Figure 18 Pulling on socks with a sock aid.

▪ ▪ FOOD PREPARATION, HANDLING AND EATING

Food preparation, handling and eating may sound like a simple task, but when you break it down into the components that go together to make even a simple meal, it becomes a complex activity. To make a meal you require sufficient mobility to be able to move in and around the kitchen. Cooking involves activities that require a great deal of coordination and motor control, like chopping and stirring. You need to plan to have the appropriate ingredients to make a meal, and ideally to have chosen nutritionally balanced ingredients. The ingredients need to be stored in a way that means that they are still fresh, nutritious and do not cause food poisoning. Serving the food requires access to the appropriate tableware and utensils.

▪ The kitchen environment

Before attempting any activities in the kitchen, the environment should have been assessed and modified according to the client's needs. Ensure that the

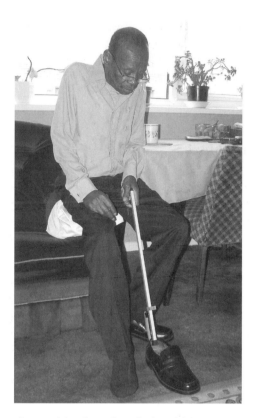

Figure 19 Putting on shoes with a long-handled grabber.

kitchen is a safe place in which to work. In particular, try to avoid risks of slipping or tripping, such as a slippery or uneven floor or loose rugs. Electrical safety is an important consideration. Be aware of frayed wires or loose plugs, or electrical cords that risk getting wet. Unsafe electrical appliances should be replaced and loose sockets fixed by an electrician or handyman. Electrical appliances that have an automatic cut-off are preferable to those that need to be watched and manually stopped when the water has boiled or the bread is toasted.

As with the bathroom, ensure that taps are easy to turn on and off and stiff washers have been replaced. Tap extensions may be necessary. Assess the quality of the lighting in the kitchen. The areas used for preparation and eating should be well lit, but free of glare.

Examine the kitchen layout and storage. Make sure that frequently used items, such as tea and coffee, are easy to access. If the client has trouble lifting their arms above shoulder height, then there is little point storing regularly used items in overhead cupboards. Heavy items, such as saucepans, should be stored in a way that limits the amount of lifting that needs to be done. For instance, storing a heavy pressure cooker in a low cupboard which is away from the stove could make it almost impossible for the client to use it. Instead, try to place them so that they require minimal moving to get from their storage place to the stove.

The client's active involvement in exploring possible solutions is essential. Small adaptations to the kitchen environment made life much easier for Vinita. The taps, door furniture, plugs and oven controls were replaced with larger controls. Storage cupboards were reorganised so that equipment and supplies were all within easy reach.

Stop and think

Pain can be demoralising, frightening and demotivating, and can lead to protective postures which produce muscle tension.

List the possible ways in which Vinita's painful wrists could impact on her ability to prepare food and to eat independently (case study 1).

If you have never come across Vinita's diagnosis of rheumatoid arthritis before, how would you find out more information?

Why might you need to know about the clinical features of an illness, and the prognosis?

Clients with poor vision or cognitive deficits may benefit from crockery in dark and light colours that contrast strongly with the colour of the food being served in them. For instance, it is much easier to see mashed potato on a black plate than a white plate. It is also useful if the crockery contrasts with the preparation surface and the dining table or tablecloth. Cutting surfaces should also be in highly contrasting colours, and sight impaired people may benefit by using pre-chopped food.

■ Meal planning and preparation

Where possible, meals should be planned around the normal routine of the client. This includes timing the meals as close to regular mealtimes for the client and their family as possible, and allowing them to dictate the types of food they normally eat.

Stop and think   Cultural and religious considerations around food preparation

Dietary and eating habits are determined largely by people's culture and will influence what people eat, when they eat and how they eat. You should not be expected to know all the different cultural and religious requirements, but you should always ask the client and their family about the cultural or religious considerations that need to be taken into account around the preparation and planning of a meal. For instance, during Ramadan, Muslims tend to fast during daylight hours. Christians may give up their favourite food during Lent, or eat fish on Fridays. Most Jews do not eat pork or pork products. Make sure that you are aware of the needs of the client groups that you are working with and build these into your intervention planning.

Enhancing function

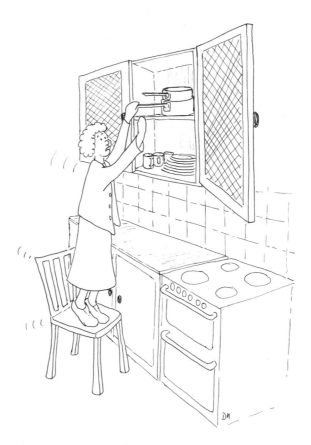

Figure 20 Ensure items are stored within easy access.

For clients in a rehabilitation programme, it is a good idea to plan meals in advance. This allows the client to purchase the majority of their food needs in a single visit to the shop, rather than having to make multiple visits to buy individual items. A well-planned shopping list will save money by allowing the client to purchase some products in bulk, and can also reduce waste. A further benefit of a shopping list is that it makes it much easier for someone else, such as a family member or neighbour, to do the shopping for the client, which may save unnecessary trips.

Meal planning should consider the client's budget, their food likes, dislikes and cultural requirements, and their ability to eat and swallow. For instance, many clients with dentures will have difficulty biting into a crisp apple. When arranging the shopping, consider the storage facilities available in the client's house. It may be possible to make more food than the client requires for a single meal and freeze some for later consumption.

Some clients will have ongoing support for the provision of their meals, for instance they might receive Meals on Wheels for their midday meal. There are private companies that will deliver pre-made meals that are frozen and delivered a week at a time. Be aware of the food that the client is receiving

Box 20 Principles of joint protection

- ■ Do gentle range of movement exercises daily.
- ■ Maintain a healthy diet and maintain ideal weight.
- ■ Adopt a work/rest balance.
- ■ Prioritise, pre-plan and organise activities.
- ■ Respect pain.
- ■ Reduce effort in daily activity.
- ■ Avoid positions of deformity.
- ■ Use larger, stronger joints for activity.
- ■ Avoid static positions.
- ■ Avoid activities which cannot be halted.
- ■ Use equipment to assist task performance.

elsewhere, and ensure that their diet is appropriately supplemented with fresh fruit and vegetables. It is also a good idea to ensure that there is a supply of easily accessible and relatively nutritious food available as a back-up. This could include a tin of baked beans, tinned fruit and vegetables, creamed rice and/or powdered milk. It may be possible to arrange regular delivery of groceries from a nearby supermarket. Again, good planning is required to ensure that the client orders the items that they need, to avoid unnecessary additional trips.

Education and practice in alternative techniques, in conjunction with advice in joint protection methods enabled Vinita to perform meal planning and preparation for herself and her family without assistance. Vinita was advised to avoid carrying wherever possible. Instead she was advised to slide objects along the work surface, to push objects rather than pull them, and to use a trolley. She was also supplied with a perching stool which allowed her to sit when preparing meals and drinks.

■ Independence in eating

When implementing a feeding programme, you need to consider:

- ▪ The dining environment.
- ▪ The choice of tableware and furniture.
- ▪ The positioning of the client.

The rehabilitation worker needs to ascertain the routine and habits of the client and family. Eating is a very personal activity, and people choose to eat their food in different ways. For some it is a quiet time for reflection, for others a social activity, others eat 'on the go' whilst they are engaged in other activities. Some cultures encourage the use of cutlery, but in many cultures finger feeding is the norm.

Enhancing function

Box 21   Independence in eating

- Clients can use a universal cuff to hold utensils to bring food to their mouth. This cuff fits around the hand and has a pocket to hold the handle of a utensil. This is particularly useful for people with muscle weakness who have difficulty grasping food.
- Built-up, lightweight handles on cutlery may help those with poor grip strength.
- People who use only one hand may benefit from the provision of cutlery such as a 'Splayd', or 'Spork' which combines the function of different pieces of cutlery into one utensil.
- Angled and lengthened cutlery can help people with a limited range of movement and restricted reach in their upper limbs.
- Swivel cutlery is available for those with limited wrist and elbow movement.
- Deep-rimmed plates assist pushing food onto cutlery.
- Plate guards are devices which clip onto plates and stop food falling over the edge.
- Non-slip placemats prevent plates and bowls moving around while cutting or putting food onto cutlery.
- Insulated mugs and plates help to maintain temperatures and protect the hands of those with sensitivity and sensation problems.

Balance, stability and positioning are important elements in independent feeding. The client should be assisted to attain and maintain the optimum sitting position. A chair with arms will provide more support than one without. Feet must be flat on a stable surface, such as the floor, stool, or foot rests on the wheelchair. A winged headrest may assist the client with limited head or neck control. The wheelchair user will require sufficient clearance under the table to prevent over reaching. A high table and chair may be required for the person with stiff lower limbs.

Special eating aids are available for people with specific problems. Any equipment provided should be as unobtrusive as possible and safe and easy to use. Careful individualised assessment is important, and a range of styles and types of equipment may need to be tried before a comfortable fit with the client is made. Clients will frequently require instruction and practice in the use of any assistive device.

In some cases, adapting equipment already in use may be preferable to providing new equipment.

Vinita was helped to become more independent in her kitchen in the ways described below. She was asked by the rehabilitation worker to keep a daily diary over a period of one week. In this diary Vinita recorded her daily activities and whether her pain, stiffness and fatigue was light, moderate or severe. Using this information, the rehabilitation worker was able to offer guidance to Vinita on changing techniques and using equipment which minimised her symptoms. Vinita was supplied with adapted cutlery with padded, lightweight handles, her keys were adapted to facilitate grip, and wherever possible her

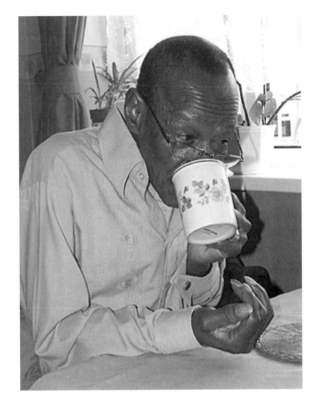

Figure 21 Client independent in drinking.

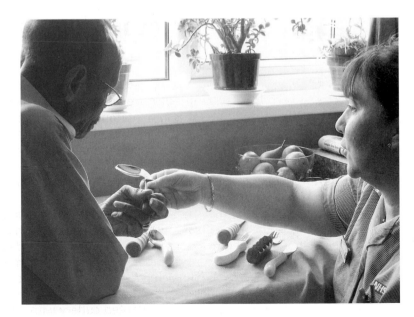

Figure 22 There is a wide range of adaptive cutlery available.

clothes were modified, with Velcro replacing small buttons, laces and other difficult fastenings. She was supplied with tap turners.

Advice was given on joint protection. The principles of joint protection were carefully explained to Vinita. She was provided with opportunities to practise techniques under the guidance of the rehabilitation worker, and she was given a simple leaflet containing illustrations as a follow-up reference. Vinita was also invited to attend a joint protection group run by the rehabilitation worker, where people with similar problems met to discuss and practise activities, and share advice and knowledge.

Vinita attended the hospital outpatient department where she was measured for and supplied with bilateral resting splints covering the forearm, wrist and hand. The aims of the resting splint were:

- To support the joints in order to alleviate swelling and pain.
- To reduce pressure on nerves by maintaining a neutral position.

During her visits the rehabilitation worker monitored Vinita's use of the splints and checked the skin for signs of rubbing.

■ Food storage and hygiene

Food that is not stored or handled properly risks causing food poisoning. Older people are particularly susceptible to food poisoning and may experience symptoms that someone younger and healthier will not experience. The most obvious symptoms of food poisoning are changes in digestion, such as diarrhoea and vomiting.

Bacteria are a common cause of food poisoning. Appropriate food handling can reduce the risk of bacterial food poisoning. Bacteria do not like very cold or very hot temperatures and will grow more slowly at temperatures below 5°C and above 60°C. In general, good food handling involves the following principles:

- Try to keep food at temperatures below 5°C or above 60°C. Reduce the amount of time that food is in the temperature 'danger zone'.
- Ensure that cooked foods are heated to a high enough temperature and when re-heating food, make sure it is steaming hot.
- Reduce the risk of cross-contamination of food (transferring bacteria from one item to another) by ensuring that cooking utensils are washed in hot, soapy water.
- Do not store raw meat next to cooked food or food that will be eaten raw. Store uncooked meat towards the bottom of the refrigerator to avoid contamination of other foods from juices. Always cover leftovers and place them on shelves above raw meat or poultry in the refrigerator. Never re-use a container that has held raw meat without washing it thoroughly.
- Always wash your hands before preparing food.
- Keep pets away from the food preparation areas.
- Wash food before you eat it.

- Buy frozen foods last, so they have less time to defrost before you get them home, then put them in the freezer immediately. Frozen foods should be stored at or below −18°C. Avoid thawing and re-freezing food where possible.
- Check the 'use-by' date on foods and discard food that has passed its best.
- Read the storage instructions on the food label and store the food appropriately. Refrigerated food should be kept at around 5°C.
- Kitchen sponges, cloths and tea towels harbour bacteria so change them frequently.

■ Nutrition and healthy eating

Eating a healthy, nutritious diet is an important component of restoring and maintaining good health. It is very easy not to eat healthily, particularly if the client has reduced mobility and is limited in their ability to access fresh food, or has difficulties eating or swallowing. Many countries have developed nutritional guidelines which may be available from the health department or the national dietetics or nutritional associations. These provide a useful guide to encourage healthy eating for specific groups of people. The Nutritional Guidelines for Older Australians are included below.

Enhancing function

Box 22 Nutritional guidelines (adapted from the Australian National Health and Medical Research Council, 1999)

(1) Eat a wide variety of nutritious foods.
(2) Remain active to maintain muscle strength and a healthy body weight.
(3) Eat at least three meals per day.
(4) Prepare and store food correctly.
(5) Eat plenty of fruit and vegetables.
(6) Eat plenty of cereal, bread and pasta.
(7) Eat a diet low in saturated fat.
(8) Drink adequate amounts of water and/or other fluids.
(9) Limit your alcohol intake.
(10) Eat salt sparingly and choose foods low in salt.
(11) Eat foods that are high in calcium.
(12) Use added sugar in moderation.

Copyright: Commonwealth of Australia, reproduced with permission.

You may be involved in shopping with or for the client, and can help to ensure that the client has access to a varied and healthy diet. It would be beneficial for you to have an understanding of basic nutrition. Adhering to the principles listed above will ensure that the client has a healthy, balanced diet. Encourage the client to read the packaging when they are purchasing goods, to look at items such as salt (sodium) and fat content of the items they buy.

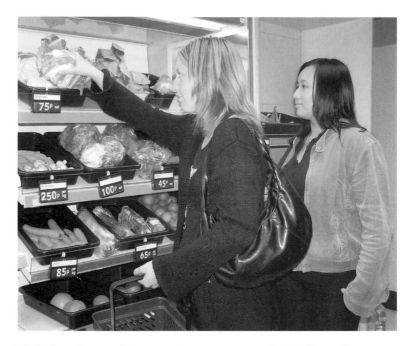

Figure 23 Fruit and vegetables are an important part of a nutritious diet.

Some rehabilitation teams will include an assessment by a dietician. If you are concerned about the client's diet, of if they have particular nutritional require-ments resulting from a condition such as diabetes, Crohn's disease or food allergies, a referral should be made to a dietician. Similarly, clients struggling because they are overweight may benefit from nutritional guidance. If the client has sudden or dramatic weight loss you should alert their GP. There are a num-ber of nutrition screening tools available that are simple to administer and will tell you if the client is at nutritional risk. Nutritional screening tools include the Nutrition Screening Initiative and the Mini Nutritional Assessment. Links to screening tools and further information about nutritional screening are provided at the end of this section.

▪ ▪ SWALLOWING PROBLEMS

An obvious, but important, component of eating and proper nutrition is being able to chew and swallow food. Swallowing problems, also called dysphagia, may occur when there is damage to sensation, strength or coordination of muscles of the head (for example cheeks, lips and tongue), neck, or chest. The causes of dysphagia include neurological disorders, such as stroke, dementia, or Parkinson's disease, or result from other diseases such as head and neck cancer or respiratory diseases such as chronic obstructive pulmonary disease (COPD). This may cause difficulties drinking, chewing/eating, controlling saliva, protecting the airway or swallowing. As a consequence, dysphagia may cause choking, chest infections or pneumonia.

Guidance from a speech and language therapist, or other professionals specialising in dysphagia assessments, can help to make mealtimes less stressful and maintain optimum health and nutrition.

▪ Normal swallowing

To understand swallowing difficulties, it is important to know how the normal swallow works. Swallowing can be broken down into four stages (Figure 24):

(1) **Oral preparatory stage**. This stage describes the senses 'getting ready' for eating and drinking. You see the food being prepared and you smell the food in front of you. This starts saliva building up in your mouth and makes your brain know you are about to eat or drink.

(2) **Oral stage**. This stage describes the food inside the mouth. The lips, tongue, teeth and cheeks work together to break up the food, mix it with saliva, and form it into a ball to be swallowed. You still have control of the food at this stage and can choose to spit it out or continue to swallow it.

(3) **Pharyngeal stage**. When the food touches the very back of the mouth and moves toward the throat it triggers you to swallow. Once the swallow is triggered you have no voluntary control over the food. The windpipe (trachea) is closed by the Adam's apple (larynx) moving upwards. Breathing is stopped for 1–3 seconds whilst the food is pushed through the throat to the gullet (oesophagus).

(4) **Oesophageal stage**. This stage starts when the food has moved past the throat and entered the gullet (oesophagus). Food is pushed down toward the stomach by muscles.

Problems can occur for many reasons in one or more stages. Common problems you may notice with clients are:

▪ Not recognising food/drink.
▪ 'Forgetting to swallow' food/drink already in the mouth.
▪ Difficulty chewing food, or moving food to the back of the mouth.
▪ Food/drink/saliva dribbling out of the front of the mouth.
▪ Too much, or not enough saliva in the mouth.
▪ Food pocketing in the sides of the mouth after eating.
▪ Food/drink coming out through the nose during swallowing.
▪ Complaining of heart burn or indigestion.
▪ Regurgitating food back into the throat or mouth.
▪ Coughing or choking on food/drinks.
▪ Gurgly/'wet' voice after eating/drinking.
▪ Facial weakness or slurred speech.
▪ Poor oral hygiene.
▪ Spitting out lumps of food.
▪ Eating very fast, or putting too much in the mouth at once.

Enhancing function

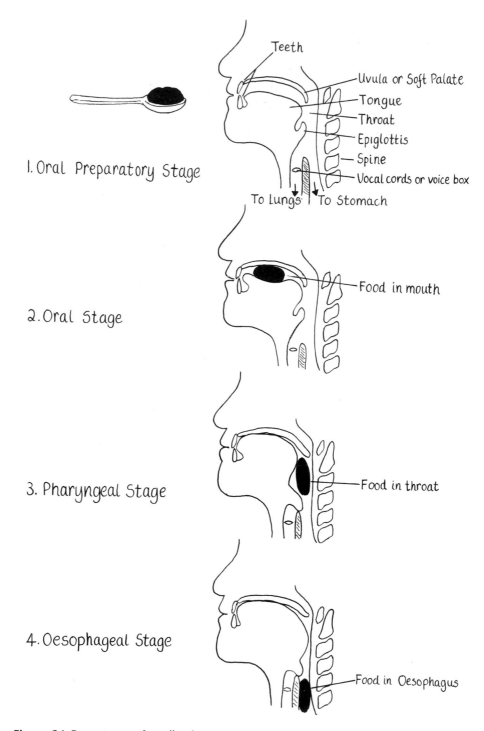

Figure 24 Four stages of swallowing.

- Refusing types of food or drink.
- Talking and eating/drinking at the same time.
- Complaining of food getting stuck in throat or lower down.
- Problems swallowing tablets/medications.
- Chronic chest infections of unknown cause.
- Becoming short of breath and/or sweaty during mealtimes.

Swallowing ability may take a long time to recover, or may not recover at all. For a person to gain the nutrition and hydration they need, discussions may occur with a doctor about placing a feeding tube (such as a percutaneous endoscopic gastrostomy or PEG) into the stomach. Food and drink may be given totally via the tube, or there may be a mixture of using the tube and some food and drink going through the mouth. If swallowing function completely recovers, the tube can be taken out.

▪ General suggestions

Here are some general tips which should aid most swallowing problems.

- Sitting in an upright chair, with supportive sides and back, to eat is better than in bed, if possible. Make sure the feet are flat on the floor or a stool. If the client must be fed in bed, make sure they are as upright as possible, using pillows to stop them from sliding down the bed.
- Head should be upright and chin tucked slightly down towards the chest. This helps the first stage of the normal swallow process.
- Certain head positions can help food move through the mouth and throat safely. If the speech and language therapist has recommended a certain head position, use it for every swallow.
- Make sure the person is awake and alert, and not drowsy.
- Ensure dentures fit properly and are not loose.
- Avoid using beakers that make the head tip back. Tipping the head back opens the throat up making it difficult to control food in the mouth.
- Avoid using syringes to administer medication or drinks orally. It can confuse a person to see a syringe going to their mouth and it bypasses the first two stages of the normal swallow process.
- Make sure the mouth is clear of food before giving the next mouthful.
- Allow time between mouthfuls. This helps breathing to return to normal.
- If food is building up in the mouth, try giving an empty spoon rather than more food. This can sometimes encourage a second swallow of the food remaining in the mouth.
- Don't chat to the person whilst feeding them, as they will try to answer your questions with food in their mouth. Tell them what food is coming next, for example 'Here's another spoon of pudding.'
- If possible, use 'hand over hand' techniques during feeding if the client cannot feed themselves. Place their hand around the cutlery or cup and

Enhancing function

put your hand over theirs to help control the item and support their hand. By using their hand in the eating process, you are telling their brain that something is coming towards their mouth.

■ If you are feeding the person, make sure you are sitting in front of them, at the same level or slightly lower, ensuring you make regular eye contact.

■ Reduce all distractions during eating. Turn off the television. Make sure that the person is facing towards a quiet section of the house (that is, not looking out of a window onto a busy street). The room should be adequately lit.

■ Crushing tablets and putting them in mashed banana or yoghurt, or ordering syrup form may make medication easier to swallow. Seek advice from your doctor to see if medications can be crushed or come in alternative forms. Some medication cannot be crushed as it has a special 'time release' coating.

■ Remain sitting upright for 30–40 minutes after eating or drinking. This makes gravity work by pushing the food towards the stomach. If you lie down straight after eating and drinking the food is more likely to come back up.

■ Any bacteria in the mouth may cause chest infections. Make sure the mouth is clean after every meal. Check that teeth are clear of food particles. Any excessive bacteria in the mouth may cause chest infections.

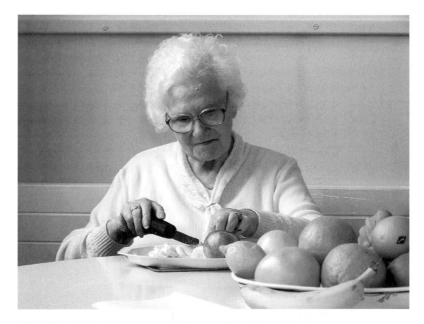

Figure 25 Client sitting in an appropriate position for eating.

■ Types of food and drink

A speech and language therapist will assess the safest types of food and drink that the person can manage. Certain types of foods and drinks may be recommended depending on what stage of swallowing the person is having problems with. If the food or drink needs to be modified the dietician may need to ensure adequate nutrition is being maintained. Foods can be classified into categories depending on how easy or safe they are to swallow. Foods can be grouped into five types:

- Normal: for example fried chicken, pastries, cakes, steak, toast, bacon.
- Soft: for example skinless sausages, pasta and sauce.
- Soft fork mashable: for example scrambled eggs.
- Pureed: for example mashed potato.
- Liquidised in a blender: for example soups.

Drinks can be naturally grouped by their thickness levels, or a specialised thickener can be added to drinks to make the thickness required. Making drinks thicker may make them easier to control in the mouth or throat, and can be grouped into four main types:

- Normal: for example water.
- Naturally thick: for example full cream milk.
- Coating: e.g. tomato juice.
- Thick drink: for example McDonald's thick shakes.

Foods that are especially difficult to eat are classified as 'high risk of choking' foods. They are:

- Mixed textures: e.g. cornflakes and milk, minestrone soup, fruit and nut chocolate, salad sandwiches.
- Stringy textures: for example cabbage, celery.
- Floppy textures: for example cucumber.
- Skins/husks textures: for example baked beans, porridge, grapes.
- Crumbly textures: for example biscuits, dry cakes.
- Small/hard textures: for example peanuts, peas, rice.

Clients who have a left CVA (leading to right arm and leg weakness) may find that their speech and language skills are affected. It may also affect their swallowing skills, leading to problems chewing and moving the food around the mouth. They may not be able to trigger swallowing as quickly as needed. If the right side of the throat is weak and not working properly, food and drink may be directed towards the lungs instead of the stomach. These clients will need a full assessment of their swallowing skills and recommendations to be followed for every swallow.

Enhancing function

Stop and think

Think about Mick (case study 4), who has chronic emphysema, and the possible impact of this on his ability to chew and swallow. His emphysema may mean that he gets tired chewing; he may have difficulty coordinating his chewing and breathing or coordinating his breathing and swallowing; or it may be that he can't coordinate swallowing and closing his airway. This is likely to be a progressive problem which will deteriorate over time and fluctuate with exacerbations. He will need to be monitored over time and reviewed during exacerbations.

Some ways to address these problems may be to provide him with education on types of food and drink that are safe to have during exacerbations. You may need to monitor and change food or fluids as his swallow deteriorates. It will be important to pace his food and drink to regain breathing coordination.

■ ■ MANAGING MEDICATION

Many clients who undergo rehabilitation will take a number of different medications. In addition to prescribed medicines, individuals may purchase medicines over the counter from supermarkets, health stores and pharmacies. Taking multiple medications can be confusing and even the most organised clients can easily forget to take their medication at the right time or in the correct dosage.

Being independent in the management of medication is an important aspect of rehabilitation. Self-administration of medication is the ability of the client to open and close containers, follow prescribed schedules and dosages, report any side effects or problems that may occur, and store the medication appropriately.

Stop and think   Medication management

When attempting to ensure that the client is independent in the management of their medication, consider the following points:

- Who usually looks after their medication?
- Do they have any swallowing problems?
- Can they read the labels?
- What medication are they taking at the moment?
- Does the client know what the medication is for?
- Does the client have any other medication stored in their home?
- Do they remember when to take their medication?
- When do they normally take their medication?

Self-medication can enable greater participation in work, leisure and social events. Combinations of interventions, such as more convenient care, reminders, reinforcement and self-monitoring, can help people to follow self-medication programmes.

▪ Adherence to medication

Adherence is the extent to which the client follows the instructions to take their medication as intended by the prescriber. Many people do not take their medication the way it is prescribed. Underlying beliefs and attitudes are important in determining adherence. Those with negative or mixed views about medication are generally less likely to adhere to treatment.

Informing the client about their medicines, how they work, the possible side effects and ongoing management is thought to improve adherence and thereby contribute to cost effectiveness, as well as being beneficial to the individual's quality of life. An information card can be valuable and may also act as a reminder chart. The chart should be updated every time the client's medications change. Typically, they take the form shown in Figure 26.

People vary in the way they interpret the instructions on labels. It is helpful to have the important points reinforced on the information sheet. Remembering to take medicines can be quite a chore, especially if there are many to be taken at different times of the day. Some people find it helpful to write down the times on a weekly calendar and tick them off each time a dose is taken (see Figure 27 below).

Another way of remembering to take medication is to use a memory aid container, a 'Webster pack', or blister pack (see Figure 29). These are containers that contain several small compartments that are divided into appropriate days or weeks, according to medication times. There are different types available. Some open and close more easily than others, which can be important for people with arthritis.

Medication	Form & strength	Frequency/time of day					Purpose	Special instructions	Possible side-effects (common ones)
		Breakfast	Lunch	Tea	Dinner	Bedtime			

Figure 26 Medication chart.

Time	Medications I need to take	S	M	T	W	T	F	S

Figure 27 Medication calendar.

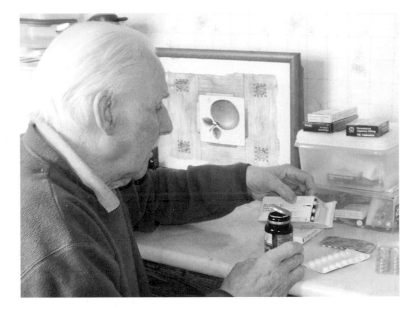

Figure 28 Clients often have to take multiple medications.

Stop and think

Research has shown that people who are depressed are less likely to adhere to their medication regime. Some conditions actually increase the risk of depression. For instance, people with diabetes are twice as likely as people without diabetes to become depressed.

Consider the case of Frances (case study 6) who has diabetes and suffers from depression. How do you think that these two conditions together may impact on her adherence to her medication and therefore her overall health and wellbeing?

■ Side effects and multiple medications

Most medications can produce side effects in some people. Some people may never experience them, whilst for others it may be worth putting up with some mild side effects if other symptoms get better.

Older people who take multiple different medications are at particular risk of adverse effects from interactions between their different drugs. Medication interactions can occur between multiple prescription medications as well as with over-the-counter drugs. Non-prescription drugs bought over the counter for symptom relief of such things as colds and flu, indigestion, constipation and headaches, can sometimes adversely interact with prescribed medicines.

Stop and think

Mrs Kalnina (case study 8) is depressed and has sleeping difficulties. She is on prescription antidepressant medication and has bought some tablets from the pharmacy to help her sleep. Mrs Kalnina needs to be aware of the risk of drug interactions between her antidepressants and the sedative medication and should ask the pharmacist or her GP before taking this combination. Alcohol may exacerbate the effects of both medications, depending on the active ingredient in each, so it would be advisable to avoid alcohol whilst taking this combination of medication.

It is also possible for medication to interact with the food that the client eats. Food can speed up or slow down the action of a medication, or suppress or increase the appetite. Certain drugs may alter the way that different nutrients are absorbed by the body.

You need to be aware of the problems of adverse drug reactions and to watch for any signs and symptoms that occur after starting a new medication, and ensure that they are quickly brought to the attention of the client's GP. The types of symptoms that may occur include:

■ Incontinence
■ Frequent falls
■ Depression
■ Fatigue
■ Constipation or diarrhoea
■ Confusion
■ Weakness or tremors
■ Excess drowsiness or dizziness
■ Agitation or anxiety

It is particularly important to identify drug-related side effects, as sometimes clients can end up taking unnecessary new medication to treat the side effects of the first drug. If you are aware of food–drug interactions, then ensure that the client avoids the offending foods.

■ Safety issues

Like food, medication has a limited shelf life. The expiry date is usually found on the container and the outer packaging. Medicines will last longer if they are kept cool and dry. The best way to avoid taking medicines that are past their expiry date is to return them to the pharmacist once they are no longer needed. Medicines should never be thrown away with household rubbish.

Enhancing function

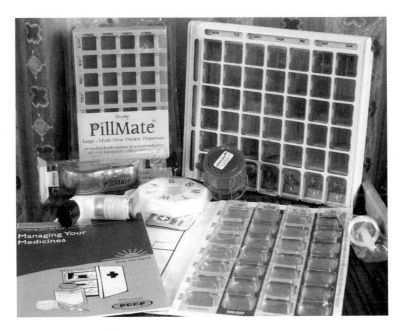

Figure 29 A variety of pill dispensers.

■ Problem solving

Practical difficulties can sometimes occur which may prevent self-medication. The rehabilitation worker is often able to offer advice and alternative options. Simply opening the medicine container can be a struggle for some people. Whilst child-resistant closures are routinely used to help reduce the accidental poisoning of children, ordinary caps can be fitted to medicine containers on request. Special winged caps may be available for people with arthritic hands. The use of a jar opener aid may also be beneficial. Some pharmacists can produce large print for labels, or Braille labels. The local pharmacist will be able to advise.

■ ■ GOING OUT

An important stage of achieving independence in rehabilitation is the ability of the client to function within their wider community or environment. This might involve going shopping, walking the dog, going to church, visiting friends or even resuming normal work activities. Going out can fulfil a range of different needs. It is a way for the client to start to feel more independent. The ability to socialise with family and friends is important. In many cases, the client will need to leave their home to meet some of their basic needs, such as shopping and banking.

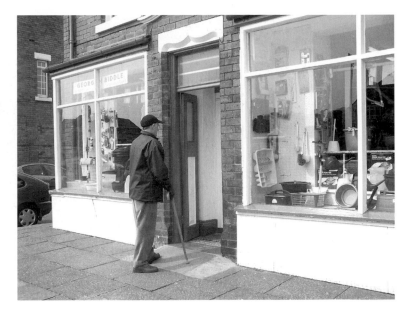

Figure 30 Client using local facilities.

Enhancing function

■ Social skills

Social skills are an essential part of going out. Social skills are comprised of attending and listening, conversation, problem solving, supporting others, and self-control. They include verbal and non-verbal behaviour, and are acquired by development, learning and practice. Disease, illness and developmental delay affect a person's social skills in varying degrees, causing some clients to have deficits or difficulties in relation to them. One of the most important areas of social skills training is teaching assertive behaviour. Assertive behaviour includes helping clients to make choices for themselves, making independent decisions, requesting information or help, and defending oneself from being taken advantage of.

The rehabilitation worker's role in social skills training is to help the client develop the specific skills necessary to perform effectively in social situations. Bob's rehabilitation programme is aimed at encouraging greater independence and expanding his social network and activities. Amongst other things, Bob needs to learn how to use public transport independently, how to abide by traffic safety rules, and how to manage his money.

Assessment

The first step in social skills training is assessment of the individual's behaviour. For example, does the client have difficulty initiating conversations, engaging in group activities, listening and understanding the needs of others, or showing appropriate feelings? In what specific circumstances do these difficulties arise?

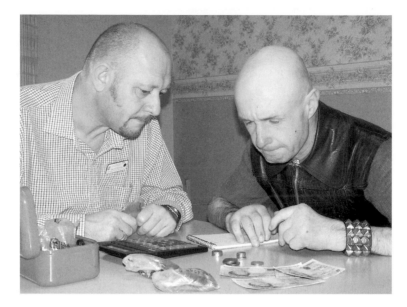

Figure 31 Client learning to differentiate currency.

For example, does the client have difficulty relating to strangers, members of the opposite sex, or people in authority? Does the individual experience stress or anxiety in specific situations, for example open spaces or noisy environments? The rehabilitation worker and the client work together in trying to understand the possible source of the difficulties. One method of identifying the source of the difficulties is self-monitoring. The client keeps a diary in which they record their emotions and behaviour. The client can note when events affect their emotions, and how these emotions influence their interpersonal behaviour. They can also record details of situations in which they felt comfortable, relaxed and confident.

Bob was unable to keep a diary because of his difficulties with reading and writing, but the rehabilitation worker was able to talk with Bob and observe his behaviour in several situations to identify the problem areas.

Programme planning

After identifying the individual's problem areas a rehabilitation programme can be implemented. The rehabilitation worker will structure and organise learning experiences and provide feedback to the client on their performance. This must be done in a way that draws upon the person's strengths. There are four steps in teaching any social skill:

(1) Educational instruction.
(2) Demonstration and modelling.
(3) Guided practice.
(4) Independent activity.

These four steps are used sequentially. The individual builds up to using the skill in real-life situations. During the period of the rehabilitation programme, structure and guidance are gradually reduced. The ability to teach at an appropriate level and to provide relevant instruction and materials is essential.

Stop and think

Refer to the case study of Bob (Case study 7, p. 66), who has Down's syndrome.

- Identify the methods of public transport Bob could use.
- Carry out an activity analysis of Bob using the train service.
- What methods could you use to teach Bob how to use the local train service?
- As well as Bob's needs and abilities you will need to consider your own manner and approach, the learning environment and the resources available.
- What risk/safety issues need to be considered?
- How would you involve Bob's grandmother in the rehabilitation programme?

■ Work and leisure

Boredom is a problem which is often overlooked, yet it can lead to frustration, low mood and lack of self-worth. Participation in work and leisure activities is an important part of life. Unfortunately, many of the people you will see have not had the opportunity to learn how to overcome the obstacles that limit their involvement in work and leisure activities.

Engagement in work and leisure provides a framework for organising daily routines. It provides people with the opportunity to meet people and form relationships, and has an important influence on how people see themselves, on their concept of personal value and identity. Different motivational forces are behind the choice of work and leisure activities. These include social acceptance and contact, a feeling of achievement, financial need, and intellectual and creative stimulation.

Stop and think

Imagine meeting somebody for the first time and one of the first questions they asked you is
'What do you do?'
Think how you would feel if you had no work or leisure activities to talk about.
What impression is this likely to give about you?

Enhancing function

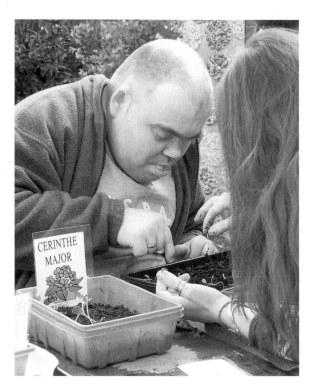

Figure 32 Bob gardening.

Rehabilitation programmes offering work and leisure activities may be aimed at helping the client to adapt to a new situation, or may be therapeutic, facilitating functional and physiological gains. Many work and leisure activities can be easily adapted to suit the individual's needs. Sports such as golf, horse-riding, swimming; office tasks such as typing; and table top games such as bingo and cards can be made enjoyable through the provision of education and assistive devices. Large print and audio books enable the resumption of reading. Gardening can be modified to include using raised beds and long-handled tools.

 Stop and think

Make a list of the possible reasons why Mrs Kalnina (Case study 8) may have lost her confidence in going outside.

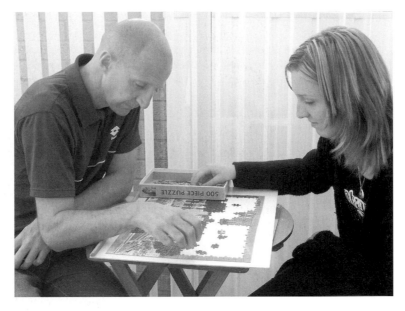

Figure 33 Previous leisure interests can help develop self-awareness.

Developing self-awareness

Both the client and the rehabilitation worker need to develop an understanding of the meaning, values and demands attributed to work and leisure activities by the client. One way to do this is to have the client describe what they particularly liked and disliked about the activities carried out in the past. Effective rehabilitation encourages the client to explore their potential, discover what suits them and make choices based on self-awareness.

Questions that may help to develop self-awareness include:

- What type of work and leisure activities has the client been interested in?
- How did the client find out about the different activities?
- What does the client say they are good at?

Mrs Kalnina reported that she liked having somewhere to go to meet people, but she found it very tiring working all day as well as having to do the household chores. This caused her to lie awake at night worrying, which increased her tiredness and affected her ability to concentrate at work. She then began to worry about her work performance. She enjoyed working in a quiet setting and said that she had a high level of literacy, numeric and clerical skills, but was not physically strong.

Once this awareness has been developed, information can be sought on suitable activities. Consider local resources such as the library, leisure centre or adult educational centre. Charities and organisations can provide specialist information and help. Some offer sheltered employment or leisure groups.

Developing habits and skills

Enhancing function

Engagement in a new activity will require a change in the individual's normal routine. Habits involve learned ways of doing things that when repeated sustain engagement in activity. Through repeated experiences people gain a kind of map for appreciating and behaving in familiar contexts. Because of habits, people know when it is time to leave for work, or what road to take to a familiar destination.

Mrs Kalnina's self-confidence and concentration were low, so a rehabilitation programme was devised with the aim of improving these. The rehabilitation worker introduced Mrs Kalnina to a local needlecraft group. The group was working on a project to produce a wall hanging display for the local community centre. There are written instructions to follow and all participants are encouraged to work at their own pace and on their own section of work, but they need to be aware of the group endeavour and need to work with other participants negotiating, sharing and cooperating.

Stop and think

By joining this group, which physical, cognitive and social skills will Mrs Kalnina be using?
How will this help her to achieve her long-term goals?
If you were the rehabilitation worker, how would you introduce Mrs Kalnina to the group?

Voluntary work provides an avenue to practise and develop skills. Advantages of volunteering are that the client can choose the hours and types of activity. However, it does not provide income and may even incur added expenses such as transportation costs.

Stop and think

After successfully completing the needlecraft project, Mrs Kalnina decided to aim for part-time voluntary work as she is eager to ensure long-term engagement in work-related activities rather than repeat the stop start pattern of the past three years.
How will part-time voluntary work help her to achieve this?
What kind of voluntary work do you think is suitable for Mrs Kalnina? Why?
How could you support Mrs Kalnina in finding and maintaining voluntary work?

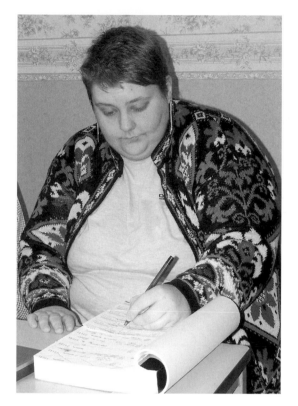

Figure 34 Voluntary work provides an avenue to practise and develop skills.

Reintegration into the community

It is becoming increasingly popular to discharge people home from hospital as early as possible. However, this creates the risk of isolation if the person lives on their own. Restoring their ability to function within a wider environment is an important component of ensuring that they do still have a sense of belonging to society.

▪ Planning the outing

Obviously, each outing will be a bit different, but generally, if the outing is part of a rehabilitation programme, it is worth considering the following:

(1) The goals or purpose of the outing.
(2) The proposed timeframe.
(3) Transport plan.
(4) How much money will be required?
(5) The facilities available at the destination (for example toilets, seating).
(6) Contact details in case of emergency (for example mobile telephone, medic alert).

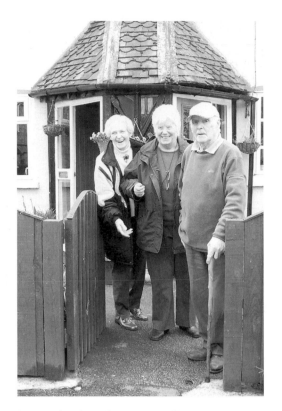

Figure 35 Clients reintegrating into the community.

(7) Known safety risks.
(8) Perceived risks or fears.
(9) How those risks or fears will be addressed.

It is also worth considering whether there are alternatives to the proposed outing, or some way of making it easier. For instance, if the purpose of the outing is to buy groceries, consider whether it makes more sense to order these by telephone or the Internet. However, make sure you keep in mind the overall goals of the client. Whilst buying goods over the Internet can help to increase independence in some aspects, it can be disempowering if the client is unable to achieve their goals.

When the client returns from the outing, reflect on the visit on what worked well and what was difficult. How did they feel about their particular fears and how could they be better overcome next time? Or, if they didn't materialise, do they feel more comfortable about the trip?

Remember to pace the trip. Don't attempt to do too much on the first outing. Build in regular stops, breaks and opportunities to sit down. For instance, if you are going shopping with a client, have a coffee break and make other opportunities to sit down away from crowds.

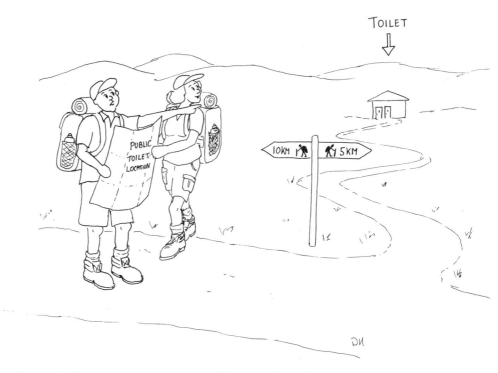

Figure 36 Find out about support facilities available before you go out.

Many large public venues now publicise factors such as their accessibility, the location and numbers of public toilets and wheelchair access, and loop systems for hearing aids, in brochures and on the Internet. It can be useful to keep these details in a resource file at your office so that other members of your team can use them, or 'bookmark' them on your computer. Making this information available to the client before they go out can help ease many of their fears about the outing. If the information is not publicly available, then telephone the venue and ask them about their accessibility, support facilities and public toilet access.

Be aware of the community resources available to support clients with hearing or visual deficits. Again, these details are normally publicised by large public venues. A number of large venues, including shopping centres and public buildings, provide access to wheelchairs, powered wheelchairs, crutches and walking frames. These can increase the mobility and safety of the client when they are on an outing. It is worth checking before you go out, to see what support is available at the venue.

Going out requires a multidisciplinary approach. It is about more than just physical function, it is about state of mind, confidence, socialising safety and resources. Ensure that the whole team are involved in the client assessment and development of the intervention plan for the client. Ensure that the client's clothing is comfortable and appropriate for the outing. There is no point wearing stiletto heels if the client has to walk a long way and is at risk of falling.

Case study 2   Mrs Heath

One of Mrs Heath's former students is making her debut performance at the Opera House, and she has been invited to attend as a guest of honour (case study 2). Mrs Heath is understandably very keen to attend this auspicious occasion. However, it is only six weeks since her fall, and she is still feeling quite nervous about walking beyond the familiar surroundings of her house. Neither she nor her husband drive, but they live quite close to a railway station from which it is about a forty-minute journey to the nearest station to the Opera House. She had planned to catch the train. The performance starts at 8 pm on Saturday night, and will finish at around 11 pm. She has been looking forward to this event for several months, but did not anticipate feeling so fragile.

Mrs Heath has had several weeks to plan for her goal, which is to make it to the Opera House on Saturday night in time for her pupil's performance. She and the rehabilitation team have been working together to try to ensure that she is able to get to the event safely and comfortably. This meant that she needed to be mobile enough to be able to get to the event, walk within the Opera House, and be able to sit for several hours.

The rehabilitation worker looked at the Opera House website and found that there is a free shuttle bus to and from the nearest station to the Opera House. The website described access to each of the theatres and the concert hall, including the number of steps within the venue. From this information they could determine that Mrs Heath would be able to move around within the Opera House.

Transport to the Opera House was a primary concern. The local railway station is only accessible by overhead bridge, which has 51 steps to walk up and down to get to the platform. The rehabilitation worker has worked with Mrs Heath to increase her confidence on steps. However, she can only walk up 15 steps at a time without needing a rest. She knows that there are escalators at the station nearest the Opera House, but sometimes these do not work, which means that she would need to go to the next station where there is a lift, and then get a taxi back to the Opera House. Fortunately, her son offered to drive Mr and Mrs Heath to and from the performance, saving them the difficulties of public transport and the high cost of a taxi.

Mrs Heath was also concerned about her incontinence. The website described the location of the toilets, which were not very accessible from her seats in the concert hall. However, the website did say that staff would be available to help if necessary. The rehabilitation worker telephoned the Opera House reception to confirm that Mrs Heath would be able to be helped to get to and from the toilets quickly during the interval.

Mrs Heath took a walking stick to improve her confidence walking, but also to alert other people to her frailty. Mr Heath agreed that he would stay nearby. Had Mrs Heath been less confident she could have made arrangements with the Opera House to use a wheelchair. However, she was confident enough of her ability to walk by this stage.

Developing a clear plan of the evening beforehand took a small amount of time and research, but, as a result, Mrs Heath knew exactly what to expect, and was able to address most of her fears before she went out. The staff were available to help her to the toilet as promised, and the performance was an enormous success. She is still cautious when she goes out, but can now manage the full 51 stairs to get to the station and is more confident about catching the train.

Conversely, it is unnecessary to feel uncomfortable wearing trainers to a wedding if the client will be accompanied the whole way, will travel by car and have little distance to walk. Consider the climate, and indoor and outdoor activities the client will be involved, in as well as the ease of removal and storage or carriage of those clothes.

Build up gradually, from simpler to larger or more complex activities. There is no point making the first visit a trip to a large shopping centre to go Christmas shopping. It is exhausting and dangerous for the fittest of us. Instead, you could aim to go to one relatively quiet department store, shop for a short time, then stop for a coffee. Ensure that there is a way for the client to 'get out' easily. Do not go for a long walk or drive where the only way to stop is to retrace your long travels. Make sure there are frequent possibilities to stop and go home, or go somewhere safe and comfortable if necessary.

Make sure that you have an appropriate amount of support. Be aware of potential risks to the client's safety at all times. If they are out alone, make sure they have a way of contacting someone who can help them if they get into difficulty. This might involve a mobile phone with some key telephone numbers programmed in, or the use of a medic alert which will trigger a response at an agency.

■ ■ SUMMARY

This section has covered much ground. Although it is impossible in one section to provide detailed information on the entire range of enablement activities, this section has presented an overview of how the rehabilitation worker may be involved in enhancing the functional ability of clients. Specific techniques and items of equipment have been offered only as illustrative examples. You will need to explore particular areas in more detail and are encouraged to follow through with the further reading.

Behind the everyday familiarity of the activities discussed in this section, such as washing, dressing and food preparation, lies complexity and challenge. We hope this section has shown something of the multi-layered and complex process of enhancing functional activity and participation. Multiple problems, choices, issues and challenges confront us in our rehabilitation work. This means simple answers and formula solutions have little to offer us. It is not enough to see the person in terms of their illness or problem. Instead, we need to see the person's hopes, skills, values and strengths, as well as knowing how they interact with family, friends and the wider community.

Any agreed rehabilitation programme must be personalised, consistently implemented and regularly reviewed. You need to know and understand the roles of colleagues and be familiar with community provision and local facilities. The demands on rehabilitation services are not static; they will continue to change and develop as circumstances change. New legislation, new technologies and developments in practice will all bring changes that we will need to respond to. Therefore, it is extremely important that we remain open to learning.

Enhancing function

It is hoped this section has helped to provide some insights, as well as some confirmation of existing skills, knowledge and good practices. But most of all, we hope that it has stimulated you to think about:

■ What you are doing.
■ Why you are doing it.
■ How you can learn and progress.

■ ■ FURTHER READING

General

www.arthritiscare.org.uk *This organisation produces a range of publications to meet the needs of people with arthritis, including pamphlets called 'Food for Thought' and 'Reaching Independence; a Guide for Living at Home for People with Arthritis'.*

Jogee, M. (2004) *Religions and Cultures: A Guide to Beliefs, Customs and Diversity for Health and Social Care Services*, 6th edition. PO Box 17249, Edinburgh EH11 2XZ, R & C Publications. http://www.religionsandcultures.co.uk *This booklet gives practical advice to ensure careful consideration around others' beliefs and customs. Copies can be ordered by contacting the publisher.*

Repper, P. & Perkins, R. (2003) *Social Inclusion and Recovery*. Edinburgh, Bailliere Tindall. *This book is based on the lived experiences of people with mental distress. It focuses on ways in which rehabilitation workers can assist people with mental health problems.*

Sladyk, K. & Ryan, S.W. (2001) *Ryan's Occupational Therapy Assistant. Principles, Practice Issues and Techniques*. New Jersey, Slack Incorporated. *The main focus of this text is for occupational therapy assistants. However, it includes a wide range of principles and interventions that are likely to be useful for rehabilitation assistants. It illustrates the main therapeutic processes using a range of disease specific case studies.*

Mobility and transfers

Aitchison, L. (1999) *Safe Handling of People in The Community*. Middlesex. National Back Pain Association.

Lloyd, P., Fletcher, B., Holmes, D., Tarling, C. & Tracy, M. (1997) *The Guide to the Handling of Clients – Introducing a Safer Handling Policy* (4th edition) Middlesex. National Back Pain Association.

Mandelstam, M. (2005) *Manual Handling in Health and Social Care : An A – Z of Law and Practice*. Gateshead, Athenaeum Press.

These three text books give good overviews of the manual handling regulations and legislation relating to the UK.

Trew, M. & Everett, T. (2003) *Human Movement. An Introductory Text* (4th Edition). Edinburgh, Churchill Livingstone. *This book contains essential information for those studying human movement for therapeutic means. The anatomical, physiological and biomechanical aspects of movement are all addressed in a readily accessible style.*

Whittle, M.W. (2002) *Gait Analysis. An Introduction* (3rd Edition). Oxford, Butterworth Heinemann. *This text book explains human walking and covers a wide range of the methods available to study gait.*

Washing, hygiene and dressing

Australasian Podiatry Council. http://www.apodc.com.au. *This website provides free access to information about a wide range of different foot care issues.*

The Disabled Living Foundation and Independent Living Centres offer equipment information and advisory resource services. More information can be found at the following websites:

www.dlf.org.uk

www.ilc.com.au/

www.cailc.ca/

Food preparation, handling and eating

Copeman, J. (1999) *Nutritional Care for Older People: A Guide to Good Practice.* London, Age Concern. *This book is written by a nutritionist and includes information about the food environment and presentation, risk factors, menu planning and recipes, cultural and religious issues, and the nutritional needs of people with specific illnesses.*

Binns, C. (1999) *Dietary Guidelines for Older Australians. Commonwealth of Australia, National Health and Medical Research Council.* http://www.nhmrc.gov.au/publications/_files/n23.pdf *This is an excellent guideline, 216 pages long, which is available online. It provides a wide range of well-researched information about the food handling and nutritional needs of older people, including the needs of older people in aged care facilities and the Australian Nutrition Screening Initiative (nutrition screening tool).*

National policy resource centre on nutrition and ageing. http://www.fiu.edu/~nutreldr/SubjectList/N/Nutrition_Screening_Assessment.htm#2 *This is a valuable website which provides links to the Nutrition Screening Initiative and the Mini Nutritional Assessment and information and resources about both of these nutritional screening tools.*

Managing medication

Bird, C. & Hassall, J. (1993) *Self Administration of Drugs. A guide to Implementation.* London, Scuturi Press.

US Food and Drug Administration, Center for Drug Evaluation and Research. http://www.fda.gov/cder/consumerinfo/druginteractions.htm *This is a useful site for information about different types of drug interactions and the effect of those interactions.*

Enhancing function

Section 3
Problem-based approach

- Communication
- Psychological aspects of rehabilitation
- Preventing falls – a key to maintaining independence
- Continence
- Memory loss
- Fatigue
- Palliative care

Communication

Kelly McPhee

Introduction

Communication plays a key role in everyday life. It provides a connection with other people in the community and is important in maintaining self-esteem and psychological wellbeing. Difficulty with communication can disrupt our social networks and relationships with our family and friends. It may lead to isolation and difficulty making choices and decisions. It is important to remember that loss of communication ability is a problem with speech and/or language, and not a loss of intelligence.

A rehabilitation worker's aim is to enable or facilitate communication for the client, not to speak for the client. You are likely to have many opportunities to support the client to practise their communication in natural settings (for example banks, shops, on the phone, on the bus, at home etc.). This approach to support may take longer in the short term, but will provide maximum benefit in the long term for both you and the client. It is your responsibility to monitor for communication failures, and identify the best repair strategy for the client. You or a family member can always help a client to communicate more effectively, no matter how severe the communication problem.

Clients who have insight into, or awareness of, their communication problems may become very frustrated with their difficulties in communicating their needs. Rehabilitation workers, friends and family may also feel strong emotions. This chapter will look at strategies to help identify areas of communication breakdown and how to repair it, therefore reducing some of the anxiety felt when not being understood. Being familiar with the client's strengths and communication style will increase communication success and decrease frustration levels of clients and/or rehabilitation workers. If necessary, your local speech and language therapist can provide a specific assessment of the client's individual ability and communication strategies. Individual therapy sessions with a speech and language therapist may be limited, so carry-over of exercises into familiar environments (such as their home) will give the client maximum potential to improve, or be understood and continue to play an active role in the family/community.

▪ What is communication?

Communication is more than just talking. In order to communicate effectively, you need at least one speaker and one listener. It is a two-way process. The speaker gets his/her message across to the listener through verbal (speaking), and non-verbal (gesturing, pointing, writing/drawing, eye contact and body language) techniques. The speaker will use a combination of verbal and non-verbal techniques during every conversation. The listener will understand the message by hearing the words/sentences, listening to the voice, reading any written words, and seeing the gestures, facial expressions and body language the speaker is producing. The speaker and listener will monitor each other and know when to start talking, or when to listen. They watch each other's facial expression and body language to learn if somebody is happy, angry, telling a joke or being serious. They will know when it is time to finish the topic and move onto another topic, or finish the conversation completely. There are four main reasons why people communicate with each other:

- ▪ **To convey needs:** 'Can I have a drink?'
- ▪ **To ask for information:** 'When does the bus come?'
- ▪ **To supply information:** 'It is cold outside.'
- ▪ **To express feelings/emotions:** 'That hurt me.'

The most basic level of communicating is through gestures, pointing and drawing pictures. This requires no knowledge of the spoken language. Slightly more difficult is reading and understanding some words spoken to you. More complex language skills are required for speaking and writing. The highest level of language skill is not only understanding and speaking in a conversation, but being able to interpret higher level language structures, such as sarcasm and humour. When a person has difficulties using and/or understanding verbal and non-verbal communication, communication breakdown, frustration and misunderstanding can occur.

Stop and think

Imagine you have arrived in a foreign country for the first time. You cannot read or speak the local language. The local people do not read or speak your language. The culture is very different from your own. You are feeling sick and need a doctor.
How do you communicate so you can find out where the local hospital is and how to see a doctor?
When you find a doctor, how do you let them know what is wrong with you?
How does the doctor convey to you what is wrong and how to fix it?
How do you ask for the medication and know when/how to take it?

Communication

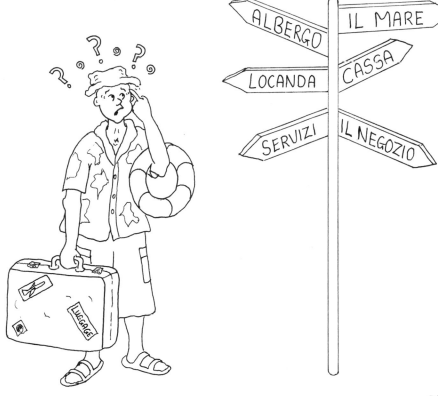

Figure 1 Communication barriers in a foreign country.

■ Communication problems

There are specialised centres in the brain that are responsible for communication. These centres can be damaged as a result of a stroke, excessive long-term drug use, head injury (such as car accidents, falls or hits to the head), cancers, or progressive disorders such as motor neuron disease, multiple sclerosis, dementia and Parkinson's disease. Depending on the extent of damage to the brain, different types of communication problems may occur, either permanently or temporarily. The difficulties can be classified as mild, moderate or severe, but to the client a mild problem can cause just as much anxiety and frustration as a severe problem.

Aphasia

Aphasia is a general medical term for many types of communication problems due to damage to specific areas of the brain. The most common cause of aphasia is caused by a cerebrovascular accident (CVA) or stroke. Aphasia can be broken down into two main types; *receptive* and *expressive* aphasia. Receptive aphasia (the receiving or input side of language) is the inability to understand what is said to you or follow instructions, and expressive aphasia (the expressing or the output side of language) is an inability to speak in well-formed sentences, with clear speech sounds. The client may show varying degrees of difficulty in one or both areas.

Clients with aphasia may or may not be aware of the mistakes they are making. They may:

■ Have difficulty following simple instructions, for example the rehabilitation worker's instruction: 'Point to your nose'; or longer more complex instructions, for example the rehabilitation worker's instructions: 'Before you go to the door, put your red hat on and get your keys from the coat pocket'.

■ Answer 'yes' and 'no' incorrectly to questions asked of them.

■ Have difficulty understanding what they are reading in cards, books, magazines or newspapers.

■ Speak in full sentences that do not make sense or cannot be easily understood by the listener. Not all the words in the sentence will be 'real' words, or may not be formed correctly. This is called *jargon speech*.

■ Use only one word during talking. The person thinks they are talking in full sentences and are making sense. However, in reality they are repeating the same word over and over again, but with complete rise and fall of how a sentence sounds. For example 'car car CAR CAR?' with rising at the end to indicate a question. The person could be trying to say 'Can you open the window?' or 'What's for lunch?'

■ Have difficulty getting words out clearly, or hesitate in finding the right word to say. Words may come out jumbled or not make sense. However, they usually know what word they want to say, but just can't 'get it out'. Therefore they may use 'filler' words, such as 'thingamajig', or 'stuff'. Or they may try and describe the word they are looking for, such as 'you drink from it' (for 'cup'). This is called *word finding difficulties*.

■ Use words incorrectly. They may make mistakes by saying words that are closely matched by category, such as 'table' when they want to say 'chair', or matched by sound, such as 'mouse' instead of 'house', or not matched at all, such as 'gate' for 'boat'. This is called *word* or *sound substitutions*.

■ Be 'stuck' on the last word they have said and repeat this word over and over again. This is called *perseveration*.

■ Have difficulty writing single words, or sentences. They may have difficulty with spelling or grammar. They may have difficulty with keeping lines straight on the page. This is called *agraphia*.

■ Repeat word for word what has just been said to them. This can be just single words or complete sentences. The client is unaware of imitating the other person's speech. This is called *parrot speech* or *echolalia*.

> **Case study** Charlie
>
> Charlie has had a stroke in the left side of his brain, causing muscle weakness on the right side of his body. This includes his right arm, right leg, as well as the right side of his face. The left side of Charlie's brain is where most of the areas for communication are situated. The assessment suggests Charlie is struggling with understanding conversations and getting his words out. This means Charlie has *receptive* and *expressive aphasia*. He may have difficulty getting words out because he is having *word finding difficulties*, or he is *dysarthric* or *apraxic*. If Charlie does not have any more strokes, his communication skills may improve, or if the stroke was severe, his communication skills may remain the same. They should not deteriorate over time. Suggestions will be given in the section entitled Ideas for successful communication to show how the rehabilitation worker/family member should monitor their own language to help Charlie understand what has just been said, and exercises for Charlie to improve his own talking.

Dysarthria

Dysarthria is a result of the muscles used to make the sounds of speech becoming damaged or weak. These muscles include the lips, tongue, cheeks, larynx (or voice-box). Breathing control is also needed in order to get the words out clearly and with enough volume. Clients with dysarthria:

- Can sound slurred (as if they are drunk), or mumbling.
- May sound as if they can't finish the ends of their sentences due to running out of breath.
- Can sound low in volume, or whispery.
- May sound like they have a cold, or nasal speech.

> **Case study** Mick (Case study 4, p. 65)
>
> Mick has been diagnosed with chronic emphysema or chronic obstructive pulmonary disease (COPD) (see Section 2: Case studies). Unlike Charlie, Mick's difficulties are not due to damage to his brain. His main difficulty is coordinating his breathing and talking. Chronic emphysema is progressive, so his difficulties with coordinating his breathing and talking will not improve. Suggestions from the speech and language therapist/speech pathologist will focus on making sure Mick has correct breathing support; muscles during breathing and talking are not tense, and he learns how to relax them; and sentences and breathing are paced, so sentences are not rushed at the end of a breath making them hard to hear and understand. The majority of suggestions will be for Mick to practise. However, some suggestions will help the family/rehabilitation workers support Mick in making talking easier.

Communication

Apraxia

Apraxia is a problem with planning and coordinating the muscles for speaking. The muscles are not necessarily weakened, but the client has difficulty getting the right sounds in the right order, due to a breakdown in the links between the brain pathways to the muscles used for speaking. This leads to sound errors, such as 'dat' for 'cat'. Often these errors are made inconsistently, as the person struggles to find the correct position of the tongue and lips for each sound in a word. Sometimes automatic or over-learned speech (such as days of the week, counting, greetings such as hello/goodbye, well-known songs and sometimes swearing) can be said more easily than newly formed sentences. The client with apraxia is usually aware of the mistakes and will try and correct them. So 'dat' for 'cat' may become 'bat', 'sat' or 'sit' after several attempts. The longer the word the more likely errors will occur. The client may also have difficulty with facial expressions when instructed, for example they may not be able to 'pucker' the lips when asked, but can automatically give a kiss when the spouse walks into the room. This is usually out of the client's voluntary control, but they may be very aware of their mistakes, which may lead to increased frustration.

Cognition

The client with cognitive problems may have difficulty with processing information given to them, remembering all the information, or sequencing ideas in a logical order. They may:

- Have difficulty attending or concentrating long enough to finish a task, such as eating a meal, or remembering the sequence of doing something as everyday as getting dressed.
- Be easily distracted from a task by busy environments or people talking to them.
- Forget family members' names, or not recognise them when they walk into the room, but may mistake new people for previously known friends/family.
- Forget what the name of an object is (for example cup), or how to use it (to drink from it).
- Have difficulty remembering new information, but can remember past events perfectly.
- Have difficulty understanding jokes, sarcasm or implied requests (such as understanding that when you say 'It's cold in here', you really mean 'Can you close the window?').
- Have difficulty with reading emotions in other people and responding appropriately (for example they may laugh when somebody is crying).
- Have difficulty staying on a topic of conversation and stray into other topics inappropriately. They may lose track of conversation, or forget what was being discussed.

The client with pragmatic or social skills problems will have difficulty following the normal social rules of conversation. They may talk too much, or not continue the turn taking process of a conversation. They may stand too close, making the speaker feel uncomfortable. Behaviour changes such as aggression, or mood swings may occur. Sometimes exaggerated emotions occur where the client can cry or laugh excessively without any control over the behaviour.

Case study Evelyn

Evelyn has been diagnosed with moderate dementia. She will have *cognitive* difficulties and, depending on the type of dementia, will experience different types of language difficulty. Dementia is progressive, which means the language skills will not improve and will deteriorate over time. It is important that the speech and language therapist/speech pathologist monitors Evelyn's dementia, and offers advice when needed. Most of the advice will be for the family/rehabilitation workers on how to use compensatory strategies with Evelyn to help her function independently for as long as possible.

Voice

The client with voice problems may have difficulty with producing a clear, strong voice. It may sound husky or breathy, or low in volume. The voice may sound unusually 'flat' or monotone, not using the normal rise and fall of natural speech.

Respiration

The client with respiration problems will have difficulties providing enough breath support to speak clearly, loudly and intelligibly. They may try to breathe from the upper part of their body rather than from their diaphragm. They may also try and put too many words/sentences in one breath, causing their speech to sound rushed.

Case study Bob (see Case study 7, p. 66)

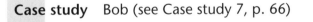

Unlike the other case studies, Bob does not have a new or acquired problem with communication. His reading, writing and speech difficulties are the result of a congenital problem (or were present at birth). Bob may have had speech and language therapy/speech pathology as a child and may have compensatory strategies that a rehabilitation worker should investigate. If this is not the case, Bob may benefit from exercises for weak facial muscles or for specific speech sounds he has difficulty producing. Depending on the level of reading and writing skills, Bob may benefit from a communication book. This is an individualised book prepared by the speech and language therapist which provides information to Bob in single words or pictures for everyday situations. Bob can use the book to converse with people in shops/streets/the doctor's etc. It may help him communicate more effectively with strangers who cannot understand him, or explain his reading and writing difficulties.

■ Ideas for successful communication

Three areas that can be addressed very quickly and easily when communicating with anyone who has a communication problem are the *environment*, the *client* and the *rehabilitation worker/family member*. Addressing these areas will ensure the best possible chance for successful communication. As each person is an individual, so are their abilities and difficulties. A speech and language therapist usually assesses the client's skills and abilities and will provide recommendations.

Environment

The environment where you communicate with the client can play a significant role in making conversation easier and more effective. This means:

- Choosing a room that is quiet, free from busy people walking in and out, barking dogs, telephone/doorbell ringing, television on or washing machine working.
- Choosing a room that does not have distractions out of the window, such as a busy street.
- Turning off the radio or television.
- Making sure the room is not too hot or too cold.
- Making sure the light is not too bright and the client is not facing into the sun (this makes it difficult to see your face).
- Making the room as clutter free as possible to avoid losing the client's attention.

Client

Making sure the client is 'at their best' will help communication be more enjoyable and successful. For instance, their glasses should be cleaned and worn if needed (make sure they have the correctly prescribed glasses). The client's hearing aids should be cleaned, the battery checked regularly, and placed correctly if needed. If dentures are worn, make sure they are clean and fit well. Make sure the client's mouth is clean and looks moist.

Find out which language the client prefers to communicate in. If the client is bilingual, they may only be able to speak or understand their first language. You may need an interpreter in this case. Try to ensure that you understand the client's cultural or religious needs.

Make sure the client is awake and alert. Work out what times of the day are better suited for intense communication, or just 'light talk'. This may relate to personal preferences (being a 'morning person', or a 'night person'), or may be due to side effects of medication. Check medication for side effects such as drowsiness, dizziness, or dry mouth. If medication is making the client feel drowsy, they will not feel like talking. Discuss the medication with their doctor.

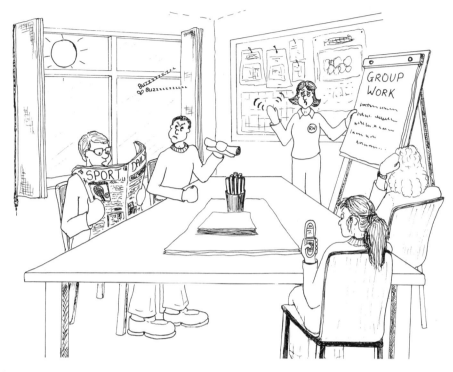

Figure 2 Inappropriate environment for communication.

Make sure the client is comfortable in the chair or bed and that the lighting and temperature are appropriate. Check that they are not hungry or thirsty and are not needing to go to the toilet. All of these factors will distract the client from clear communication.

Rehabilitation worker or family member

By following some basic rules in conversation, the rehabilitation worker or family member can facilitate conversation and bring out the best in the client.

General tips

- Avoid speaking to others about the client whilst they are in the room, or within earshot.
- Involve the client in conversations as much as possible.
- Avoid speaking for the person.
- Try to have only one person speaking at a time. People speaking at the same time can be confusing.
- Encourage and motivate the client to be part of the conversation.
- Be aware that the client may be tired, hungry, or uncomfortable.
- Speak slowly and clearly without shouting.

- Give the client enough time to respond to a question. This can sometimes take a while, so be comfortable with silences.
- Don't rush. Make sure you have given enough time to allow the client to get his/her message across.
- Encourage the client to speak slowly and clearly. Prompt the client to use fewer words per breath if they sound rushed or become out of breath before finishing the sentence.
- Always face the client at the same level. This helps the client hear you and see you.
- Make conversation as relevant and interesting for the client as possible. Find out what their hobbies and interests are.
- Discreetly model correct speech or sentence structures if the client is struggling with words or sentences.
- Discreetly keep the client on topic or task, or help them remember jobs/events about to happen or which have occurred in the past.
- Use all types of communication and accept all types of communication to get the message across. This could be a combination of pointing, or gesturing, or writing the word down, with speech, or one of these methods alone.

Specific tips

Here are some specific ways you can shape your own language and monitor answers from the client to facilitate a more successful communication interaction.

You should aim to keep instructions or conversations at the right level for enabling the client. This may be by breaking down multiple steps from one sentence into many single steps, or allowing time in between sentences. For example:

> Rehabilitation worker: 'You will need to have a shower today because we are running late for your doctor's appointment this afternoon, so before that go and have your breakfast and I'll sort your clothes ready on your bed so you can make your bed later.'

This can be too much information at once and can be confusing. The same information can be broken down into smaller steps:

> Rehabilitation worker: 'Good morning. Do you feel like breakfast? . . . OK, breakfast is finished, now have your shower . . . Here are your clothes to put on . . . OK, let's make the bed . . . Now we are ready to go to the doctor's.'

The rehabilitation worker should avoid using abstract language. Keep conversation in the 'here and now', that is, talk about today's events *today*, and tomorrow's events *tomorrow*. Keep conversation 'concrete' and to the point. For example, say 'I was angry' instead of 'I hit the roof', or say 'Close the window' instead of 'It's getting cold in here.'

Stop and think

It is easier for a client to understand your message if your body language and facial expression match your voice and the words you are using. Which of the following drawings in Figure 3, would convey to the client that the rehabilitation worker is REALLY happy and having a good day?

There are three main ways to ask a question, which allows for different types of responses from the client. The rehabilitation worker can ask a variety of questions in these three ways, depending on the ability of the client.

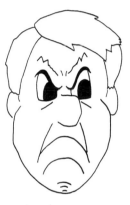

I'm having a
wonderful day

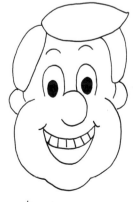

I'm having a
wonderful day!

Figure 3 Which face accurately reflects the caption?

Open ended questions: These types of questions are the hardest to answer as there are no restrictions on the choice of answer. For example:

'What do you want to do today?' or 'What would you like to make to eat?'

Multiple choice questions: These types of questions are slightly easier to answer because the answer can be chosen from a restricted choice. For example:

'Do you want to go to the shops or the park today?' or 'Would you like porridge or scrambled eggs for breakfast?'

Yes/no questions: These are the easiest types of questions to answer as they require only a yes or no response. For example:

'Do you want to go to the shops?' or 'Do you want porridge?'

Throughout your conversation with the client, make sure they have understood what you have said to them. If you notice the client did not understand you, try repeating what you have just said in a different way. For example:

'Do you want three or four sugars in your cup of tea?'

This may not have been understood; therefore say something like:

'Your cup of tea . . . three sugars?'

Another way to make sure the client has understood you is by asking the same question in a different way. This confirms that you have the right answer. For example:

Rehabilitation worker: 'Do you want to go to the shops before dinner?'
Client: 'Yes.'
Rehabilitation worker: 'Should we eat first then go to the shops?'
Client: 'No.'

If you do not understand what the client has just said to you, reinforce that what they are saying is important to you, and ask them to repeat *the word* you misunderstood. For example:

Client: 'Tomorrow I want to go to the . . .'
Rehabilitation worker: 'Sorry, I missed that, you want to go WHERE?'
Client: 'Bank.'
Rehabilitation worker: 'OK, you want to go to the bank tomorrow?'
Client: 'Yes.'

If the client is having difficulties getting the right word out, you can encourage them to use as many clues or prompts as needed to find the right word. This can be achieved by:

- Pointing to the object if it is near.
- Writing down the word/first letter.
- Using a gesture, for example pretending to drink from a cup.
- Describing the object/word. For example:

> Client 'You drink from it.'
> Rehabilitation worker: 'A cup?'
> Client: 'Yes, a cup.'

Sometimes clients can communicate more effectively by pointing at pictures/photos, alphabet boards or written words to get their message across. If you know the word the client is struggling with, tactfully try to help the client retrieve the word by providing different levels of prompts. Always start with the lowest level of prompting/support and move through the hierarchy as the client needs more help. This makes the client work for the word/sentence, and will provide maximum practice.

Lowest level of support: Provide the first letter of the word. For example:

> Client: 'It's on the —.'
> Rehabilitation worker: 'It's on the t—.'
> Client: 'Table.'

Second level of support: Provide a phrase for the client to complete to prompt the word. For example:

> Client: 'Can I have the —?'
> Rehabilitation worker: 'You want the salt and —?'
> Client: 'Pepper, yes, can I have the pepper?'

Third level of support: Provide a forced choice. For example:

> Client: 'Let's go in the —.'
> Rehabilitation worker: 'Car or bus?'
> Client: 'Car.'

Highest level of support: Provide the word the client is struggling with. For example:

> Client: 'I want the —.'
> Rehabilitation worker: 'Scarf?'
> Client: 'Scarf, I want the scarf.'

Provide a 'language stimulation' environment. For example, get the client involved in preparing meals and drinks, or organising the food list for shopping. The client can look for items missing in the cupboards or find items in the supermarket. You could ask the client to tell you the next step in cooking. Discuss what is going to happen and has happened during the day.

Stop and think

Make an audio-visual recording of any interaction with the client (after obtaining consent of the client and anyone else appearing in the video). Make the recording for a minimum of an hour. It could be during a mealtime, during a visit from friends or family, or just a normal hour in the sitting room. When you are watching the tape, use the ideas above to guide your observations and ask yourself the following questions:

How many times did the client/rehabilitation worker/family start a conversation?
How many times did the client/rehabilitation worker/family respond to questions?
What types of questions did the client/rehabilitation worker/family ask?
Is the communication partnership equal? In other words, does each person initiate and respond in equal portions?
Does the client look comfortable?
What is happening in the room? Are there any distractions?
Where is the rehabilitation worker/family sitting when talking to the client?
How long are the sentences the rehabilitation worker/family is using?
Can you understand what the client is saying?

■ Further reading

Bauby, J.D. (1997) *The Diving Bell and the Butterfly.* London, Fourth Estate. *Jean Dominique Bauby suffered a severe stroke, leaving him unable to control any muscles except his eyelids. He writes a personal account of his stroke by blinking at individual letters from a communication board.*

Connect – The Communication Disability Network. Retrieved on 15 November 2005 from www.ukconnect.org

Parr, S., Byng, S., Gilpin, S. & Ireland, S. (1997) *Talking about Aphasia: Living with Loss of Language after Stroke.* Philadelphia, Open University Press.

Rayner, H. & Marshall, J. (2003) Training volunteers as conversational partners for people with aphasia. *International Journal of Language and Communication Disorders*, **38**(2), 149–64. Taylor & Francis Ltd.

Sacks, O. (1998) *The Man Who Mistook his Wife for a Hat: and other clinical tales.* New York, Touchstone. *Oliver Sacks is a neurologist (who also wrote Awakenings) who discusses unusual and interesting cases he has seen clinically. This book is more medically based and explores the neurological reasons behind difficulties seen in strokes, Parkinsonian and memory disorders.*

Sienkiewicz-Mercer, R. & Kaplan, S.B. (1989) *I Raise My Eyes To Say Yes.* Boston, Houghton Mifflin. *Ruth Sienkiewicz-Mercer was diagnosed with encephalitis at five weeks of age, and later with cerebral palsy. She became wheelchair bound, unable to speak and was misdiagnosed as mentally retarded. Through family and rehabilitation workers understanding Ruth's communicative intent, Ruth was able to learn to communicate by using communication boards. This is her life story.*

Communication

Tipton-Dikengil, A. (1994) *Communication Carryover for Adults: Caregiver Information and Instruction*. Communication Skill Builders. London, The Psychological Corporation.

The following websites offer support and advice for specific conditions such as stroke, Alzheimer's disease and Parkinson's disease. Use the Internet search engines for information on specific conditions or support groups in your local area.

(1) www.speakability.org
(2) www.alzheimers.org
(3) www.parkinsons.org
(4) www.stroke.org
(5) www.strokeassociation.org (USA)

Communication

Psychological aspects of rehabilitation

Bob Spall, Darren Perry & Hannah Barratt

Introduction

There are many psychological factors to consider when you are working with clients who require rehabilitation. For instance, what is the personal impact of the client's illness or disability? How much does the client understand about his or her condition and the therapy required? To what extent is the client experiencing the common reactions of low mood, depression and anxiety? Does the client perceive that he or she has any control over the outcome of rehabilitation or feel that this depends solely on the skills of the staff?

Some clients may have to cope with multiple stresses in life in addition to their illness, or disability and rehabilitation. This chapter highlights these and other important psychological issues and describes a framework for providing non-specialist psychological care that can be used by rehabilitation workers.

The wider view of the client's life

Imagine that you only had access to partial information about some of your clients. For example, you may not have known that 65-year-old Judy is a widow, or that her only child has moved abroad and that she appears to have no social support. This contextual information is potentially very important and may account for her depression. Her low mood may make it difficult for her to engage in rehabilitation and so it would be important to address this. You might consider interventions that increase her social support and enable her to talk about her husband or the lack of contact with her only child.

In extreme circumstances it can be very clear that rehabilitation is going to be difficult if other issues are not addressed. For example, Edith experienced a stroke a short time after her husband died. While she was on the rehabilitation ward her adult son also died, which had implications for whether she would be able to go home. It was important that she had specialist psychological help to enable her to work on these issues, otherwise her chances of benefiting from rehabilitation would probably have been slim. Even in far less extreme situations it can be very important to take a wider view of a client's life.

Consider the case of 85-year-old Phyllis, who cares for her husband. She was alert and quite active prior to breaking her hip. Now, she is unable to cook and clean the way she used to. She is very house-proud and it worries her that she cannot maintain her previous high standards of cleanliness, or care for her husband as effectively as before. Such anxiety may cause Phyllis to overdo things, or if she feels anxious a lot of the time, it may interfere with rehabilitation.

It can be helpful to enquire about the client's personality by asking questions like 'What kind of person would you say you are?' You might give prompts, such as 'happy-go-lucky', 'a worrier', or 'practically minded' if the client is not very forthcoming. An alternative question might be 'How would a friend or relative, who knows you well, describe your personality?' It is important to know if a client has always been a worrier and gets anxious easily. Many clients are likely to be worrying about the current situation and wondering 'Will the rehabilitation work?' 'Will I be able to cope independently?' 'I don't want to be a burden on people'. Clients who think this way would probably benefit from psychological care that addresses their anxiety.

Stop and think   The importance of knowing the client

Imagine that you have a virus that will develop in 24 hours. Once the symptoms develop, you will be unable to communicate your needs to anybody for some considerable time. You will be unable to do any tasks for yourself. You will be completely reliant upon staff in the residential service to which you will be moved. Write down important things that you want your carers to know about you:

- Your usual daily routine.
- People who you want to visit you.
- Your likes and dislikes.
- Things you want to have around you.
- Any specific things that the carers need to know about you.

This will be the only information that your carers have about you.
Now tear the list in half and throw one half away, so that your carers will not be aware of some of the things you have written.
Reflect on this:

- What would it be like to realise that your carers only had partial information about you?
- Would you find it distressing that your carers didn't know particular things on your thrown away list? If so, why?

■ Psychological reactions to physical ill health

Sometimes clients are referred to a psychologist because they appear upset or anxious. In this scenario a discussion may take place about what kind of emotional reactions can be expected in relation to physical ill health. Feelings of low mood and anxiety are common and often these emotional reactions are normal. Sometimes just listening to clients talk about their feelings and offering reassurance that many other people have similar feelings can be helpful.

Psychological reactions to physical ill health can be viewed in a similar way to the experiences of people who are bereaved or dying. Clients may feel shocked or numb and disbelieve that they have a chronic illness. They may ask 'Why has this happened to me?' They may yearn for a return to their previous healthy state. The phantom limb experience of people who have had a leg amputation (that is, feeling that the leg is still there) is similar in some ways to the experience of bereaved people who think that they have seen or heard the person who has died.

There may be anger directed at other people, for example 'If they hadn't caused me so much stress I would never have developed this illness,' or 'The doctor should have advised me to reduce my cholesterol sooner.' The anger could be directed at oneself: 'I should have got more exercise,' or 'I should have stopped smoking years ago.'

People may feel guilty about things they have done in their life and think that the illness is a punishment. Some people may engage in bargaining and tell themselves 'If I make a good recovery from this illness I'll be a better person and do more for other people.' There may be concerns about having to adjust to a different lifestyle, about learning to do new things, or about having to do things differently. Again, you can play a role in listening to these thoughts and feelings and reassuring clients that such reactions are a natural response to major changes in health.

■ How do psychological difficulties affect independence?

Low mood or depression can affect the client's engagement in rehabilitation because they may be pessimistic and find that it is too much effort to get started on anything. For instance, they may think that it is no good doing rehabilitation because things are never going to be as they were before the illness. See Box 1 for possible indicators of low mood or depression.

Clearly, if several of these symptoms persist for some time, it may be necessary to involve staff with specific expertise, such as a clinical psychologist, a psychiatrist or a cognitive behavioural therapist. However, this is unnecessary for many clients. Because you have regular contact with the client, you are in a good position to notice changes in the client's mood, and monitor whether he or she seems more withdrawn.

> ### Box 1 Possible indicators of low mood or depression
>
> - A noticeable change (deterioration) in mood from how client normally seems.
> - Less talkative than usual, more withdrawn.
> - Increased difficulties with sleeping.
> - Reduction in appetite.
> - Feeling too tired to engage in rehabilitation.
> - Expressed general negative thoughts, for example 'I don't feel I'm getting anywhere.'
> - Specific expressed negative thoughts, for example 'At my age I don't see any point in carrying on.'
> - Inability to concentrate for very long.
> - Showing little interest in anything.
> - The rehabilitation worker feels that the client is having a depressing effect on his/her own mood.

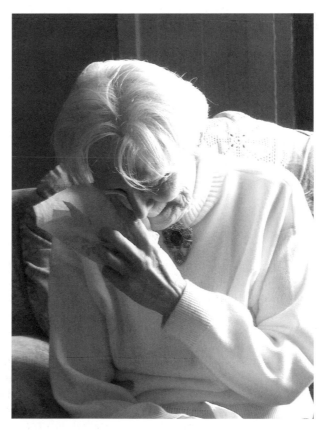

Figure 1 Client feeling dejected.

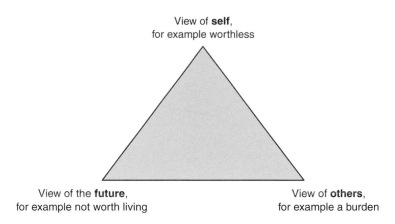

View of **self**,
for example worthless

View of the **future**,
for example not worth living

View of **others**,
for example a burden

Figure 2 Cognitive triangle of depression.

The cognitive triangle of depression (see Figure 2) illustrates how a client may be feeling about his/her situation. A depressed way of thinking might be: 'I am worthless, others will view me as a burden and the future is not worth living.' In contrast, someone who is not depressed but just experiencing sadness about the situation might think: 'I am impaired but others will support me and I can still gain fulfilment in the future.' This cognitive triangle idea of depression can be helpful when working with a client who is depressed, as it suggests different areas for the rehabilitation worker to be aware of when engaged in discussions with the client.

Anxiety can also affect independence; for example a client who has experienced a fall may restrict his or her attempts at walking for fear of having another fall. Several falls may be viewed by others as an inability to cope and the client may fear that others will then start suggesting the need to consider residential care.

In rehabilitation it is important that anxious clients are required to engage in carefully graded tasks so their confidence can gradually be developed. They should be given feedback about their progress, and a 'pat on the back' at every stage. If anxiety disrupts the client's engagement in rehabilitation then more specific support may be necessary. You may be able to suggest simple relaxation or breathing techniques and should work with other members of the team (see a suggested text in the Further reading section, and the simple relaxation exercise in the Fatigue chapter). If the problem continues then it would be appropriate to seek more expert help.

Cognitive impairment will also affect independence and it is important to be aware of some of these factors when engaging a client in rehabilitation. For example, perceptual difficulties such as visual neglect would determine from which side the rehabilitation worker should approach the client. Depending on the type of impairment the client may cope better with instructions delivered in a particular modality (for example, verbal, written or pictorial). Some of these issues are discussed in other chapters.

Psychological aspects of rehabilitation

If a client is not engaging fully with rehabilitation there could be various reasons for this. See the Stop and think box below for some possibilities.

Stop and think   Possible reasons why a client may be reluctant to engage in rehabilitation

Your (male) client is reluctant to engage in rehabilitation. Consider these points:

- Does he think that however hard he tries, he will not make any significant improvement?
- Is he feeling depressed and just can't be bothered or can't make the effort?
- Is he feeling anxious, for example, that he might fall, sustain an injury and make things even more difficult?
- Is he finding it difficult to come to terms with something unrelated to physical ill health, for example a bereavement?
- Is he finding it difficult to adjust to the possibility of having to give up his home and maybe enter residential care?
- Has he previously been the person who gave the orders, for example at work or at home?
- Does he understand the nature of his condition and the necessity for specific kinds of rehabilitation efforts?
- Does he understand the nature of rehabilitation, that is, that achievements are usually made in small chunks, or is he expecting improvement to be quick?
- Does he have any cognitive problems such as problems with following verbal instructions or difficulty with switching from one task to another?

Difficulty in adjusting to physical ill health can directly impact on the client's independence. To take an extreme example, a male client may still believe that he will walk again after rehabilitation when it is the opinion of all members of the multidisciplinary team that this is very unlikely. The client may feel that he would improve faster if more physiotherapy or occupational therapy were available, or that if a second medical opinion were sought, then there would be a more positive prognosis (that is, a more positive view about the likelihood of improvement in function). This psychological state is sometimes referred to as 'denial'. It indicates that emotional adjustment is going to be difficult because the client is unable to accept the reality of what has happened. Denial has implications for the acceptance of advice. For instance, if the client thinks he will walk again, he is unlikely to want to discuss adaptations to his home. As time passes it becomes more difficult for denial to be maintained and it can be useful to ask questions like: 'Do you ever think, even for a moment, that your rehabilitation is not going to work out as you expect?' or 'Have you ever thought about how you would cope in the worst case scenario, that is if you weren't able to walk again?'

Another important issue that seems to impact on adjustment, and therefore independence, is 'continuity'. If a client perceives that there will be some continuity from the pre-illness life to how life will be in the future, then he or she is likely to cope better. Corporal Smith used to be in the Parachute Regiment and enjoyed walking a lot before his stroke. It was very important to him that he was able to engage in some form of physical exercise in the future, albeit much reduced compared to his previous levels of activity. For many clients an anticipated return to previous activities symbolises recovery, and re-engagement in these activities can restore meaning to life. When it is not possible to re-engage in these old activities then it is important to identify alternative meaningful and achievable interests.

■ The importance of the psychological environment

For clients to overcome some of the psychological blocks to effective rehabilitation it is crucial that their psychological environment encourages and facilitates the expression of their thoughts, feelings and concerns. From some research with nurses it is known that they can at times engage in distancing tactics (see Stop and think box).

Stop and think

Have you experienced any of these factors in yourself, your colleagues or the clients that you have worked with?

Factors that may limit psychological care:

Staff member's fear of:

- Unleashing powerful emotions in the client.
- Making the client feel worse.
- Facing difficult questions.
- Taking up too much time.
- Getting too close emotionally.
- Having to carry 'emotional baggage' (that is, take on emotional burdens of client).

Common distancing strategies used by staff:

- Ignoring.
- Avoiding getting into conversation.
- Premature normalising (that is, informing client too soon that such emotional reactions are common).
- False reassurance.
- Leaving it for someone else to do.
- Changing the subject.
- Jollying along.

Client's unhelpful perceptions about emotional expression:

- Problems are inevitable – cannot be alleviated.
- Should avoid burdening staff.
- Will be judged to be weak if show emotions.

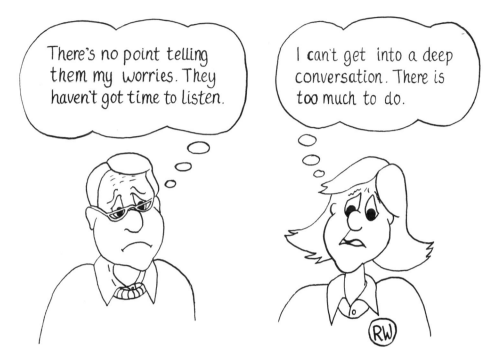

Figure 3 Two-way barriers to psychological care.

It is thought that distancing strategies are used to help protect the worker from some of the stress of caring. Unfortunately, this is at the expense of not meeting the client's psychological needs. Clients may not be inclined to share their concerns because they view the staff as being 'too busy' or think that their concerns are less important than others with more serious health problems. Sometimes clients perceive that health workers must have other people who need their help more. A discussion might then take place including the observation that everyone is an individual and has the right to assistance in overcoming his or her difficulties.

In some environments staff will indeed be busy. However, it is crucial that time is made for discussing clients' concerns with them. If they perceive that staff are always too busy to have more than a very brief conversation with them, or are on the receiving end of some distancing tactics used by staff, it is highly unlikely that clients will 'open up' with their concerns.

Some people perceive that psychological work can be done while carrying out physical tasks such as helping a client to wash. However, if psychological care is to be taken seriously, some time should be set aside just for discussing the client's feelings and concerns.

Some clients may be moved between several different care settings, such as hospitals, respite care and residential care. It is good practice to discuss the move with clients, including what to expect and what the new environment is like. For a more permanent move, such as into residential care, it is important that the client is fully involved and has some control over the process. One of the authors

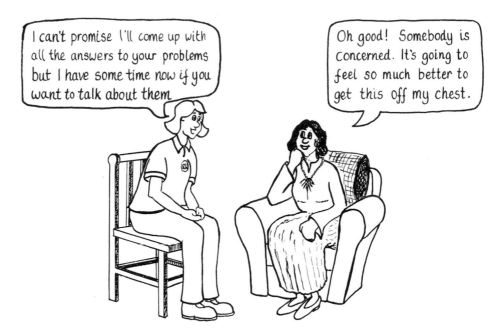

Figure 4 Promoting psychological care.

Box 2 Assessing challenging behaviour

- Monitoring antecedents (what was happening just prior to behaviour?).
- Where was client?
- Who else was around?
- What consequences followed the behaviour (for example reactions of staff and others)?

---

was once involved in discussions with staff at a residential home that was closing and all the clients were moving to a new purpose-built home. Clients were taken to the site of the new home as it was being built and photographs were taken, they were involved in deciding colour schemes for their new rooms and collectively chose a name for the new home. This level of involvement appeared to ease the transition to the new home for many of the clients.

The psychological environment is also important when working with clients showing challenging behaviour, such as verbal or physical aggression. See Box 2 for some aspects of the assessment process. The assessment may show, for example, that the behaviour is more likely to occur at a particular time of day (such as afternoons) and that this behaviour is an effective way for the client to gain attention from staff. Changing the psychological environment may involve giving the client extra attention in the afternoons, at times when he or she is not showing challenging behaviour. With this kind of approach it is important that the psychological environment is consistent and all staff adopt the same approach.

Other aspects of the psychological environment may be important in relation to particular clients. For example, some clients may be more impressed by perceived status and therefore be more responsive to staff they think are more important. Some clients may relate better to men or women, or to younger or older members of staff. It is important that these individual differences are considered and viewed as aspects of the client's personality or preferences, rather than as a slight on particular members of staff. It is helpful if staff do not take the views of such clients personally.

More generally, the day-to-day interactions between staff and clients can be a measure of the quality of the psychological environment. For example, a visitor to a ward or a day unit may notice that some staff talk to older clients as if they were children or observe staff talking in the presence of the client as if the client was not there.

■ Some key psychological ideas

The idea of continuity has already been referred to above in relation to adjustment to physical ill health. There are some other psychological ideas that can be very helpful in understanding the process of clients working towards independence.

Self-efficacy

Self-efficacy refers to people's beliefs about their capabilities to perform at a given level in a way that will influence their lives. People with a strong belief in their capabilities approach difficult tasks as challenges to be mastered rather than as threats to be avoided. They attribute failure to insufficient effort or lack of knowledge and skills which could be acquired, and quickly recover after failures or setbacks. In contrast, people who doubt their capabilities tend to avoid difficult tasks and view them as personal threats. When faced with such tasks they may think about their personal weaknesses and of the obstacles they will meet. They tend to blame performance on limited ability and are slow to recover their sense of efficacy following failure or setbacks.

One way of applying this to rehabilitation is for clients to observe other clients who are in similar situations to themselves, who put in a lot of effort and make good progress in rehabilitation. This is likely to strengthen their beliefs about the possibility of good progress. Some people may respond to persuasion and encouragement that they have what it takes to succeed by putting in stronger effort and maintaining it. There is clearly a role here for the rehabilitation worker to motivate people by helping them to believe in their own abilities. Sometimes it can be helpful to discuss how the client has coped and got through difficult experiences in the past and then to think about how these skills can be applied to their approach to rehabilitation.

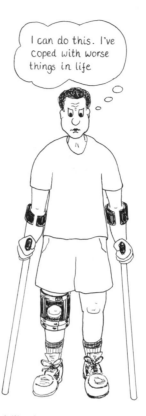

Figure 5 Self-efficacy and rehabilitation.

It is important in terms of improving self-efficacy to structure situations so that success is extremely likely. In rehabilitation, this may involve selecting carefully graded tasks that are achievable and not too difficult. Feeling anxious and stressed during rehabilitation tasks may reduce clients' belief in their own abilities, so it is important that this is addressed. Relaxation and breathing exercises may be beneficial. You could also encourage positive self-talk such as 'I'll do better if I just concentrate on what I am doing,' or 'My rehabilitation worker has said I'm doing very well, I just need to keep calm.'

Locus of control

'Locus of control' refers to the perception of whether rewards depend on the individual's own behaviour or depend on external forces. If outcomes are perceived to be connected with the individual's own behaviour then the individual is said to have an 'internal locus of control'. If the client believes that outcomes are dependent on external forces such as fate, chance, or powerful others, the individual is referred to as having an 'external locus of control'. These different orientations may have implications for rehabilitation. For example, clients with

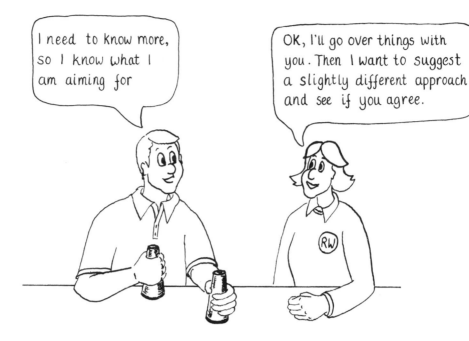

Figure 6 Internal locus of control in rehabilitation.

an internal locus of control are likely to respond best to a highly collaborative approach in which they have a lot of input into the rehabilitation process.

In contrast, clients with more of an external locus of control might respond better to more direct advice and guidance about the process of rehabilitation. People with an external locus of control may also need more support and encouragement from the rehabilitation worker in order to maintain a positive self-concept.

It is thought that people with internal and external locus of control differ in observable ways. For example, people with internal locus of control are more likely to actively seek out information and knowledge about their health problems, whereas people with external locus of control are less likely to do this and are more likely to accept the information that is given to them. People with internal locus of control are more likely to be self-confident and set realistic goals, whereas those with external locus of control are more likely to lack self-confidence and be unrealistic in goal setting. So it should be possible for the rehabilitation worker to get an idea of the client's tendency to either internal or external locus of control.

Learned helplessness

'Learned helplessness' is the situation in which a person believes that nothing in his or her power will make any difference or bring any pleasure or enjoyment. It is closely linked to depression. It is interesting to consider how learned helplessness could develop, as these are the kinds of things that a rehabilitation worker would want to avoid when working with clients.

Feelings of helplessness can arise by attributing a loss of control to global, internal and stable attributes. An example of this would be 'I can't do the exercises that the rehabilitation worker is asking me to do because basically I am a thick, not very intelligent person.' If this prevents the client from engaging in rehabilitation exercises, then from the client's perspective there is very little chance of changing things. Helplessness is also promoted by providing the client with no choice about what they are doing in rehabilitation and making things unpredictable so that they don't know what is going to happen or when. Rewarding helpless responses and punishing controlling responses also facilitate feelings of helplessness. An example of this is when informal carers (usually relatives) insist on doing things for clients rather than letting them try for themselves. Finally, agreeing with clients in their acceptance of a helpless self-concept further encourages feelings of helplessness.

So what are the implications of this in relation to rehabilitation (see Box 3)?

Ideally, we want to encourage clients to think about their rehabilitation difficulties in terms of factors that are temporary and specific, and to tell themselves that everyone has off days. Involving the client in the rehabilitation process is important, but as mentioned above, people who tend towards an external locus of control may like more direct guidance. It is worth noting that clients who perceive that they have some control over the rehabilitation process are likely to find it less stressful. Although you, as a rehabilitation worker, are unlikely to reward helpless responses or punish controlling responses, you may work with relatives who tend to take this approach. For example, while acknowledging that it may be quicker and easier for relatives to do things for the client, you could suggest that it would probably be better in the long term for the client to become as independent as possible. Giving positive feedback to clients needs to be consistent with the rehabilitation worker's personality. For example, if you are usually naturally bubbly and enthusiastic, then saying something like, 'Extremely well done, you're doing really well!' would seem natural to clients. Alternatively, if you are more reserved, then it may be more appropriate to say something like 'I'm very pleased with what you've achieved today.'

Box 3 Rehabilitation and avoiding the development of learned helplessness

- Look for temporary causes for 'off days' for example poor sleep on previous night, not feeling very well.
- Involve the client in rehabilitation, for example explaining what is going to happen and the reasons for attempting particular tasks, giving client a choice of tasks.
- Ensure as far as possible that rehabilitation takes place as planned.
- Support relatives to encourage client's efforts at gaining independence.
- Give positive feedback for small achievements.

■ Some useful skills for enabling clients

Psychological care

To get an idea of what good psychological care might involve, it is helpful to describe poor psychological care. The use of distancing tactics as a way of avoiding conversation that might lead into emotive territory has already been mentioned. Poor psychological care is characterised by the development of relationships with staff in which clients feel unable to discuss how they are feeling about their current circumstances. They may feel that they should put on a brave face, keep a stiff upper lip, bottle up, or suppress their emotional responses because they will otherwise be considered to be weak, melodramatic or a burden to staff. These suppressed emotions may become increasingly powerful and eventually preoccupy the client. Ultimately, the lack of emotional engagement may cause them to feel resentful of, or disenchanted with, the rehabilitation programme or the staff personally. Clients in rehabilitation are likely to do better if they have ready access to information, support and understanding. Two important aspects of psychological care are informational care and emotional care.

Informational care

The main objectives of informational care are to:

■ Encourage realistic expectations.
■ Reduce the fear, stress and confusion caused by uncertainty.
■ Promote participation in treatment and self-care.

Poor informational care is easy to spot. It includes providing information in an inappropriate context, such as in a noisy room where there are several distractions. It may involve unclear information using jargon or complicated language, providing too much information or too little information. One approach to informational care is the IIFAR scheme (see Box 4).

Although this scheme was originally devised with regard to the imparting of important information like that required after a diagnosis of a chronic illness, the ideas can be applied in general information giving situations, including the giving of information relating to rehabilitation.

Emotional care

Emotional care involves giving clients support and companionship as they deal with thoughts and feelings associated with illness. The objectives of emotional care are to offer understanding and acceptance, encourage emotional expression and facilitate adjustment and recovery. Emotional care can be blocked because staff make false assumptions, such as 'only expertly trained

Box 4 The IIFAR approach

Initial check

- **Check** the emotional and cognitive state of the client.
- Is this a suitable time/setting to offer information?
- **Check** they actually want the information.
- **Check** what they already know.
- Ask them to explain, in their own words, what they know already.

Make a judgment about what information is needed and what language and level of complexity is to be used (to enable understanding).

Informational exchange

- Provide information in short 'chunks'.
- Use repetition, questions, discussion and pauses (occasionally check that you are not overloading client with information).
- Make notes/diagrams to support information.
- If offering a leaflet, look through it with the client and check that they understand it.

Final **A**ccuracy check

- Ask the client to give you a summary of the key points you have discussed. For example, 'So, what will you tell your wife about this later if she asks?'

Reactions

- Explore the thoughts and feelings invoked by the information: ask clients how they feel about the information you have given.

The IIFAR approach (after Nichols, 2003).

people can deal with emotional reactions', or 'emotional care is only necessary when there is strong and significant distress'. A basic outline of emotional care in practice follows (assuming a male client).

Invitation

Invite the client to talk, but only proceed if he recognises the need and thinks it will be helpful. Inform the client of how much time you have and whether there is the possibility of a follow-up discussion at a later time.

Appropriate environment

Try to ensure a quiet, comfortable and private setting. Ask other people not to interrupt and consider putting up a sign to this effect.

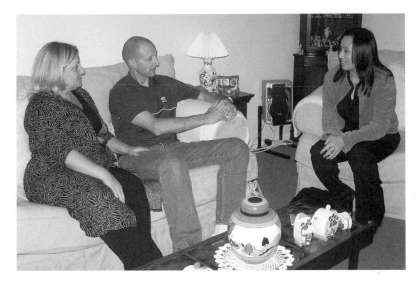

Figure 7 Rehabilitation worker with the client and his partner carrying out emotional care.

Who is present

There would usually only be one member of staff with the client. You may want to consider asking the client whether he would like to invite a relative to sit in, for instance if it helps him to feel more secure to have a familiar, trusted person who can chip into the conversation.

Narrow the social gap

Try to drop the 'professional persona' and make the interaction more 'person to person'. Sit close, but not so close that it intimidates the client. If you are not already aware of how the client likes to be addressed, check whether it would be all right to use first names.

Communicate safety through relaxed acceptance

Pay attention to the character and tone of your reactions. Avoid evaluations or judgements, or the use of blocking tactics. Maintain a relaxed, supportive atmosphere and try not to think that you always have to say the right thing. Maintain natural eye contact. Demonstrate understanding and empathy (the ability to put yourself in the other person's shoes) by the use of non-verbal gestures such as nodding your head and making statements such as, 'I understand', or, 'Tell me a little more.' Occasionally, reflect understanding back to the client by briefly summarising what has been said.

Ending the encounter

Finish with a summary of the discussion, as this makes it clear that you've listened with interest and allows you to check that you've understood. You may want to thank the client for speaking to you and ask if he found it helpful. If you are going to make any notes about the discussion you should check with the client that he has no objections to this. If necessary, offer further opportunities to talk.

When undertaking emotional care it is important to consider your own need for support. This could be obtained through formal systems such as clinical supervision and informally from colleagues doing the same kind of work (see Section 4: Teamworking and supervision for more information about supervisory support).

Basic counselling skills

Some basic counselling skills have already been mentioned above in relation to emotional care, including verbal and non-verbal behaviours that show you are listening. There are some key requirements for effective counselling:

- The client feels that the counsellor is on his/her side (acceptance).
- The client feels able to say anything without being judged (unconditional positive regard).
- The counsellor is being real with the client and not pretending (congruence).
- The counsellor tries to see the world through the client's eyes and conveys an understanding of what the client is trying to say (empathy).

Active listening involves paying attention not only to what the client says but also to non-verbal cues such as tone of voice and posture. Reflection is the basic skill of reflecting the content of what the client is saying back to him/her. This conveys the message: 'I am listening carefully to what you're saying and am trying to understand. I will indicate this by letting you know that I heard what you just said. Did I get it right?' For example, if a client seems to be indicating that rehabilitation is difficult, a reflection statement might be 'you seem to be finding the rehabilitation work hard?' Questions should be asked in a way that encourages the client to talk. Closed questions are less helpful in this respect as they can usually be answered in a yes or no type of response, for instance, 'Would you say that you are an anxious person?' Open questions leave the options for answers wide open and they usually start with words like 'how', and 'what'. For example, 'How do you usually feel in that situation?' Counselling has developed a lot as a profession in itself in recent years, but there are courses that you could take to enhance your use of counselling skills in day-to-day work. See the 'Further reading' section for basic counselling texts.

Monitoring the effectiveness of psychological work

One client was finding it difficult to even attempt an exercise that involved her standing for about 30 seconds at a time. In order to encourage her, a simple chart was devised consisting of two columns for the date and day of the week and a third column on which she entered a tick if she attempted the exercise on that particular day. The chart was kept at the end of her bed on the ward. She found it helpful to peruse the chart and see how she was progressing. Her daughter also found it helpful to be able to look at the chart when she visited. Keeping a written record of rehabilitation activity for the client is one method by which staff can provide concrete feedback and encouragement. In this example, the fact that the client was attempting the exercise was evidence that she was beginning to overcome her block to engaging in rehabilitation.

If a goal was to reduce a client's anxiety during rehabilitation sessions, the anxiety could be assessed by observation. Are there bodily signs of agitation such as tensing up? Is the client making worrying comments such as 'I don't think I can do this?' Also, self-report ratings of anxiety could be used, such as one of those below.

1	2	3	4	5
Not anxious at all	A little anxious	Fairly anxious	Very anxious	Extremely anxious

The client could be asked to give a rating of how anxious he/she is feeling mid-way through the rehabilitation session and the appropriate number from the above scale could be recorded.

Not anxious at all   Extremely anxious

With this kind of scale (which is 10 cm long) the client is asked to mark off the point on the line which indicates how anxious they are feeling, so for example, a mark through the line near the right-hand end would indicate that the client is feeling very to extremely anxious (an accurate measurement can be made with a ruler in order to compare different ratings).

One of these forms of ratings could be recorded during each rehabilitation session and used as a measure of progress or lack of progress in relation to reducing the client's anxiety. Such ratings could be used to assess other things, such as how positive clients feel about their progress in rehabilitation.

Short questionnaires can also be helpful to monitor changes in a client's psychological state, for example the Hospital Anxiety and Depression Scale (HADS). This is a 14-item self-report measure and doesn't take long for the client to complete. It includes questions such as 'I feel tense and wound up' (with four possible ratings ranging from 'most of the time' to 'not at all') and 'I have lost interest in my appearance' (with four possible ratings ranging from 'definitely' to 'I take just as much care as ever'). See Further reading for information on accessing various measurement scales.

Psychological aspects of rehabilitation

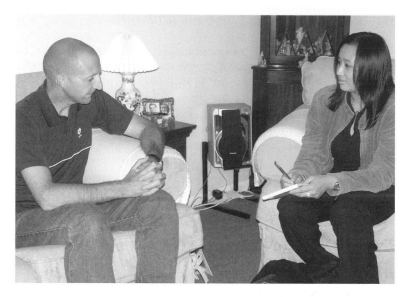

Figure 8 Rehabilitation worker and client completing an anxiety rating scale.

Conclusion

This chapter has highlighted the importance of taking a wider view of the client's life and of appreciating that various psychological reactions to physical ill health are common and can affect independence. Consideration was given to the importance of the psychological environment and some key psychological ideas that are relevant to the process of rehabilitation. Also, thought was given to ways in which rehabilitation workers might apply psychological care to their work with clients, including informational care, emotional care and basic counselling skills.

Further reading

Bowling, A. (2004) *Measuring Health: A Review of Quality of Life Measurement Scales* (3rd edition). Maidenhead, Open University Press. *A good guide to measures of health and quality of life, including functional ability, psychological wellbeing, social networks and social support. Includes an appendix detailing a selection of scale distributors and useful addresses.*

Burnard, P. (2005) *Counselling Skills for Health Professionals* (4th edition). Cheltenham, Nelson Thornes; *Explores basic principles and theory of counselling and practical skills, including attending and listening, use of questions, reflection and approaches to exploring feelings. Includes some useful counselling skills exercises.*

Fitzgerald Miller, J. (1999) *Coping with Chronic Illness: Overcoming Powerlessness* (3rd edition). Philadelphia, F.A. Davis. *A useful book that applies ideas relating to the psychology of coping, control and learned helplessness to helping people with chronic illness. It includes chapters relating to people with specific chronic illnesses, for example end stage renal disease, arthritis, multiple sclerosis.*

Frankland, A. & Sanders, P. (1995) *Next Steps in Counselling: A Students' Companion for Certificate and Counselling Skills Courses.* Ross-on-Wye, PCCS Books. *Covers some theory and the core conditions for counselling. Helpful in relation to counselling skills, for example listening and exploring, appropriate use of questioning. Suggests useful activities for the reader and includes general, fictional case vignettes.*

Morrison, P. & Burnard, P. (1997) *Caring and Communicating: The Interpersonal Relationship in Nursing* (2nd edition). Basingstoke, Palgrave Macmillan. *Covers some useful aspects of caring, including psychological care and the caring attitude from the perspective of both nurses and patients. Also, two chapters on counselling, and basic communication and counselling skills, and a chapter on self disclosure by nurses.*

Nichols, K. (2003) *Psychological Care for Ill and Injured People: A Clinical Guide.* Maidenhead, Open University Press. *Useful for health care professionals of all disciplines who have regular contact with clients recovering from physical illness or injury. A very readable combination of theory, practical advice and case observations that clearly outlines the potential psychological impact of impaired physical functioning and the importance of good psychological care.*

Niven, N. (2000) *Health Psychology for Health Care Professionals* (3rd edition). London, Churchill Livingstone. *Includes sections on interpersonal skills, attitudes and behaviour change, pain and stress, life transitions and crises, and health behaviour. Also, stresses the importance of the environment for both clients and staff. Includes some useful 'new research' boxes and case histories.*

Payne, R. A. (2004) *Relaxation Techniques: A Practical Handbook for the Health Care Professional* (3rd edition). Edinburgh, Churchill Livingstone. *A useful text that brings together various methods of relaxation and provides a practical introduction to their use. It covers methods involving physical tension and exercises, for example, progressive relaxation training, and cognitive techniques, for example use of imagery and visualisation.*

Payne, S. & Walker, J. (2004) *Psychology for Nurses and the Caring Professions.* Maidenhead, Open University Press. *Discusses the influence of psychological factors in health care and includes chapters on applications of theories of learning, stress and coping, pain, and the development of social relationships and loss. Includes useful exercises and case studies to help the reader think about psychological issues and their application in health care. Also, a useful glossary of terms.*

Zigmond, A.S. & Snaith, R.P. (1983) The hospital anxiety and depression scale. *Acta Psychiatrica Scandinavica* **67** (6), 361–370. *Describes the development and evaluation of this short self-assessment scale with seven questions relating to anxiety and seven to depression. The scale enables an estimate of the severity of anxiety and depression (mild, moderate or severe, or within the normal range). (NB Copies of the scale can be obtained from NferNelson, Swindon, SN2 8BR, UK.)*

Preventing falls – a key to maintaining independence

Keith Hill, Lindy Clemson & Freda Vrantsidis

Who do falls affect?

How often have you found that one of your older clients had a fall, was hospitalised, and even after returning home, lacked confidence while walking? Did you know that one in three older people aged 65 and over report falling at least once a year, with some reporting numerous falls? For those who fall, at least a quarter suffer injuries that reduce their mobility and independence. Hip fractures are one of the most common serious injuries sustained. Falls can lead to a fear of falling even if an injury does not occur. This fear can lead to avoidance of some activities, which can lead to muscle weakness, further increasing the risk of falling. Falls are also a common reason for admission into long-term care.

In the UK in 1999, almost 650 000 accident and emergency attendances, over 200 000 hospital admissions and 4800 deaths were due to fall-related injuries in people aged 60 and over. The total estimated cost to the Government (National Health Service and personal social service for long-term care) from unintentional falls was almost £1 billion. The substantial health care costs, and the negative impact on the older person's independence and general wellbeing makes falls prevention a major health issue for older people, their families, the health care system and the wider community.

Older people often dismiss falls as being due to external causes, such as tripping on a step, or put them down to rushing or not paying attention. These excuses may be the cause in some instances, but often there are other underlying health issues substantially contributing to the individual's risk of falling.

■ How to identify the risk

There are many factors which can increase a person's risk of falling. These are broadly grouped into two main categories, intrinsic and extrinsic factors:

Intrinsic falls risk factors

These relate to the effects of age or disease on the parts of the body involved in maintaining effective balance. Although age is a factor, it is not the major contributor to falls risk for older people. There are many fit and active people in their eighties and even nineties who are living independently in the community. Instead, it is the health problems that affect the body systems involved in balance that are the main intrinsic factors contributing to risk of falling. Examples are shown in Table 1.

Table 1 Falls risk factors, cues to indicate presence of the risk factor, and suggested management strategies to reduce risk of falling.

Intrinsic falls risk factors	Markers/indicators of risk	Options to consider to reduce risk
History of previous falls	Review circumstances of falls and look for common themes	Use a self screening checklist (for example Figure 1) Medical review of causes Discuss circumstances of recent falls with the older person
Leg weakness	Difficulty standing up from chair without using the arms	Medical review of causes Strength training/general exercise programme Refer to physiotherapist for assessment and development of individualised strength training programme
Balance problems	Unsteady/veering during transfers and walking/near falls	Medical review of causes Group exercise programmes that include balance training Home exercise programme that includes balance training Refer to physiotherapist for assessment and supervised balance exercises Consider use of walking aid

(Continued)

Preventing falls

Table 1 Continued.

Intrinsic falls risk factors	Markers/indicators of risk	Options to consider to reduce risk
Impaired walking	Unsteady/veering during transfers and walking	Medical review of causes Refer to physiotherapist for assessment and balance/walking exercises Consider use of walking aid
Functional impairments	Difficulty with bed mobility, transfers, dressing, other personal activities of daily living	Medical review of causes Refer to an occupational therapist for assessment/ provision of aids and appliances/retraining Refer to physiotherapist for assessment and exercise
Visual problems (for example cataracts, glaucoma)	Hesitant gait, bumping into furniture, trips, falls involving environmental hazards or stairs	Medical review of causes Ensure regular eye checks (at least every two years) May need to consider avoiding use of bifocal glasses for outdoor walking (wearing distance glasses instead) Use of strategies to cope with low vision (may need occupational therapy or low vision clinic referral)
Postural hypotension	Unsteady/giddy when first stands up Can also be a problem soon after eating	Medical review of causes Encourage standing up slowly, and waiting a short time before walking May benefit from pressure stockings
Cognitive problems/ dementia	Poor planning/ judgement/safety monitoring Poor ability to follow instructions (for example to use walking aid), or difficulty learning safety instructions	Medical review of causes Frequent reminding about safety issues Ensure safe environment Review by physiotherapist regarding most appropriate walking aid, and whether client will be able to use it safely Review by occupational therapist to consider training or compensatory strategies/assistive devices Hip protectors Vitamin D and calcium supplementation

(Continued)

Preventing falls

Table 1 Continued.

Intrinsic falls risk factors	Markers/indicators of risk	Options to consider to reduce risk
Incontinence	Urinary or bowel accidents Strong odour of urine Falls when going to the toilet Needing to rush to the toilet	Medical review of causes Specialist assessment and treatment Use of a commode at night Continence aids Review timing and amount of caffeine intake
Multiple medications (four or more) or high falls risk medications (sedatives/)hypnotics/ antidepressants	Any problems (for example unsteadiness/dizziness) soon after a change in medication Falls at night	Medical review of medications and possible contribution to falls risk Review night-time medication use Use of commode at night Trial of options to improve sleep without medication, such as avoiding caffeine at night, avoid naps during the day, and use of relaxation strategies
Chronic medical conditions such as stroke, Parkinson's disease, arthritis	These conditions commonly affect balance and mobility Sensation and perception can sometimes be altered Walking and balance performance commonly worsens over time	Intermittent review by physiotherapist or occupational therapist, with implementation of an exercise programme and appropriate aids can increase safety and independence Hip protectors Vitamin D and calcium supplementation
Acute health problem such as urinary tract infection, pneumonia, delirium	Rapid change or deterioration in function These conditions often cause a short-term increase in unsteadiness and falls risk	Urgent medical review Acute medical care Additional safety strategies while unwell
Osteoporosis (low bone density)	History of fractures Family history of osteoporosis Low bone density identified by bone scan	Vitamin D and calcium supplementation Hip protectors Possible use of anti-resorptive medication
Osteomalacia (low vitamin D)	Vitamin D levels	Nutritional assessment Vitamin D and calcium supplementation Sunlight exposure Hip protectors

Preventing falls

A very important additional intrinsic risk factor for falling is a previous fall or injurious fall. Even a fall that may not cause an injury doubles the risk of falling again in the near future. However, most people who fall do not report the fall to their doctor or other health professionals, particularly where no serious injury was sustained. If a fall goes unnoticed or is not reported, there will be no investigations to determine why the fall occurred, and therefore no actions taken to reduce the future (increased) risk of falling.

Stop and think

A key role of the rehabilitation worker is to be aware of signs of changes in balance/walking/confidence, or whether a fall has occurred. Examples include observing:

◾ Unexplained bruising.
◾ Increased unsteadiness in walking.
◾ A change in walking aid used.
◾ A reduction in activity level or walking.

Further examples of these type of cues are described in Table 1. Each of these should prompt sensitive and careful discussion of what may be contributing to the observed change. Where possible, the rehabilitation worker should aim to support the older person by discussing these issues with their local doctor, other health professionals or the case coordinator.

A useful strategy to determine if a client is at increased risk of falling is to provide them with a self-checklist of risk factors for falling (Figure 1). This checklist can be used in several ways:

◾ It can be left with a client, who can work through it in their own time, and then discuss it with the rehabilitation worker on their next visit, or take it to their next doctor's appointment.
◾ A rehabilitation worker could work through the checklist with the client. This will provide opportunity to expand upon issues raised, and to look for subtle clues in answers provided that might indicate additional issues to explore.

If the checklist has one or more items ticked, it is recommended that the client should go to the doctor to discuss ways to reduce the risk of falling.

Case study   Joe

Joe is an 87-year-old widower who lives alone in his small suburban home. He has a number of medical conditions which have affected his independence and mobility, including:

■ A mild stroke four years ago, causing slight weakness in his left arm and leg, and a little unsteadiness. He walks slowly with a single point stick inside and outside the home (to the local shop, about a block away, once each week).

■ Diabetes, which has caused peripheral neuropathy (poor sensation in his feet) and reduced vision.

■ Moderate arthritis in both knees, causing pain when he goes up or down stairs.

■ A total hip replacement for his right hip five years ago, with good recovery.

Joe takes seven different types of medication each day, including a sleeping tablet. He has recently been having some difficulties remembering to take his medications.

Joe has had four falls in the past six months. Three of the four falls occurred at night, when he was getting up to go to the toilet at the end of a long corridor from the bedroom. Usually he didn't turn on a light until he reached the toilet. The other fall involved tripping over a loose mat in the kitchen.

Joe usually wears loose-fitting slippers at home, and was wearing these during each of his falls.

Joe has not injured himself in the falls other than bruising, and he has not seen his doctor about the falls. His rehabilitation worker visits the day after the most recent fall, and notices a bruise on Joe's face. When questioned about it, Joe admits to having the fall, and also describes the other recent falls.

Stop and think

■ Use the self-checklist (Figure 1) to identify some of Joe's risk factors for falls.
■ List any other things that might be contributing to Joe's risk of falling and why.
■ Keep this list to refer to in section on Community hazards, in this chapter.

By using the checklist, risk factors contributing to Joe's increased risk of falling are:

■ Previous falls.
■ Multiple medications.
■ Limited amount of exercise.
■ Past history of stroke and arthritis.
■ Frequent need to go to the toilet at night.
■ Some unsteadiness when walking.

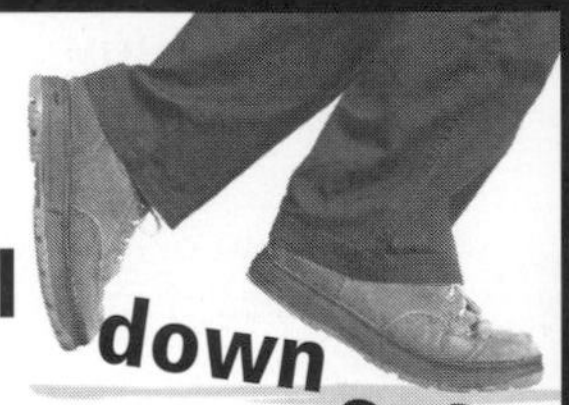

Preventing falls

How many of these questions do you fall down on?

When you're 60 or over, a fall can have shattering consequences on your mobility, independence and lifestyle.

Did you know....

- One in four people aged 60 or over fall at least once a year.
- Falling is not a normal part of ageing – falls can be prevented.
- Only a small proportion of falls are caused by tripping, slipping or "not being careful" – most are the result of health or lifestyle factors.

Try this checklist to determine your risk of falling ...   Yes ☑

	Yes
Have you had a fall in the last year?	☐
Having previously fallen increases your chance of falling again	
Do you do less than 30 minutes of physical activity a day?	☐
Are you unsteady on your feet, do you find it difficult to get up from a chair or do you have trouble walking?	☐
Many falls are the result of muscle weakness and/or impaired balance	
Are you taking three or more medicines?	☐
Are you taking sleeping tablets, tranquillisers or anti-depressants?	☐
Has it been more than 12 months since your GP reviewed your medicines?	☐
Some side effects and combinations of medicines can increase your risk of a fall	
Do you have diabetes, arthritis or Parkinson's Disease?	☐
Have you had a stroke or do you have problems with your heart or circulation?	☐
Has it been more than 12 months since your eyes were tested or your glasses checked?	☐
Do you experience dizziness, light headedness, unsteadiness, drowsiness, blurred or double vision or have difficulty thinking clearly?	☐
Many health conditions can increase your risk of falling	

If you answered "yes" to one or more of these questions you are at risk of falling.
The good news is that there are steps you can take now to reduce your risk.

If you answered "no" to all of these questions, but are aged 60 or over, you should still take falls seriously and take action to stay mobile and independent.

To find out how to prevent falls before they happen, ask for a FREE copy of the Stay On Your Feet WA™ booklet from your GP or pharmacist. Or call HealthInfo on 1300 135 030.

www.stayonyourfeet.com.au

Government of Western Australia — Department of Health — Stay On Your Feet WA™

HP 2571 April 05 20163

Figure 1 Self-checklist for screening risk of falling (reproduced with permission from the Injury Prevention Unit, Department of Health, Government of Western Australia).

As well as the factors on the checklist, other possible falls risk factors include his loss of feeling in his feet/legs; his reduced memory, possibly affecting correct use of medications; lack of a night light when getting up to go to the toilet; loose mats on the floor being possible tripping hazards; and unsafe footwear. All of these factors should be discussed, with a recommendation that

Joe should in the first instance discuss his falls and what can be done with his local doctor.

Extrinsic risk factors

These include hazards within the environment, such as poor lighting, obstacles or uneven surfaces that might cause a slip or a trip, as well as behavioural risk factors – performing activities that have a high risk of falling associated with them relative to the person's balance capabilities (for example standing on a chair on a table to change a light bulb).

Brief environmental and behavioural checklists illustrate some of the more common hazards associated with falls (See Figures 2 and 3). Screening tools such as these may identify that some hazards are present and, along with a history of falls or other 'markers' of risk, will indicate whether a full home safety assessment is required. In particular, older people recently discharged from hospital, or those with a history of a fall in the past year can benefit from a home visit by a health professional, such as an occupational therapist, who will perform a home safety assessment and discuss the risk of falls. These assessments may also be useful for those feeling less confident with their walking, or those experiencing near falls.

For the more active person at risk of falls, things like ladder safety, not leaving obstacles on steps, or enhancing skills in community mobility may be most relevant. For the less mobile person things like loose mats and the absence of a secure handrail that extends to the bottom step could be more relevant. When someone has poor vision the environment can be more hazardous, and this is often less obvious when people are in familiar surroundings. A marker of poor vision can be that the standard of cleanliness about the home has deteriorated, resulting in increased clutter.

Stop and think

Observing the home environment and how the client interacts/copes within their environment will help identify activities that are causing them concern. Listening to the person will help reveal their personal fall experiences, their beliefs about what causes falls and their attitude to taking action to prevent falls.

Ask yourself whether there are any 'markers' to suggest that environment or behavioural factors could contribute to the client's risk of falls. 'Markers' for specific risk factors are described in Table 1.

Falls also occur away from the home. At risk are those who have reported tripping, have a history of falls, lack confidence walking amongst crowds or when

	Yes	No	Comments
(1) Are there are any floors that are slippery when wet or dry?			
(2) Are there obstacles in traffic-ways (that is, the routes the person takes to get from place to place), on stairs, in areas of access to the home, or on outside pathways?			
(3) Is the lighting dim, poorly lit or shadowy in living areas, traffic-ways, access areas and stairwells?			
(4) Are steps and stairs slippery, do they lack contrast, have worn coverings or lack a grab-rail?			
(5) Are floor mats slippery, loose or do they have curled edges?			
(6) Are floor coverings worn or loose?			
(7) Is the person unsafe with reaching or climbing, or do they use unstable furniture or equipment when climbing?			
(8) Does footwear fit poorly, have poor fastenings, have slippery soles, high heels, or no room for the toes?			
(9) Are outdoor pathways uneven, broken, loose or mossy?			
(10) Are there cords on the floor?			
(11) Are there spills on the floor? Is cleaning equipment inaccessible or difficult to use?			
(12) Are medications difficult to open, poorly remembered or do they have instructions that are difficult to read and understand?			

If there are any 'yes' responses, the rehabilitation worker should consider discussing an occupational therapy home assessment with their manager, as well as with the client.

Figure 2 Home hazard screening checklist (modified from the Westmead Home Safety Assessment, Clemson, 1997).

out and about, and those with vision or mobility problems. Muscle weakness and balance loss can contribute. Environmental factors that cause falls in the community include:

■ Uneven pathways/surfaces.
■ Slippery floors in shopping centres.

Preventing falls

How often would you do the following in your daily life?	Never	Sometimes	Often	Always	Comments
(1) I talk with someone I know about things I do that might help prevent a fall.					
(2) When I stand up I pause to get my balance.					
(3) I bend over to reach something only if I have a firm handhold.					
(4) I hurry to answer the phone.					
(5) I use a light if I get up during the night.					
(6) I adjust the lighting at home to suit my eyesight.					
(7) When I walk outdoors I scan ahead for potential hazards.					
(8) I avoid ramps and other slopes.					
(9) I go out on windy days.					
(10) I avoid walking about in crowded places.					
(11) I ask my pharmacist or doctor questions about side effects of my medications.					

Often/always denotes protective behaviours except for items 4 and 9 which are reversed. The person's physical and functional status needs to be taken into account when determining degree of risk. This modified FaB may be used to raise discussion and awareness of fall risk associated with behaviours, and in conjunction with the environmental hazard screening tool, can indicate the need for referral for a home assessment or a community mobility assessment.

Figure 3 Behavioural factors and falls (modified from the Falls Behavioural [FaB] Scale for Older People, Clemson et al., 2003).

- Unmarked steps.
- Changes in levels.

Behavioural factors include hurrying, not noticing hazards, not scanning ahead, not lifting feet when walking or climbing steps and stairs, misjudging the environment because the correct glasses are not being worn, and fatigue.

Preventing falls

Preventing falls

Case study Nancy

Nancy is 85 and lives with her husband, Ned, 87, in a first-floor flat in a retirement village. Nancy is bright, alert and quite active and thought falls just happened to frail old people. But Nancy fell over a month ago while she was putting out the rubbish and broke her hip. She was on her way out, all dressed up in her woollen suit and high-heeled shoes, looking forward to lunch with her daughter. But Nancy noticed Ned had not put the rubbish out so decided to do it herself quickly. She knew her cataracts were getting worse and her feet were becoming increasingly sore, and although she was in a rush she thought she had taken extra care on the steps. She walks a lot and considered herself fit, but somehow she lost her balance. She grabbed the handrail, it wobbled and she fell. Nancy also had a fall about six months ago – climbing on a chair to reach the large saucepan in the top cupboard. Although shaken, she thought that was an accident and, anyway, she didn't hurt herself, so she didn't see anyone about it.

Stop and think

Use the home hazard screening checklist (Figure 2) to determine possible extrinsic risk factors contributing to Nancy's falls.
Keep this list to refer to in section on Community hazards, in this chapter.

Using the screening checklist, the loose handrail, and wearing high heels were the two main extrinsic risk factors present. Nancy is also increasing her risk by some of her actions, such as standing on a chair to get saucepans out of high cupboards. In addition, several intrinsic risk factors were also present, including her cataracts and her loss of confidence in walking.

■ What can be done?

Nancy and Joe's stories show that the causes of falls can be multiple and different for every person. Making one change to one important risk factor can dramatically reduce their risk of falls. Often people need a number of strategies to address each of the risk factors present. Each of the main risk factors for falls are described below, together with examples of actions that will help reduce the risk of future falls. Table 1 summarises some of the main recommendations to address specific intrinsic falls risk factors.

Multiple medications, sleeping tablets, tranquillisers and antidepressants

Taking multiple medications can increase a person's risk of falls because there is a greater chance of an interaction between drugs, of accidentally taking the wrong dosage, or just a higher chance of taking a drug that can cause falls. People aged over 65 should have their medications reviewed by their local doctor at least annually. A medication review card can be useful for keeping track of medications.

Sleeping tablets, tranquillisers and antidepressants can make people drowsy or impair balance, and are best avoided or taken in as low a dosage as possible. Short-term usage might be useful but problems arise when used over the longer term. For the majority of older people, these medications substantially increase the risk of falls and hip fracture. Reducing use of these medications has been shown to have a strong effect in reducing falls. Alternatives to these medications which may improve quality of sleep include increasing activity during the day, use of relaxation or imagery exercises at night, and establishing good sleep patterns/routines. If these medications cannot be avoided then the older person needs to take extra care and have other strategies in place that will compensate for the increased falls risk.

Poor balance and muscle weakness

Balance problems and reduced muscle strength reduce the effectiveness of a person's attempt to save themselves when a fall or near fall is about to occur.

Exercise programmes that improve balance have been shown to reduce falls among older people, even those with a number of pre-existing falls risk factors. Exercises to improve balance involve moving in ways that work the balance system. Exercises can include walking, high stepping, changing directions, moving the head or catching a ball while walking, and negotiating obstacles. A number of programmes combine balance and strengthening exercises, including both home exercise programmes and group programmes. Examples of these type of programmes that have been shown to reduce falls include those found on the following websites:

http://www.monash.edu.au/muarc/projects/nofalls/
http://www.acc.co.nz/injury-prevention/growing-and-living-safely/older-adults/
preventing-falls/otago- exercise-programme/

T'ai chi is another form of exercise that has been shown to reduce falls (Figure 4).

Help clients make exercise part of their weekly routine but not a chore. Share stories about the benefits of exercise. Support people to focus on changing habits by starting with small, easy-to achieve goals: 'Start low and go slow', and by parking the car further away from the shops and walking or using the stairs instead of the elevator.

For high falls risk clients, an assessment by a physiotherapist is recommended to determine the most useful and safe approach to exercise for the individual. Physiotherapists can tailor a programme specifically for an older person who has muscle weakness or balance problems, including how to safely upgrade the exercises. Physiotherapists can also help design a community group programme with the correct falls prevention elements.

For clients with balance problems a walking aid can improve stability. Walking aids give varying levels of support. A single stick or cane provides least support, a tripod or four-prong stick provides intermediate support, and a frame (pick-up or wheelie) provides the greatest support. It is important that the most appropriate

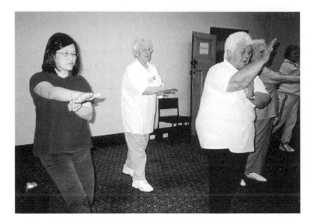

Figure 4 T'ai chi has been shown to be an effective form of exercise in reducing the risk of falling.

aid (that is, the one which gives the necessary amount of support and is the correct height) is used and that it is used correctly (for example, a walking stick should be used in the hand opposite the most affected leg). A physiotherapist can provide this advice and determine whether an exercise programme would also be useful to improve balance.

Visual problems

Good eyesight is essential for the body to sense and avoid obstacles or hazards in the environment. Regular eye check-ups with an optometrist or eye specialist are recommended at least once every two years. Rehabilitation workers can encourage older clients to do this, and to wear their prescribed glasses. About 50% of eye problems are preventable or can be fixed with the correct prescription glasses, a simple measure that can prevent falls. Early referral for cataract surgery or other treatment to improve vision can also reduce falls risk.

If the visual problem cannot be improved, strategies to help clients manage safely can be implemented. This can include better lighting, using contrast to make objects and furniture easier to see, keeping pathways free of clutter, avoiding slippery surfaces, and training in scanning and other mobility techniques.

Specialty services are also available, including low vision clinics, orthoptist assessments to recommend equipment such as magnifiers and task lighting, and home and community mobility training from vision or mobility officers or specialty occupational therapists. (Useful website: http://www.rnib.org.uk/xpedio/groups/public/documents/code/InternetHome.hcsp)

Footwear and footcare

Feet and footwear provide the interface between you and the support surface in any situation where a fall might occur. Good footcare and footwear can improve stability and are likely to reduce the risk of falling.

Preventing falls

Ask clients what they were wearing during their fall. If worn, slippery shoes or slippers contributed to a fall, clients may be prepared to think about safer shoes. Major features of safe shoes include plenty of room for the toes, secure fastening (laces or elastic), low broad heels, textured (non-slippery) soles, and they should fit snugly but not tightly.

Foot pain and foot problems are risk factors for falls and should be attended to. This includes applying emollient creams to dry heels, toe grasping exercises to maintain foot mobility and function, ankle exercises, treatments for bunions and other foot problems, and a referral to a podiatrist or physiotherapist.

Postural hypotension

Postural hypotension is a reduction of systolic blood pressure by more than 20 mmHg when standing up from lying. Under normal circumstances, automatic adjustments ensure that any change in blood pressure with these positional changes is limited. However, when these mechanisms are not working effectively, standing up can cause light-headedness, dizziness, or unsteadiness, which predispose the person to falling. A medical review of the cause of the postural hypotension is required. Other strategies, such as foot exercises before standing up, standing for longer before walking, and elastic support stockings might reduce the magnitude of the problem of postural hypotension. Gradually increasing time spent walking and standing, especially after a period of bed-rest, can also be beneficial.

Cognitive problems

Cognitive problems, such as reduced memory, impaired planning, poor judgement and monitoring of performance with respect to safety all increase the risk of falling. Most common causes include Alzheimer's disease, multi-infarct dementia, and delirium. Delirium is a reversible condition, often triggered by another acute health problem. Sudden changes in cognition need urgent review by a doctor.

People with mild cognitive problems might still benefit from some of the standard falls prevention activities such as supervised exercise. Environmental modification is extremely important to minimise exposure to hazards. Injury minimisation approaches, such as the use of hip protectors (see section on Protection from injury associated with falls) might also be useful to reduce the risk of hip fractures if falls do occur.

Acute and chronic health problems

Chronic health problems such as stroke, Parkinson's disease and arthritis can all affect balance, mobility, and increase a person's risk of falling. People with these conditions often benefit from regular exercise or activity, particularly exercises which can improve balance performance. Some improvements can be achieved even many years after onset of the chronic health problem.

Acute health problems such as pneumonia, urinary tract infection, or even acute onset pain can affect a person's balance and mobility, and increase their risk of falling. Delirium, or an acute confusional state, can also cause impaired thinking, planning and monitoring of safety, which can cause falls. Early recognition of a change in health status, prompt review by a doctor, and early management programmes can reduce duration and severity of the acute condition, thereby reducing the risk of falling.

Incontinence

Incontinence can increase falls risk in a number of ways. When in a hurry to get to the toilet (urgency), a person may not concentrate as much on their balance, increasing their risk of falling. Having to get up to the toilet a number of times overnight (nocturia) often means walking when not fully awake. Additionally, if a urinary accident occurs, it can create a slipping hazard. Continence problems should be investigated by the doctor, and often strategies can be implemented to improve continence. Environmental modifications such as use of a commode for night-time use may also improve safety overnight.

Home hazards

People tend not to see hazards or notice that they have developed risky behaviours in their familiar home environments (see Figure 5). Review of the home environment by occupational therapists and instituting safety recommendations have been shown to reduce the risk of falling in older people with a history of falls. However, even in studies where positive results were achieved not all recommendations

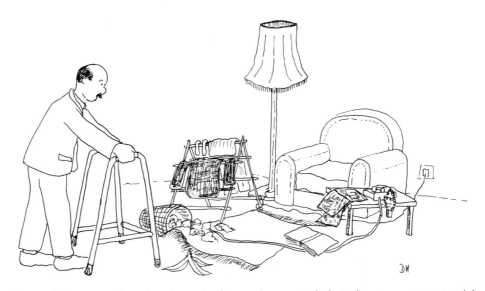

Figure 5 Loose cords and mats, and other environmental obstacles can cause potential tripping hazards.

were implemented by the older person. Perception of risk, costs, availability and aesthetics all influence whether the older person will follow through with the recommended environmental and behavioural modifications. Clients often need to be encouraged to make changes to their environment or the way things are done to increase safety. Support by rehabilitation workers in reinforcing and assisting with recommended environmental changes could be instrumental in improving outcomes.

Explore options when considering solutions. Mats have a purpose, ranging from aesthetic to practical. The person often needs to believe it is a danger before they will remove part of their personal surroundings. Other options can be to replace with a heavier, non-slip mat or secure with double-sided tape. Engage a family member who can reinforce and prompt follow through of planned changes.

Independent Living Centres often provide demonstration of useful aids and appliances that increase home safety, and provide phone or website information on products. Local councils or health centres may also provide home modification information and services.

Community hazards

Falls in public places can result in being less active, walking less and having less confidence in managing steps, gutters, road crossings and public transport. Occupational therapists and physiotherapists or other aged care workers may offer graded mobility training to increase confidence and competencies in tackling different terrains and situations. Clients may need support, or even to be accompanied, in their local community to practise. If community hazards are observed they should be reported to the relevant authority, to prevent the hazard being the cause of someone else's fall.

Stop and think

▪ Refer back to your list of falls risk factors developed when completing the self-checklist (Figure 1) for Joe.
▪ Describe actions that might be useful to help Joe reduce the risk of future falls.

First, Joe needs to see his doctor to discuss his recent falls. The doctor will most likely conduct a detailed assessment of the factors contributing to his risk of falls. A number of actions are likely to be recommended, including:

▪ A medication review, perhaps reducing the number of medications being taken. In particular, the doctor may wean Joe off the sleeping tablets, suggesting some alternative strategies to help with sleep. A dosette box may help Joe manage his medication better.

Preventing falls

- Increased exercise, including more frequent walking, and referral to a physiotherapist for supervised and home-based exercises to improve balance and strength.
- Adequate pain control and exercises to control the arthritis in his knees and maintain joint flexibility and muscle strength.
- Review possible causes and treatments for Joe's frequent toileting at night.
- Referral to an occupational therapist for a home safety assessment and modification recommendations (for example night light, and removing loose mats), and to help Joe undertake activities at home and away from home in a safer manner.
- Suggesting Joe wear safe shoes and avoid wearing his slippers.
- Addressing any of these risk factors will reduce Joe's risk of falling: the more that can be addressed, the greater the reduction in his risk of falling.

Stop and think

Refer back to your list of falls risk factors developed when completing the home hazard screening checklist (Figure 2) for Nancy.

- What can Nancy do to reduce her falls risk?
- How could you support her to follow through with these things?

After her hip operation, Nancy spent three weeks in hospital. She returned home to the retirement village walking slowly on a single point stick. The falls risk factors identified earlier, and her reduced balance and mobility since her hip fracture surgery mean that she continues to have an increased risk of ongoing falls. Following her return home, Nancy should visit her doctor to review her ongoing risk of falling. A number of actions are likely to be recommended, including:

- A referral to an occupational therapist for a detailed home assessment, with particular emphasis on stabilising the loose rail, and other safety strategies. Re-organising items in her kitchen and bedroom cupboards so that most commonly used items are within easy reach will reduce the need for over-reaching.
- A referral to a physiotherapist for group or home exercise programmes to improve her balance, strength and mobility, and to improve her confidence in walking. The rehabilitation worker can support the exercises by asking regularly about progress, and reinforcing improvements seen in walking and function over time. Exercising with a friend can also help maintain motivation for exercise in the longer term.
- A referral to have her cataracts removed. Home hazards are particularly problematic for people with vision impairment.
- A referral to a podiatrist to assess and manage the painful feet and discuss safer footwear.

The rehabilitation worker can reinforce the importance of implementing each of these recommendations.

■ Protection from injury associated with falls

Some people will continue to have a high risk of falling, despite the range of actions implemented. Furthermore, people who have osteoporosis (softening of the bones related to change in the structure of the bones) or osteomalacia (low bone strength due to vitamin D deficiency) are at high risk of fractures, even from fairly minor falls. The following actions can help reduce the risk of fractures from falls:

- Use of hip protectors, specially designed undergarments which have protection over the hip areas, so that if a fall onto the hip occurs, the risk of fracturing is substantially reduced. Various types are available, including hard shields over each hip in specially designed undergarments which act to spread the force of impact to tissues away from the hip, and soft hip protectors that work by absorbing some of the impact of the fall.
- Vitamin D combined with calcium supplementation, and sunlight exposure. Many older people are vitamin D deficient, which can cause a moderate weakening of bone strength and an increased risk of fracture. Vitamin D and calcium supplementation (in combination) can slow down the rate of loss of bone strength, and reduce the risk of fractures. Sunlight exposure of the face and limbs for about 20 minutes on most days can also help to prevent vitamin D deficiency, and is therefore likely to reduce the risk of fractures as well.

People with increased risk of falling should be encouraged to develop an action plan in case a fall does occur. This includes how to call for help, how help can reach them, and knowing how to get up after a fall if they are able to. Physiotherapists and occupational therapists can train older people to get up from the floor, as well as helping to develop strategies to seek assistance if unable to get up after a fall. Examples include the use of personal alarms linked to a central call centre, having phone numbers of nearby family/friends on speed dial, carrying a mobile phone at all times or having family/friends call on a regular basis.

■ Making it work – falls prevention is everyone's responsibility

Because of the multifactorial nature of falls, an approach where all causes are reviewed and addressed by the health professional best qualified to deal with them is necessary. This will usually require involvement of the doctor and a number of other health professionals such as physiotherapist, occupational therapist, podiatrist, dietitian and psychologist.

It is vital that the older person is actively engaged in the entire assessment and management process as they are the ones who will act on (take up and follow through long term) the advice given by health professionals. They need to know what their specific risk factors are and how the recommendations aim to reduce these risk factors and therefore the possibility of future falls. They need to understand that many falls can be prevented and that by preventing falls they are maintaining their independence and wellbeing. Providing consistent and accurate information and health promoting messages is the responsibility of all health workers. Engaging family members is also important because they can help support the older person in their falls prevention activities.

Box 1   Nancy's story 6 months later

'I have to admit I'm feeling a lot more confident now. I have a lot of people helping me. My doctor's removed my cataracts. I can't believe the difference. My hip is mending well. I am now only using my stick when I am walking outside, and am continuing with the exercises the physiotherapist prescribed – they are helping me walk more confidently. I'm getting stronger and feel my balance is improving. Ned makes sure I do my exercises every day and walks with me, so this keeps me motivated. I have removed much of the clutter from my home and pathways, and I now buy higher wattage bulbs to improve lighting around our unit. I feel I am much more aware of things around me that could make me fall. The podiatrist has made me some orthotics for my fallen arches. With the orthotics and my new shoes my feet don't hurt any more. My daughter bought me the shoes for my birthday, just like the ones my podiatrist recommended. We also reported the wobbly handrail to the retirement village management so that's been taken care of as well. *I feel I have control over my life again. I'm even planning to get back to my bowls. . . .'*

Box 2   Falls prevention and independence

- All falls should be reported to the doctor and investigated for possible treatment or referral to reduce the risk of future falls.
- There are often a number of contributory causes to a fall – the more that are able to be addressed the more the risk of future falls is reduced.
- Many falls can be prevented.
- Risk of fractures from falls can also be minimised.
- Being accurately informed will help the older person make decisions to minimise their risk of falls.
- Incorporating a range of strategies to actively involve the older person in decision making about the specific actions they will undertake to reduce their risk of falling will maximise likelihood of implementing the recommended actions.
- Being aware of slippery surfaces and other obstacles is a good habit to develop.
- Regular exercise can reduce falls risk, as well as improve general health and wellbeing.
- *Falls prevention is everyone's responsibility (the older person, their family, the doctor, other health professionals and the rehabilitation worker). Falls are not inevitable, and you can make a difference.*

The rehabilitation worker has an important role because they see the older person in their home environment, and are in a position to provide information and look for environmental hazards or for cues that may indicate there is a problem (see Table 1). Effective communication between rehabilitation workers and their manager/agency and the doctor is vital.

People tend to validate their decisions with others. It can come in the form of a question or as part of conversations, just a small aside 'do you think that this will really work?' Validation is part of the decision making process we all go through when weighing up alternatives or determining if something is really worthwhile for the person to do, will it really make that much of a difference. Your casual response could make a difference to whether or not value is placed on the recommendation, and therefore whether or not it is followed through.

As people often do not think that falls can be prevented, the role of rehabilitation workers in helping their clients be informed, giving people guidance and support to initiate and then follow through with falls prevention strategies can be extremely valuable in minimising the client's risk of falls, and maximising their independence and wellbeing.

Further reading

American Geriatrics Society, British Geriatrics Society, Academy of Orthopaedic Surgeons, panel on falls prevention (2001) Guidelines for the prevention of falls in older persons. *Journal of the American Geriatrics Society*, **49**, 664–72. *Summarises the research evidence available for prevention of falls and injuries for older people living at home.*

Campbell, A. (1997) Preventing falls by dealing with the causes. *The Medical Journal of Australia*, **167**, 407–8. *A review of the risk factors for falls, and strategies to reduce risk of falls for older people.*

Campbell, A., Robertson, M., Gardner, M., Norton, R., Tilyard, M. & Buchner, D. (1997) Randomised controlled trial of a general practice programme of home-based exercise to prevent falls in elderly women. *British Medical Journal*, **315**, 1065–9. *A randomised trial that demonstrated that home exercise programmes targeting balance and strengthening exercises can reduce falls.*

Campbell, A.J., Robertson, M.C., Gardner, M.M., Norton, R.N. & Buchner, D.M. (1999) Psychotropic medication withdrawal and a home-based exercise program to prevent falls: a randomised, controlled trial. *Journal of the American Geriatrics Society*, **47**, 850–3. *A randomised trial that demonstrated that weaning older people from use of psychotropic medications can reduce risk of falls.*

Clemson, L. (1997) *Home Falls Hazards and the Westmead Home Safety Assessment*. West Brunswick, Co-ordinates Publications.

Clemson, L, Cumming, R.G. & Heard, R. (2003) The development of an assessment to evaluate behavioural factors associated with falling. *American Journal of Occupational Therapy*, **57**, 380–8. *Documents the development of the Falls Behavioural Scale for Older People.*

Clemson, L., Cumming, R.G., Kendig, H., Swann, M., Heard, R. & Taylor, K. (2004) The effectiveness of a community-based program for reducing the incidence of falls in the elderly: a randomised trial. *Journal of the American Geriatrics Society*, **52** (9), 1487–94. *An evaluation of Stepping On, a multifaceted falls prevention programme that uses a small group learning environment over seven sessions. This programme was effective in reducing falls by 31% and improving confidence in community mobility activities.*

Clemson, L. & Swann, M. (2006) *Staying Power. Tips and Tools to Keep You on Your Feet.* Balmain, NSW, Limelight Press. *A small book written for the older community-residing person. Discusses the risk of falling, explores attitudes towards falls prevention and suggests a range of fall prevention strategies.*

Day, L., Fildes, B., Gordon, I., Fitzharris, M., Flamer, H. & Lord, S. (2002) Randomised factorial trial of falls prevention among older people living in their own homes. *British Medical Journal*, **325** (7356), 128. *A randomised trial that demonstrated that group exercise incorporating balance, strength, coordination and fitness exercises can reduce risk of falls for older people.*

Feder, G., Cryer, C., Donovan, S. & Carter, Y. (2000) Guidelines for the prevention of falls in people over 65. *British Medical Journal*, **321**, 1007–11. *Guidelines based on the research evidence describing successful approaches to falls prevention for older people living in the community.*

Hill, K. & Schwarz, J. (2004) Assessment and management of falls in older people. *Internal Medicine Journal*, **34**, 557–64. *A review of the research evidence and best practice recommendations for reducing risk of falls and falls related injuries.*

Lord, S., Sherrington, C. & Menz, H. (2001) *Falls in Older People: Risk Factors and Strategies for Prevention.* Cambridge, UK, Cambridge University Press. *A comprehensive book, reviewing risk factors for falls, their assessment and management approaches.*

Tinetti, M.E. (2003) Clinical practice. Preventing falls in elderly persons. *New England Journal of Medicine*, **348**, 42–9. *A review of best practice based on available research evidence in reducing the risk of falls among older people living in the community.*

Preventing falls

Continence

Julie Vickerman & Christine Sutton

Introduction

Incontinence is an unpleasant and distressing symptom, both for the person who is experiencing it and for those who live with them or are involved in their care. Those affected often feel embarrassed, ashamed and alone. Many people with continence problems will take extraordinary lengths to hide their problem from family, friends, health and social carers, and even from themselves.

In recent years there has been a shift of emphasis in the provision of continence services, from one of managing incontinence or 'mopping up' to a more positive, proactive approach of promoting continence. There has been increased emphasis on the role of the multidisciplinary team in promoting continence rather than the traditional nursing and medical role.

As a rehabilitation worker, you are ideally placed to assist in the assessment of continence and implement any interventions, because you see people in their home environment and see the impact that having a continence problem has on their activities and wellbeing.

The aim of this chapter is to provide practical advice about some of the issues around helping people who have incontinence.

What is continence and who is affected?

Many of us take for granted the ability to be continent. It is something that we usually give little conscious thought to. Few people wake up in the morning and think about how they will remain dry during the course of the day.

Anyone can become incontinent, regardless of their age or ability, but incontinence is more commonly found in older people, women and people with disabilities. It is not automatic that this group of people will become incontinent; however, the statistics show that they are more at risk of developing incontinence.

Box 1 Incidence of incontinence

Did you know that about *one in four women* and *one in eight men* will experience some incontinence at some point in their life?

How do we become continent and stay that way?

None of us are born continent. Continence is a skill which is acquired at varying ages during our childhood development. To be continent you need to be able to:

- Recognise the need to pass urine or faeces.
- Identify the appropriate place to go to empty your bladder or bowel.
- Have the ability to reach that appropriate place.
- Have the ability to hold on until you reach that place.
- Be able to sit or stand safely to enable you to void.
- Pass urine or faeces when you initiate the process.

A breakdown in any one or more of these skills can result in incontinence.

Stop and think

Think about your clients who have a continence problem. Can you identify where the continence process has broken down in their particular situation?

Box 2 Suggested reading

It may be useful for you to have a basic understanding of normal bladder and bowel functioning to be able to help clients with continence problems.
Find out:
Where the bladder and bowel are positioned and how they work. What are their main functions?
Where the pelvic floor muscles are and what their role is in maintaining continence?

What can go wrong with the bladder?

It is useful to be aware of the main types of urinary incontinence. You may then be able to recognise a person's symptoms and help to find out why they are incontinent.

Table 1 The different types of urinary incontinence, possible causes and the symptoms they present.

Types	Signs and symptoms	Possible causes
Urge	Sudden, uncontrollable urge to pass urine, and great difficulty 'holding on' Needing to go to the toilet more frequently, possibly more often than the times the carers visit, and often at night-time Passing frequent but small amounts of urine May have recurrent urinary tract infection	Weak pelvic floor muscles and change of abdominal pressure Disturbance with the bladder and brain's ability to put off passing urine
Stress	Leakage of urine on exertion, for example when coughing, sneezing, lifting, going up/down hill or stairs, or even when rising from a chair Leakage without feeling need to empty bladder	Weakened pelvic floor muscles and urethral sphincter muscles Women, mostly during pregnancy, following childbirth and during or after menopause Men, damage following prostate surgery Obesity, constipation, chronic cough
Overflow	Passing small but frequent amounts of urine Often waking at night to pass urine Straining to void, urgency, or post micturition dribble Increased risk of recurrent urinary tract infections, because bladder is never emptied completely	Obstructed urethral outflow, often due to an enlarged prostate gland, constipation/impaction, urethral stricture, or damaged nerves through disease or injury, weak or underactive bladder muscle
Functional	*No specific symptoms but contributing factors are:* An impaired mental status Impaired mobility/physical disabilities Impaired dexterity An unsupportive environment Medications	Person has normal bladder and bowel functions, but may become 'incontinent' when unable to reach the toilet in time or cope with toileting
Reflex	Sudden voiding inappropriately without warning	Detrusor instability Neurological damage, for example spinal injuries, multiple sclerosis

(Continued)

Continence

Table 1 Continued.

Types	Signs and symptoms	Possible causes
Nocturnal enuresis night-time bedwetting (children and adults)	*Contributing factors may include* An 'unstable' bladder Infection Stress or anxiety Production of urine at a constant rate Childhood/'lifetime' habit where brain has never learnt how to control the bladder Medication, for example sedation/sleeping tablets	Cause often unknown

What can go wrong with the bowel?

As with the bladder, there is wide variation from one person to another in the frequency of bowel actions. It can be considered 'normal' to open your bowels from as many as three times a day to as little as once every three days. Only when this 'normal' individual variation changes in any way, that is going to the toilet more or less frequently than is usual for you, should medical advice be sought.

There are two main types of bowel dysfunction: constipation and faecal incontinence. The latter is less common, but very distressing and more difficult for carers to deal with. Faecal incontinence may be a presenting symptom of disease in the colon or rectum and therefore should never be ignored.

Your role in observing and reporting progress of a client may be ongoing, to evaluate whether treatment or management is effective. You may need to report on colour, amount and consistency of faeces, and whether pain is experienced during the incontinent episode. These facts will help to define why there is a problem, and how to manage and treat it most effectively.

Psychological effects of incontinence

Imagine the embarrassment associated with incontinence, and how it could really affect a person's self-esteem and confidence (see Figure 1). Take some time to consider how you would broach the subject if you suspected that your client was having some difficulties. Perhaps there is an offensive odour as you enter the property, or you can smell some signs of urine or faeces when close up to them or maybe on their clothes. This would obviously need a very sensitive and tactful approach.

Table 2 The different causes of faecal incontinence, description and contributing factors (adapted from Hunt 1994).

Cause	Description	Examples of contributing factors
Symptomatic diarrhoea	Increased intestinal movement causing frequent defecation of liquid stools	Diverticulitis, ulcerative colitis, diabetes mellitus, Crohn's disease, carcinoma or papilloma of the rectum
Neurogenic	Impaired ability of the brain to inhibit ('put off') defecation, with loss of sensation and voluntary control	Dementia, neurological disorders, for example multiple sclerosis
Faecal impaction	Hardened faeces remain in part of the bowel, but can present with 'runny diarrhoea' as liquid seeps past hard faeces	End result of chronic constipation
Loss of anorectal angle	Weakness of the pelvic muscles as result of degeneration of fibres of the external pudendal nerve	Prolonged or traumatic childbirth, habitual straining at stool, descending perineum and loss of anal reflex
Anal sphincter damage	Damage to sphincter	Childbirth, trauma, anal surgery

A continence problem may cause many of the following feelings and reactions in the sufferer:

- Embarrassment and shame.
- Stress and anxiety.
- Fear and panic.
- Low mood and low life satisfaction.
- A poor body image.
- Anger and disgust.
- Personal and social isolation.
- Avoidance of sexual activity.
- Poor relationships with others.
- Constant tiredness due to disturbed sleep, or attending to personal care.

They may find it extremely difficult to talk about their problems, and if they are feeling ashamed or embarrassed, they may try to hide the problem.

When someone has a mental health disorder, it can be difficult to determine whether this is making the continence problem worse, or if the person is withdrawn and depressed because they have a continence problem.

Continence

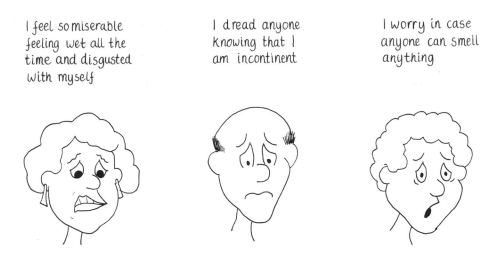

Figure 1 Psychological effects of incontinence.

Stop and think

Consider the impact on *YOUR lifestyle* and how you would feel if you were to develop problems controlling your bladder or bowel. How might you need to *readjust your lifestyle* to cope with the problems incontinence can bring?

Carer attitudes

Attitudes to continence problems can vary. Some people can be quite critical and be unable to hide their disgust. Alternatively, they can appear to give 'permission' for incontinence to continue by saying 'it doesn't matter, don't worry, it can be cleaned up'. The rehabilitation worker may need to give advice to carers on changing their approach. Building up a rapport with the client and their carer is vital, so that potentially embarrassing discussions can occur in an atmosphere of trust, sympathy and confidentiality.

Tips on how to approach the issues

■   Be empathetic, and sensitive to 'clues'. A person may be trying to raise the subject of their problem indirectly.
■   Don't interrupt. It can be tempting to 'fill in' what feels like an awkward silence, but you may be suppressing what they want to say. An unhurried approach conveys that you have time to listen.
■   Be sensitive to the use of terminology. Many people don't like to admit to being 'incontinent' but are prepared to say they 'have accidents',' leak' or 'wet themselves'.

▪ Encourage a positive approach. Much can be done to tackle continence issues.

▪ Factors that affect the client's ability to stay continent

It is important to consider that many people who have incontinence problems generally manage to cope with the resulting difficulties, but there can be added factors which make the problem greater.

Changes in routine

Many people find that a period of change in their life can affect their usual bladder and bowel routine. You may notice yourself that when you go on holiday your bowel habits change. Some people can suffer with constipation due to changes in diet, fluid intake or levels of exercise. The period of time following discharge from hospital or admission to a rehabilitation unit can also have an influence on bladder and bowel habits.

Different routines can easily cause upset and worry the client, which can in turn affect the bladder and bowel and tend to make them more 'sensitive' or 'irritable' (for example exam nerves). These changes can mean the client has to rely on carers for the first time. A person may have difficulty in 'holding on' and reaching the toilet in time if they are feeling anxious. Many of these worries are temporary in duration. Problems often settle once the new routine is established.

Infections

A urinary tract infection (UTI) can often go undiagnosed, particularly with the elderly. They are sometimes only identified when a person develops symptoms of urinary urgency and frequency. This occurs because an infection can irritate the bladder and urethra. If a person has difficulty getting to the toilet quickly then they may well become temporarily incontinent. Having an incontinence problem can also increase a person's risk of developing urinary tract infection.

Tips

▪ Check if antibiotic treatment is required – the client will need to see their GP.
▪ You may need to encourage increased fluid intake to help flush through 'low-grade' infections.
▪ Consider temporary solutions, such as a commode, if the client becomes 'incontinent' because they are unable to make the necessary frequent toilet trips.
▪ Confusion may develop due to the infection.

Continence

Medication

Taking more than one medication is common in older people and those who have multiple health problems. Different types of drugs can affect mobility, general alertness, increase the risk of falls and affect continence. Some medications can have side effects that impact on the bladder, and some may cause constipation, which can lead to urinary or faecal incontinence. For instance, diuretics can exacerbate an already existing urgency and frequency problem and can lead to constipation.

Tips

■ If a person tells you they have started to experience continence problems shortly after starting a new drug, advise them to see their doctor.

■ All clients should have their drug regimes regularly reviewed by their doctor to determine if any medication is influencing continence.

Dietary factors

Many clients reduce their fluid intake thinking that this will help to reduce visits to the toilet but in fact too little liquid can:

(1) Make the faeces harder.
(2) Lead to constipation.
(3) Make the urine more concentrated, irritating the bladder.
(4) Increase the risk of developing a urinary tract infection.
(5) Lead to dehydration and cause confusion.

Tips

■ Recommended fluid intake is at least 1.5 litres (8 cups or 6 mugs) a day. Look at ways of achieving this for people with reduced mobility, for example leaving flasks and jugs within reach.

■ Certain fluids containing caffeine, that is tea, coffee, cola and fizzy drinks, and alcohol, can irritate the bladder. Encourage the client to reduce or avoid these if possible.

■ Consider the timing of drinks. For people who need to void several times during the night, the majority of fluids should be taken during the daytime and reduced in the evening.

■ Some people may have developed a habit of drinking very large amounts, which can exacerbate a continence problem. A slow programme of reducing the amount they drink each day will help, for example drinking one cup less per day for a week.

■ A diet of mainly refined or processed foods with few fruits and vegetables predisposes a person to constipation because there is insufficient bulk to stimulate movement through the intestines.

- Generally, the common advice of aiming to eat five portions of fruit and vegetables a day helps to keep the bowel healthy.
- Eating a well-balanced diet and range of foods requires a good set of teeth and a pain free mouth. If this is a problem, the client should be encouraged to see a dentist.

Constipation

As well as the increased risk of developing faecal incontinence, constipation can make an urge urinary problem worse. It is also likely to make a person feel generally unwell and possibly confused. Being active and exercising can influence the movement of faeces into the rectum and improve appetite. Certain medicines, inadequate dietary and fluid intake, and lack of privacy for toileting can all contribute to constipation.

Tips

- Where possible, encourage the client to go to the toilet when the urge is felt. Ignoring to the 'call to stool' on a regular basis may result in constipation.
- Allow privacy and time when a person is toileting.
- Encourage the consumption of fruit and vegetables and an appropriate volume of fluids.
- If you suspect that the client is constipated, request a district nurse assessment.

Emotional wellbeing

Incontinence can occasionally result from psychological problems. A person's wellbeing can affect their motivation. For example, when someone suffers from depression they may neglect their bodily functions. Consequently, they may develop continence problems because they become indifferent, lack concentration or motivation. It is also important to remember that tiredness is a common symptom of many neurological conditions, so when a person gives the impression of being 'lazy' it may be because the effort of going to the toilet is just too much for them.

Tips

- Try to find practical solutions to make the task less demanding.
- Seek advice if you are concerned about a person's general mental health. This could be making the continence problem worse.

Continence

Environmental factors

For many people, a poorly adapted or unsupportive environment can exacerbate an existing continence problem or can actually render someone incontinent if the difficulties are great.

Tips for improving the home environment for people with incontinence

Whilst working with the client in their own home, you need to consider whether the home environment could be improved to promote easier, quicker and safer access to the toilet. There may be several hindering factors. Consider the following:

- Chairs and bed: are chairs and beds at the correct height? Is the client exerting a lot of effort in standing up? Would it help to position their chair nearer to the toilet? Would a bed rail help? Can the bed/chair be raised in height?
- Bedding: are sheets and blankets tucked in too tight? Would a quilt be easier?
- Toilet: how easy is it to get to the toilet? Is the pathway clear of obstacles? Is the distance too far? Would equipment/rails help?
- Lighting: is there adequate lighting and can switches be reached? Would a touch lamp beside the bed help?
- Signs: would signs, line drawings or photographs on the doors help someone who is confused or disorientated?
- Floor coverings: are they slippery? Are there holes in the carpets where feet or walking aids could become entangled?
- Stairs: would an additional rail help? Is carpet fixed down properly?

Consider whether a referral to the community or social services occupational therapist is required if there are several issues that need addressing. A downstairs toilet adaptation or improved access to the upstairs toilet/bathroom may be required.

Mobility and functional factors

Stop and think

Falls and incontinence are often related. Consider how one can impact on another and what you might do to help the situation. Refer to the 'preventing falls' chapter for more information

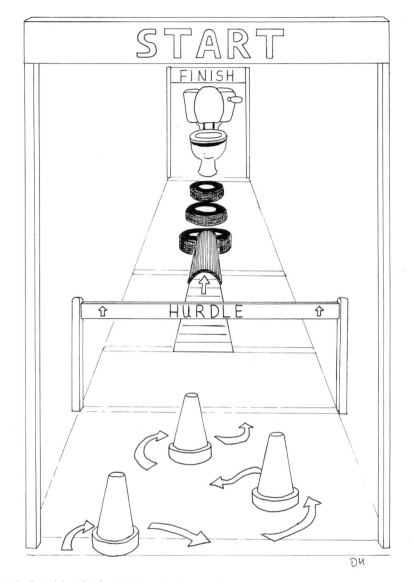

Figure 2 Consider the barriers to staying continent.

Table 3 Factors that may be affecting the ability to remain continent, and possible solutions.

Typical problems	Possible solutions and advice
General weakness and balance problems	Shorten the distance by transporting client nearer to toilet or using commode/urinal in discreet place Is a physiotherapist referral needed for assessment or exercise?
Lack of confidence	Refer for physiotherapist assessment; if home-based programme is advised, assist client to follow this Increase confidence through practice, increasing distance walked each day
'Urgency' problems	Assist speedily to toilet on mobile toilet commode or wheelchair, and then encourage walking back to chair afterwards
Pain on movement	Seek appropriate assessment to determine cause of pain Consider review of medication
Nocturia/noctural enuresis	Consider need for commode or urinal, or protective bed covers Men with an enlarged prostate can empty their bladder more effectively when standing, which can reduce risk of infection. Consider need for walking frame or bed rail if they have problems standing Women generally have difficulty passing urine in a traditional bedpan. Consider a commode, or an alternative style of urinal (refer for assessment if necessary)
Risk of falling at night	Improve the environment to promote safety and confidence Review medication
Unable to stand and sit long enough to completely empty bladder and bowels.	Grab-rails and supporting toilet equipment may help Ensure ideal 'squat position' is achieved necessary to open bowels effectively, that is knees higher than hips Raised toilet seats can sometimes hinder this 'ideal' position
Problems wiping self	Use individual tissues or moist cleansing wipes; bottom wipers may help with reaching problems

Continence

Problems with dexterity

Arthritis, tremor, weakness and general slowness will impede a client's general mobility. Encourage the client to try and use facilities that are as close as possible. A person who has problems with grip, strength, manipulative and dexterity skills may be slower and clumsier at unfastening buttons, zips and adjusting clothing. These can make the difference between someone maintaining continence or becoming incontinent.

Tips

- Look out for soiled underwear. This could be due to temporary illness, long-term changes in body, environmental factors, or simply because they are unable to manage their clothing in time.
- You need to observe a client closely when they are toileting, and pass on any useful information to the professional who may be carrying out an assessment.

Clothing issues

It is difficult to maintain continence if clothing is too tight to unfasten or there are too many layers to manoeuvre to go to the toilet quickly.

Tips

- Observe if a person is struggling with clothing, especially if they suffer from urgency and need to access the toilet quickly.
- Clothes can be adapted for easier access (Figures 3 and 4). Examples include:
  - extended zips in trouser crotches to facilitate the use of urinals
  - wrap over skirts with back openings are useful for people who are chair-bound
  - larger buttons, elasticated waists or velcro fastenings, rings or tabs on zips
  - 'drop front' style underpants, trousers or skirts
- Nightshirts/nightdresses may be easier than pyjamas.

It is important to preserve a person's dignity and individuality. Clothing should be attractive and not 'label' a person as suffering with incontinence. Adaptations should be discreet. Consider the style of clothing to allow easy access to use a urinal or continence product.

Dementia, confusion and memory problems

Some people assume that if a person has dementia then they will inevitably have incontinence. 'True' incontinence can occur quite late in the progression of

Continence

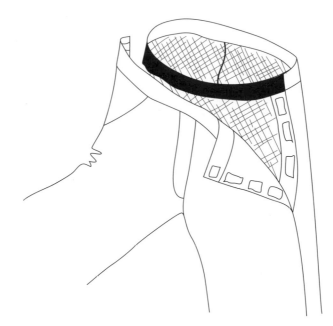

Figure 3 Drop front trousers for people with incontinence.

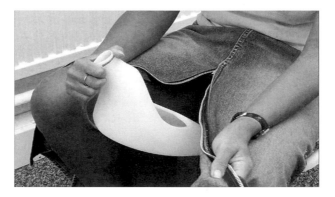

Figure 4 Adapted skirt and female urinal.

dementia, and some people with severe dementia remain continent, probably because they have established lifelong toileting habits. Assessment is crucial in establishing whether incontinence is due to any of the other contributory factors.

Where a client uses inappropriate receptacles or environments this is not really 'true' incontinence, because they have not lost awareness of the need to empty their bladder or bowels, but lost the ability to recognise the toilet.

Continence is a 'taboo' subject and difficult to approach with anyone. Imagine if you suffered with continence problems and also had difficulty with communication. Both problems together could compound the situation.

■ Issues to consider if there are communication difficulties

When a person cannot express themselves, or is unaware of their own needs, the following advice may be useful:

(1) If a urinary tract infection (UTI) is present, there may be pain or burning when passing urine. Notice if the client shows an expression of pain and look for cloudy or offensive smelling urine.
(2) People can forget to drink or be reluctant to do so.
(3) If a person is unable to tell you that they need to use the toilet, be aware of the signs such as fidgeting, wandering, or pulling at clothing.
(4) Get to know a person's habits. Often the bladder and bowel actions have some pattern to them.
(5) When trying to establish a regular toilet regime, decide it, keep to it, and inform other relevant carers and health professionals.
(6) Discuss and monitor any changes in routine, as this may help prevent them becoming larger problems.
(7) Allow adequate time to empty their bladder or bowels, to promote complete voiding where possible.
(8) If a person has a hearing or sight deficit, these factors may exacerbate any existing problems around communicating toileting needs.
(9) Seek expert advice on how to support the client.

Stop and think

When someone suffers with confusion or dementia they may benefit from following an individualised toilet programme. You may be required to assist them with this. Consider:

■ How would you reward and reinforce the desired behaviour?
■ How would you discourage inappropriate behaviour?

■ Cultural issues

It is extremely important that you have an awareness and respect for the cultural or religious practices a client may need to follow and how these can impact on toileting issues.

Continence

Consider the following factors

(1) For Hindus and Muslims it is regarded as 'unclean' to use the same hand that is used for toileting, for eating, greeting people or performing religious ceremonies.

(2) You may need to bear in mind that Muslims are required to abstain from eating and drinking (including water) between the hours of dawn and sunset during Ramadan, although usually people who are ill and the elderly are excused.

(3) Remember that some Sikh, Muslim and Hindu women keep their legs and upper arms covered at all times.

(4) A vegetarian diet may be the main diet, as is the case with Hindus.

For progress to be achieved in rehabilitation, you need to be able to communicate effectively and overcome language barriers.

■ The role of the rehabilitation worker in the assessment of incontinence

A comprehensive assessment is essential for effective treatment and management of incontinence. A suitably trained health professional will probably carry this out, such as a continence adviser or district nurse. However, all health workers should contribute to the assessment process, as this needs a consistent team approach.

As a rehabilitation worker you are ideally placed to contribute, making many important observations whilst you are assisting with personal activities. Become aware of bladder and bowel habits and other issues facing the client.

Your specific role may involve:

- Assisting the client to record information, for example completing baseline charts, bowel or bladder diaries, collecting samples to be tested by the district nurse or continence adviser.
- Implementing the recommended advice, for example prompting the client to go to the toilet at agreed time intervals.
- Observing, monitoring and reviewing progress.
- Reporting back to the appropriate professional.
- Advising and monitoring a balanced diet and correct fluid intake.
- Assisting the client to void in the appropriate place or receptacle.
- Supporting the client and family to overcome emotional factors.
- Encouraging safe use of prescribed equipment, which may include alternatives such as urinals.
- Encouragement to follow a pelvic floor exercise regime.

A baseline chart helps to establish the frequency of urination, episodes of incontinence and volume of urine passed. A person may be asked to complete a record of this information over a period of 3–5 days and you may need to assist the client to do this.

Bladder training may be used to deal with symptoms of urgency and frequency. Following completion of a baseline chart, the aim is to restore normal bladder function by teaching the bladder to 'hold on' for longer periods. This may take some time before positive results are seen, so you will need to give lots of encouragement.

Individualised toilet programmes are used particularly with clients who have dementia or confusion. You will need to reinforce the preferred pattern of behaviour and prompt the client to use the toilet when the bladder is almost full, but before accidents occur. These times will be identified from the baseline chart that the health care professional will use to design the programme.

Urinals are an alternative option when using the toilet is a problem. There are increasingly more types now available, particularly for women. Some are available on prescription. If necessary, consider a referral to the occupational therapist or continence adviser for assessment.

Pelvic floor muscle exercises are recommended for stress and urge incontinence to strengthen pelvic floor muscles and help a person to learn how to 'hang on'. Much encouragement may be needed to persevere with these exercises.

■ Living with continence problems

Living with incontinence can impact on all areas of life, such as work, relationships, socialising, holidays, travelling, and sport and leisure activities. Activities often need to be planned around the necessity to access toilets. Any anxieties may affect a client's confidence to engage in these activities, and avoidance may be seen as the easiest answer, whereas there may be easy solutions. Where people continue to be incontinent despite all interventions, careful planning can help give reassurance and confidence to overcome fears.

Stop and think

How would being incontinent affect the activities *you* carry out on a regular basis? Select such an activity and take a few minutes to consider all the factors you would need to take into account when planning and carrying out this activity.

Your role may involve helping a person to think how they can plan any activities outside their home. For instance, when planning to travel or go on holiday these tips may be helpful. Some advice may also apply to other activities:

(1) Loose fitting clothes for the journey are more comfortable.
(2) A small bag containing a 'clean-up kit' may be a good idea. for example, change of clothes, pads, disposable gloves, small mirror, handwash, wet wipes and plastic bags.
(3) Check if products that will be needed are available at the destination.

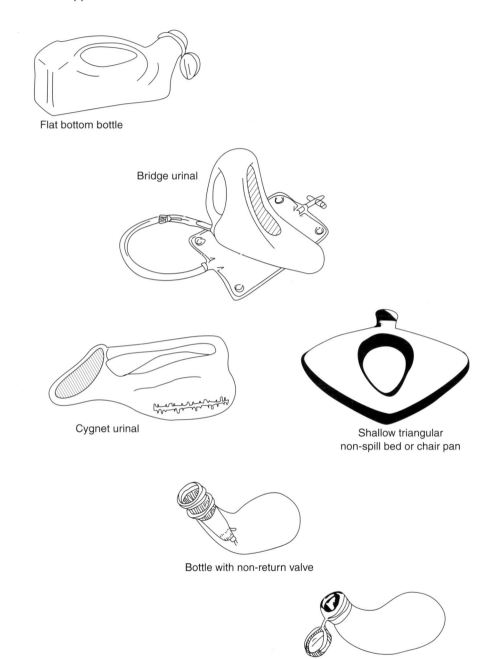

Flat bottom bottle

Bridge urinal

Cygnet urinal

Shallow triangular
non-spill bed or chair pan

Bottle with non-return valve

Male bottle with snap-on lid

Figure 5 Commonly used male and female urinals.

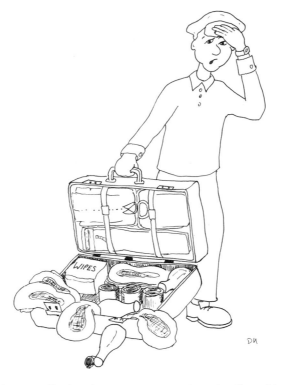

Figure 6 Organising supplies in advance can prevent overloading of luggage.

(4) Take adequate supply of all products required. Order extra supplies needed for the trip in plenty of time.
(5) If possible, post some supplies ahead. This will save on luggage space.
(6) Most companies are willing to allow extra luggage allowance if there is a medical reason. Enquire with airline or coach operators.
(7) Check which medical supplies are allowed to be carried in hand luggage. Some items, such as enemas, can explode in the hold of an aeroplane. A doctor's letter may be necessary, outlining any requirements, to assist with security checks.
(8) Wheelchairs or aisle seats nearest to toilets can be pre-booked.
(9) Find out what facilities are available at stations or on trains. Staff can assist in getting on and off the train if booked in advance. Checking of facilities and access will apply when planning all activities.
(10) If flying, remember to take extra supplies in hand luggage to allow for delays.
(11) Before leaving home, contact the hotel to find out about laundry and washing facilities.
(12) If a change in method of managing a continence problem is being considered whilst away, it is advisable to try it out at home first (like switching from intermittent catheters to an indwelling catheter).

(13) Ask the doctor for a course of antibiotics in case of a urinary tract infection whilst away, if prone to infections, a bulking agent in case of diarrhoea, or mild laxative in case of constipation.

(14) If using an indwelling catheter, a spare one should be taken. A larger drainage bag may be useful for the journey. For mobility difficulties, attach a catheter valve to the catheter before the leg bag. The leg bag can then be detached and emptied.

■ What can be done to manage a person's incontinence?

Use of products

Thousands of products are available to manage incontinence, and selecting the right product to meet the individual's needs is crucial. If you find that the prescribed product is not satisfactory refer back to the assessor for review and advice. It may be worth considering the impact that the product and the care provided by health professionals and carers can have on an individual's sexuality, emotions, relationships and sexual identity. Choosing to use a product in particular situations, for example when going to a social gathering, can give confidence or reassurance.

Tips

Pads and pants

- Available in a wide range of shapes, sizes and absorbency levels, disposable or reusable (washable). Measurements should be taken to ensure suitable fit.
- Washable products include Y-fronts, boxer shorts, male briefs, lacy knickers and thongs.
- The 'ideal' pad is the smallest one to deal with the problem.
- Ensure underwear worn with disposable pads fits well to prevent leakage.
- 'Cup' the pads before inserting to ensure more effective fitting and absorbency.
- Store pads in the appropriate manner (dry environment) to maintain absorbency properties.

Bed and chair pads

- Available to protect surfaces and give people reassurance.
- Available as washable or disposable types, in various sizes and colours. Many are discreet in appearance.

Sheaths and body worn urinals

- Available for men. A sheath is fitted over the penis to collect urine and is attached to a drainage bag, usually fitted to the client's leg.

- Body worn urinals consist of a cone that fits over the penis, a flange, a drainage bag and a belt, or pant system that secures the items to the body.
- Correct assessment and measurement is essential by the appropriate professional. Seek advice on how they should be fitted.

Catheters

- Indwelling catheter, stays in place for a few weeks and is then changed and replaced. Follow standards and procedures if you are involved in the aftercare of the product.
- Intermittent catheter, is inserted into the bladder several times each day to drain any residual urine. People can be taught how to manage this procedure themselves.

Drainage bags

- Used with catheters, sheaths, body worn urinals and some hand-held urinals. Available with many different styles of opening taps for emptying.
- Observe if the person is able to open these. If not, alternative types can be tried.
- Different types and sizes of bags and tubing are available, some more discreet than others. Ask for advice.

Skin care

This is a *crucial aspect of observation* when assisting a person with personal activities. Most people who are incontinent do not get sore skin if pads are changed often and skin is washed and dried well. People who have severely restricted mobility are more at risk of developing soreness.

Tips

- Frequent repositioning can help, whilst seated in a chair and in bed.
- Use unperfumed or pH balanced soap after an episode of faecal incontinence. Use in minimal amounts, rinsing areas thoroughly to remove any residue.
- When skin becomes wet with urine alone, cleanse with water.
- If a person has dry or sore skin, their nutritional and fluid intake should be assessed.
- Avoid vigorous rubbing, gently 'pat' skin until dry.
- Don't apply talcum powder to groin areas. It can become encrusted causing skin damage.
- Certain creams should be avoided unless medically prescribed. Seek advice.
- Seek medical advice if there is no improvement, or deterioration occurs in skin condition.

Continence

Hygiene

It is extremely important for both you and the client to prevent infections spreading from one client to another. Always wash your hands after attending to a client before you start working with the next following the recommended 'infection control procedures'. Assist the client to access their washing facilities too.

Odours

Fresh urine should not smell nasty. If it does, there may be an infection. Urine only starts to smell if it is left out in the air. The smell from faecal incontinence is less easy to hide, but special deodorants are available to help.

Tips

■ Prevent smells by use of air fresheners and assist the client to change pads or clothes as soon as possible.
■ Use the correct continence product, so that urine does not leak onto furniture or clothes.
■ Fresh air in a room is one of the best ways of getting rid of any smell.

■ Conclusion

As a rehabilitation worker you play a key role within the multidisciplinary team, to help clients maintain or regain the skill of continence or appropriately manage their incontinence. Incontinence is not inevitable for older or disabled people, but they are more at risk of developing this problem. New treatments and products are constantly being developed and so it is important to keep up to date with these as a way of improving client care.

By adopting a positive approach to incontinence issues, together with developing an appropriate level of knowledge, skills and advice, the rehabilitation worker could make all the difference to someone, in helping them overcome what can be an embarrassing and life-changing problem.

■ Additional information and useful contacts

For information on clothing:

■ Yellow Pages telephone directory may help identify local suppliers of suitable clothing.
■ The Disabled Living Centres Council (DLCC) will have details of all the Disabled Living Centres in the UK. Many centres have a clothing advisory service (www.dlcc.org.uk).
■ You could contact your local occupational therapist or Disabled/Independent Living Centre, who may be able to advise you regarding local services.

- AWEAR offers information about clothing adaptations and retailers for people with disabilities or special needs (www.awear.org.uk).

For information on continence services and products:

- RADAR (The Royal Association for Disability and Rehabilitation) run the national key scheme which offers independent access to over 4000 locked public toilets in the UK, many adapted for people with disabilities (www.radar.org.uk).
- PromoCon, Disabled Living, Manchester, UK, provide detailed, impartial information about the many different types of continence products, equipment and services available (www.promocon.co.uk).
- Worldwide continence organisations can be found via the website: www.continenceworldwide.org.
- International Continence Society includes clinicians and other multidisciplinary members representing most countries worldwide (www.icsoffice.org).
- Incontact is a leading national charity providing free support and information to people affected by bladder and bowel problems (www.incontact.org).
- 'Urgent cards' can be carried by people who have a need to access toilets quickly, and used to show others, for example in shops and restaurants. Available from The Continence Foundation. 'Just Can't Wait' cards also available from Incontact.
- The Continence Foundation of Australia http://www.contfound.org.au/
- The Australian National Public Toilet Map http://www.toiletmap.gov.au/
- The Canadian Continence Foundation http://www.continence-fdn.ca/
- New Zealand Continence Association http://www.continence.org.nz/
- The Continence Foundation (UK) will give details of your local continence advisory services (www.continence-foundation.org.uk).

■ Further reading

Department of Health (2000) *Good Practice in Continence Services*. London, Department of Health. http://www.doh.gov.uk/continenceservices.htm. *This document forms the framework, which all UK continence services are working towards. Interdisciplinary working is extensively promoted.*

Getcliffe, K. & Dolman, M. (eds) (1997) *Promoting Continence: A Clinical Research Resource.* Edinburgh, Baillière Tindall. *A useful book which contains practical and theoretical knowledge about continence problems for many client groups.*

Hunt, S. (1994) *Promoting Continence in the Nursing Home.* Victoria, Continence Foundation of Australia.

Squires, A. & Hastings, M. (eds) (2002) *Rehabilitation of the Older Person: A Handbook for the Interdisciplinary Team* (3rd edition). Cheltenham, Nelson Thornes. *This book brings together the skills and experience of experts in several fields of rehabilitation, to provide knowledge of how to manage older people in whatever environment or specialty they present.*

Continence

Memory loss

Gail Mountain

Introduction

Everyone experiences poor memory from time to time. Forgetting where we have put items like keys, wallets and documents is a frequent problem for many of us. Trying to locate the lost object can be both time consuming and stressful, and if the item cannot be found a range of other coping strategies have to be used to manage what we wanted or needed to do. Another common example of transient memory loss is forgetting people's names. This can be embarrassing, but is usually overcome with humour and generally has minimal consequences for the forgetful person. We generally manage to cope with brief episodes of forgetfulness, while at the same time making a mental note to try and ensure that it does not happen again.

Imagine, then, what it must be like to have profound and/or permanent memory loss. The disabling effects of impaired memory can be catastrophic for those who experience it, as well as for those who are close to the individual and have to cope with its impact. Living with a situation where one's memory is so

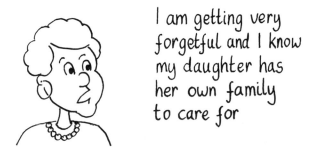

Figure 1 Memory loss can impact on family and friends.

poor that a lifetime of established habits and routines cannot be recalled, where the names of friends and relatives are forgotten, and where familiar places and situations become unfamiliar is extremely distressing.

This chapter begins with a short explanation of the different forms of memory loss in older age. This is followed by illustrations of the ways in which rehabilitation workers can help to minimise the distress experienced by older people and their carers as a result of memory loss. Finally, examples are provided of the different therapeutic interventions that can be used by rehabilitation workers to help to minimise the effects of poor memory in the people they work with.

■ Reasons for memory loss

There is no one definition or experience of memory loss; it is an umbrella term for a number of problems that reveal themselves in many ways. Furthermore, the extent of memory loss experienced by the individual can vary significantly from day to day and during the different stages of an illness. It is also a common feature of normal ageing. Examples of some of the most common underlying reasons for memory loss in older age are given below.

Age-associated memory loss

Age-associated memory loss causes significant problems. However, older people with this difficulty usually manage to continue to cope on a day-to-day basis, often with some assistance from friends and relatives, as their ability to perform functional tasks is not usually significantly impaired. Therefore, most people with age-associated memory loss will continue to live independently in the community. A well-known aspect of this type of memory loss is an increasing ability to be able to clearly recall events in the distant past. This type of memory loss is one that we are all most familiar with in older people we interact with and know personally.

> **Case study of memory loss**   Mrs Stuart
>
> Mrs Stuart is 80 years old and physically very fit for her age. She has been widowed for a few years now, but continues to live independently in her own home supported by her children and grandchildren. Mrs Stuart's family have become rather concerned recently as she has locked herself out of her house on a number of successive occasions and seems to keep losing important items. She also has obvious difficulties remembering phone numbers. However, she continues to shop and cook for herself, and do some gardening, and her home is kept in reasonable order.

Memory loss

Dementia

The term '*dementia*' includes a number of illnesses which are not a normal part of ageing. Even though a qualified medical practitioner will be able to recognise the type of dementia a person has by the symptoms they are experiencing, the course the illness takes will vary from person to person. For example, some people will decline rapidly, whereas in others the symptoms of the illness will become apparent over a longer period of time. Some will have an associated decline in physical health and others will remain physically fit. The most commonly recognised initial signs of the illness are poor memory, confusion and disorientation.

There are three main types of dementia:

(1) **Alzheimer's disease:** this is the most common form of dementia. It occurs most frequently in people over the age of 65 years. However, a smaller number of younger people each year are diagnosed as having Alzheimer's disease. This is called *pre-senile dementia.*
(2) **Vascular dementia:** this occurs as a result of a stroke, and may happen out of the blue, causing a sudden decline in the person's abilities.
(3) **Lewy body dementia:** in addition to confusion, this form of dementia has symptoms similar to Parkinson's disease; for example shuffling gait, difficulty starting movement and mask-like face.

Twenty per cent of older people aged 80 years and over have some form of dementing illness. The effect of the dementing illness upon a person can be mild, moderate or severe. However, only around one third of people with a diagnosis of dementia are at the severe end of the scale, requiring constant supervision. The common portrayal of dementia on television is the severe form of the illness. This can influence our perceptions of the illness. Also, memory loss can vary in the same individual; some days will be better than others. Finally, some causes of memory loss can be treated successfully. Nevertheless, it must also be acknowledged that in its most severe form, dementia can destroy the entire fabric of the person's life with the degree of memory loss being a major symptom.

Case study of dementia Mrs Slade

Mrs Slade is 70 years old. She lives alone in a first-floor flat. She has long-standing partial hearing loss in both ears, and has become increasingly forgetful over the past five years. As well as having increasingly poor memory, particularly for recent events, she is easily distracted, frequently not completing what she is doing. These problems have been getting worse over the last year. Most recently she has been found wandering in the street at night, not able to provide a rational explanation for her behaviour. She also often uses the wrong words for what she is describing. She has been diagnosed with moderate dementia. Her family are concerned to get her moved into accommodation where she can be assisted and supervised.

Memory loss

Delirium

Delirium is a significant problem for older people, occurring in 30% of all older people admitted to hospital. The person becomes suddenly confused and disturbed. Delirium can be due to dementia, but is more likely to be due to a treatable physical condition such as urinary tract infection, or cardiac disease. Therefore, when the acute illness is treated, the delirium will diminish in some people. However, in others the confused state persists even after the acute illness has been treated. The delirium syndrome is one that staff working with older people in general hospital settings will be familiar with.

Case study of delirium   Mrs Jones

Mrs Jones is 82 years old. She lives with her 85-year-old husband, and even though they are becoming increasingly physically frail due to their age, they were still managing to get the most out of life and enjoying their time together. However, recently Mrs Jones fell and fractured her hip and as a result had to be admitted to hospital. Whilst in hospital she became suddenly and severely confused. She could not remember who her husband was when he visited and had no idea why she was in hospital. Her confusion and disorientation were so severe that she had to be constantly supervised by nursing staff for her own safety as she kept trying to get up out of bed despite her physical injury. The medical staff diagnosed a urinary tract infection and treatment was prescribed for this, resulting in rapid improvement in her mental state. However, she remains generally far more vulnerable and frail than previously. Also, the episode upset her husband so much that he is considering residential care for them both.

As a consequence of other illnesses and conditions

Memory loss can be associated with a number of other illnesses; for example a stroke, Parkinson's disease and diabetes, where the brain has been damaged by the illness. When this occurs, the person and their carer have to manage the effects of dementia, in addition to those of the original illness.

Poor memory and confusion can also occur as a result of medication that the older person may be taking. Clients may have a bad reaction to some medication, be taking a cocktail of prescribed medicines that do not mix, or have purchased over the counter medication that does not mix with what they have been prescribed. Alternatively, they may be taking tablets at incorrect intervals. Again, the picture can be complicated, as taking medication incorrectly is a frequent symptom of poor memory.

Finally, even though it is not often readily acknowledged as being a problem of older age, we cannot overlook the effects of alcohol abuse upon the memory and cognition of older people.

Memory loss

> ### Case study of memory loss as a consequence of other illness
> #### Mr Conway
>
> Mr Conway is 67 years old, and prior to his illness lived alone. He has only recently retired from his work as a self-employed builder. He was enjoying his retirement when he became ill and was diagnosed with vascular disease. Three months ago he had a sudden stroke affecting his left side. While he has recovered from the physical effects of the stroke, his memory and mood remain severely affected. His mood fluctuates from being aggressive and angry to tearful and depressed. His anger and frustration are provoked by his extremely poor memory for recent events. There have also been further deteriorations in his memory due to a number of mini-strokes. His married daughter is currently looking after him and he attends day care. His daughter is struggling to cope and seeking residential care for her father.

As Figure 2 indicates, the impact of memory loss is only severe for a small proportion of older people. Most of those with poor memory manage to remain living in the community, assisted by family and friends. However, we must always bear in mind the impact of the condition upon the person's life and that of their family, relatives and friends, irrespective of degree of severity.

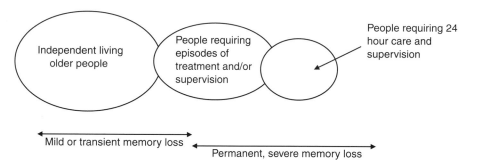

Figure 2 Impact of memory loss upon older people.

■ Symptoms of memory loss

As already indicated, memory loss can manifest itself in a number of ways, for example:

(1) Denial of problems, an unwillingness to recognise or admit to failing memory, covering up.
(2) Agitation and distress.
(3) Wandering.
(4) Forgetting who people are, key events, dates etc.
(5) Confusion and disorientation; not being able to accurately recall the time, where they are and who they are (a person who cannot recall who they are is described as 'disorientated in person' and will be suffering from severe memory loss).

Memory loss

(6) Paranoid, accusatory behaviour, often due to forgetting the location of objects and accusing others of having moved or stolen them.
(7) Personal neglect, due to forgetting to attend to own needs such as meals or hygiene.
(8) Some difficulty learning new skills.

Other factors, in particular poor hearing and eyesight, and environmental factors like poor lighting can significantly contribute towards the level of confusion and disorientation a person experiences.

A number of measures can be used by health care practitioners to diagnose the range and extent of the memory related problems a person is experiencing. The most common of these is the Mini Mental State Examination (MMSE), which is frequently used by medical practitioners and others to determine the level of memory loss and disorientation a person is experiencing.

■ The contributions that rehabilitation workers can make

Rehabilitation workers can assist people with memory loss in two main ways. First, through an approach towards the person and their carers that is both caring and supportive. This is an essential quality for all those working with older people and their carers. Second, through a number of interventions to assist with coping and trying to provide some experience of life quality. These two aspects are now described in some detail.

A caring and supportive approach

Why do you need to learn about how to approach and reassure older people with memory loss? After all, people who have chosen to work with vulnerable older people must be aware of the importance of an approach that is sensitive and understanding. Unfortunately, the past observations of the author have revealed a very different picture at times. It is all too easy for both qualified and unqualified staff to lapse into a range of behaviours and responses to older people with memory loss that are unhelpful and in some instances cruel. If we are under pressure ourselves, for example if we feel unwell, stressed or angry due to something that happened before we got to work, it can be difficult to be patient with an older person who continually repeats the same question or wanders away. It is also very easy to be distracted by conversation with other staff, rather than trying to pursue a discussion with a confused older person who appears both unresponsive and unable to comprehend. In some care settings without good leadership, workers have been observed mocking older people with dementia, having completely forgotten to respect the vulnerability, needs and individuality of the people they are working with.

All workers who come into contact with older people with memory loss should aim to assist the person to cope or help them to become less agitated, bearing in mind how distressing memory loss can be. All workers need to develop insight into their own behaviour so that they can withdraw if a situation is

---

Box 1   Being supportive and minimising distress

- Do not raise your voice to try and enhance understanding.
- Talk to the client in a quiet, reassuring manner, facing them while you do so.
- Use short, easily comprehensible sentences.
- Give the person time, do not rush the client or their carers.
- Ensure that the person's dignity is preserved at all times; do not use inappropriate humour.
- Laugh with the person and their relatives, not at them.
- Find out about the person; their life, how they like to be referred to, their preferences. If necessary get this information from family and friends.
- Use distraction if the person is becoming distressed.
- Try and engage the person in conversation and simple activities of interest to them.
- Do not allow yourself to be distracted by gossip and other activities in the area.
- If you feel that you are not coping in any way, seek assistance immediately.

---

proving too difficult to cope with for whatever reason. This is a challenging, demanding task and in common with other staff, rehabilitation workers will need assistance from colleagues to be able to deliver a quality service. For more information about ensuring that your own supervision and support needs are met, see Section 4: Teamworking and supervision. The ways in which rehabilitation workers can help older people with memory loss and minimise distress are summarised in Box 1.

Communicating clearly and effectively

It can sometimes be difficult to communicate with people with memory loss. Communication problems can arise from comprehension difficulties, poor memory, slow responses, and the client's inability to find the right words to express what they want to say. Communication difficulties are compounded if the client has poor hearing as well. More hints on effective communication can be found in the chapter on Communication. Make sure you use direct, clear communication and state exactly what you would like the client to do. Use words that are familiar to the client, for instance, 'dinner' instead of 'lunch'. You do not need to raise your voice, but do use short, clear sentences.

Supporting carers and helping them to cope

Older people with memory loss often have a member of the family or a friend who is the main carer. The older person will be extremely reliant upon that person, with the relationship between the two often referred to as the 'patient/carer dyad'. The needs of older people with memory loss are so great that the carer will be fully involved, and they often become protective and concerned, as well as stressed, as a result. They may have to neglect their own needs in order to be able to cope with the person they are caring for, for example the partners of older people with memory loss and confusion frequently cannot find time to pay attention to their own health needs. Daughters who are carers may have had to give up paid work. This means that when you work with the older person, you also have to take the needs and views of the carer fully into account.

A final word of caution here; families always have a history which will impact upon their ability to cope with the person with memory loss. Long-standing poor relationships, including those between married partners, can be stretched to the limit by the behaviour of the person with memory loss. Also, if the carers themselves have problems their coping ability will be limited, for example it is commonly recognised that abuse of older people can be triggered by alcohol abuse on the part of the carer. It is therefore essential to remain alert to possible problems between the older person and their carers, so that timely help can be provided. However, ensure that any information you supply to staff is conveyed confidentially, in a private office. Section 4: Working with clients and carers to enable independence provides more information about how to work with carers.

■ Delivering effective interventions

Rehabilitation workers are employed to work with older people in a variety of settings including people's own homes and other community settings, as well as day care, respite, residential and nursing homes, and acute hospitals. This section will describe some of the interventions that you might provide in these different settings.

It must be emphasised that irrespective of the treatment location, time must be taken to build a relationship with the older person and their family. This is an essential step and is likely to take more than one session. First, it is essential to gain an accurate picture of the life of the older person through taking time to talk with them and their relatives. This is likely to form part of the initial assessment, but the rehabilitation worker must also participate, particularly if they are to be the main worker for the person.

Second, workers have to develop a picture of extent, nature and patterns of memory loss and how this is impacting upon the life of the person and their carer, prior to suggesting means of coping; for example:

■ Does extent of memory loss vary from day to day, or over the day?
■ Are there any particular activities that are becoming problematic due to the extent of memory loss?
■ Are relationships with family, friends and neighbours being affected by the memory loss?
■ What are the things that the person really enjoys doing and are they being prevented from continuing to participate for any reason?

This information must provide the foundation upon which decisions about what to advise and suggest to the person and their carers is built.

Memory loss

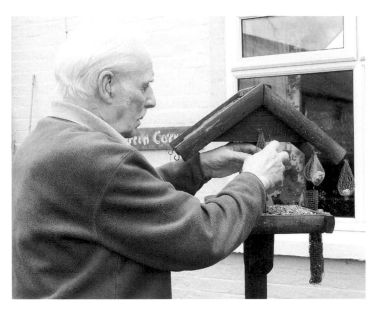

Figure 3 Clients should be encouraged to continue activities that they enjoy and, where possible, maintain their normal routine.

Working with people with memory loss in their own homes

The rehabilitation worker can be instrumental in helping the client to develop strategies to remain independent in their own home. Referrals may be received from primary care, social services or from hospitals if the person has been an in-patient or attended day hospital.

Suggesting suitable interventions

The aim should be to support the person to maintain routines and activities that work well for them and that can be maintained in the short term. It is also necessary to understand the contribution of the main carers. It would not be helpful to make suggestions that contradict existing methods of coping. The client should also be encouraged to continue with activities that they enjoy. A number of suggestions are given below.

Maintaining cognitive abilities

Keeping alert and active is a proven way of maintaining brain function. Through understanding the life of the older person, the rehabilitation worker can help to identify cognitive activities that may be of interest to that individual, for example:

- Word and other puzzles.
- Listening to favourite radio and TV programmes.

Memory loss

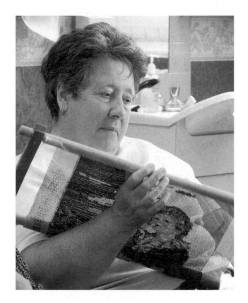

Figure 4 People with memory loss should be encouraged to continue their hobbies and interests.

▪ Reading: library books, newspapers and magazines.
▪ Playing card games.
▪ Undertaking hobbies and interests (this may necessitate suggesting new pastimes, as undertaking established activities at a poorer standard can sometimes lead to distress).

Continuing with activities of daily living

Older people with memory loss may wish or need to continue to undertake activities of daily living, such as personal care, cooking, shopping and housework. This can become increasingly difficult if the memory loss they have is due to a progressive illness. However, retaining a level of independence for as long as possible is important. This includes maintenance of established routines, as well as demonstrating to the person that they are still coping. The negative consequences of lack of confidence cannot be underestimated. Simple strategies can be adopted by the person to try and minimise the effects of their memory loss, for example:

▪ Use a diary for appointments.
▪ Always place keys and documents in the same place.
▪ Make lists, for example tasks for the day.
▪ Make sure that orientation cues in the house are accurate, clocks, calendars, etc.
▪ Place items around the house to prompt an activity; place pills in the bathroom by a regularly used object like a toothbrush or shaver, small change by a shopping bag.
▪ Use tricks like verses to help memorise particular things.

Memory loss

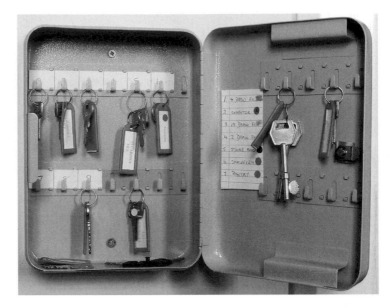

Figure 5 Clear visual clues are a valuable way to reduce the impact of memory loss.

Maintaining physical health

The rehabilitation worker can do a lot to help the older person to look after their health in a variety of ways, for example:

- Help the person to access and eat a balanced diet.
- Encourage some physical exercise like gardening, walking and shopping if their health allows.
- Alert other services if it is suspected that glasses and hearing aids need attention.
- Draw the attention of the client and their carers to any situations in the home that might lead to accidents or injuries.

Participating in social activities

It is important for the established social activities of the person to be maintained if at all possible. The continuation of long-standing friendships and social circles must be encouraged. If the client is no longer able to join in the social activities they were participating in previously, new ones should be introduced. The social needs of the carer also have to be considered.

Monitoring use of enabling technologies

An ever increasing range of technologies is being introduced to help people with failing memory to continue living in the community for longer. Examples

> **Box 2** Working with people in their own homes, pointers for practice
>
> ■ Check your facts: how is the home managed, who is providing care and assistance, are there any visitors and established social routines?
> ■ Always remember that you are a visitor in the person's home.
> ■ Decisions about the nature of the interventions and levels of acceptable risk taking must be taken with a qualified staff member.
> ■ Remain aware of changes in the person's mental state and abilities, and report back to other staff. This is particularly important if the person has become paranoid about losing items around their home or is at risk of accident or injury.
> ■ Take into account the help that might be available to assist, both from family and friends and from paid carers such as home care. There is little point in pursuing some activities when the older person is reluctant or unable to engage and assistance is readily available.

include community alarms, detectors to monitor the movement of an older person in their own home, devices to enable safe use of devices like cookers and fires, equipment to alert the person to a potentially overfull bath, and lighting to guide the person to the toilet and back into bed at night.

Community alarm systems have been available for over a decade and are the technology most likely to be encountered by rehabilitation workers in the short term. The user wears a small trigger, usually on a pendant. When the button on the trigger is pressed, it sends a radio signal to a telecommunication unit in the house, usually part of a telephone system. Operators at a central control point communicate with the caller to assess the urgency of the call and whether or not a visit is required from paid or unpaid carers.

All workers are going to have to become familiar with the use of these technologies as they become more commonly available. Rehabilitation workers will increasingly find themselves assisting older people to use these forms of technology in their homes. One new role will be helping to determine their usefulness for the individual.

Working with people with memory loss in treatment and care settings

Treatment and care settings provide the opportunity to work with older people in groups. However, the fact that not all older people enjoy group settings should not be forgotten.

Some of the well-known interventions provided in health and social care settings are described in the next table.

Groups can be effective in helping older people to remain orientated if they are well run and managed.

Table 1 Commonly used interventions in treatment and care settings.

Intervention	What it means	How it is used
Reality orientation therapy (RO)	Providing cues and reminders to prompt the person with poor memory	There are two main ways of providing RO prompts: By talking with the person either individually or as part of a group By providing cues in the environment
Reminiscence therapy	Assisting a person to recall events that have occurred during their past	Can take place on a one-to-one basis or with a group of people (see Figure 6)
Validation therapy	This is the opposite to reality orientation: the worker does not correct inaccuracies in what the person is saying but seeks to discuss further	On a one-to-one basis only; there are 14 ways of undertaking validation therapy correctly
Life review and personal story books	Allowing the person to talk about their present and previous life experiences including family, friends, working life, and leisure and social interests	On a one-to-one basis, often includes the assembling of life story books; aspects of the individual's life history are recorded in a book together with pictures and other memorabilia (see Figure 7)
Multi-sensory environment	The use of equipment that stimulates sight, hearing and feeling in an attractive, non-demanding manner	Dedicated rooms containing multi-sensory equipment with the aim of creating a relaxing environment that can be enjoyed and explored by the individual
Music	Music to stimulate the senses, promote reminiscence and reality orientation	Many and varied, for example: Community singing/choir Listening to music/asking people to select their favourite songs Inviting performers

Running groups with people with memory loss: pointers for practice

- Identify where you will hold the group. The venue needs to be quiet and not easily disturbed, for example a side room can be better than a day room.
- Identify at least one other worker to run the group with you. This is the minimum requirement; ideally you need a number of co-workers so that the participants each get the amount of attention they require, and toileting, wandering and poor attention can be managed with minimum disturbance to the group overall.
- Ensure that all the other workers you run the group with are involved in planning the session.
- Decide who will be invited to the group. Groups will be more successful if participants have similar levels of ability, or alternatively where there are plenty of staff available to assist those who are less able.
- Decide upon a structure for the group; the topics you are going to talk about and in what order.

Memory loss

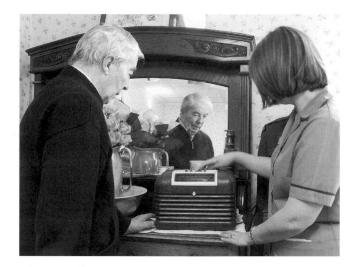

Figure 6 Clients should be encouraged to reminisce about their past.

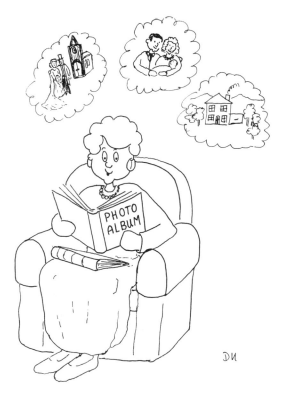

Figure 7 Life review using a photo album.

- It can be both pleasant and helpful to introduce a social element in the form of tea and cakes.
- Have plenty of materials available to prompt orientation and stimulate all senses, for example visual aids such as pictures and photographs, music, fabrics and objects to touch.
- It can often be more appropriate to make and gather your own materials, tailoring them to the past and present lives of the older people you seek to engage, rather than relying upon commercially available material. It will also be much cheaper to make your own materials.

Try to be realistic about the length of time you are able to maintain people's engagement. It is better to end a session sooner on a positive note, rather than trying to keep things going when your participants are losing concentration.

Helping to maintain daily living tasks in residential settings

Even when older people are admitted to residential care settings, some still wish to undertake personal activities for themselves, as well as engaging in activities such as making drinks, cooking, dusting and gardening. In residential settings, the emphasis should be upon maintenance of routine and the social aspects of involvement in daily living tasks within the requirements of local policy.

Leisure and recreation

This is an area where a person-centred approach really is essential. Continued engagement in aspects of life that we enjoyed in the past, or new interests and pastimes are essential for the wellbeing of all of us, wherever we live. Leisure and recreation with older people with memory loss must take into account the residual faculties of the individual, as well as what they enjoyed previously. An example would be that quizzes would not be successful with people with moderate to severe memory loss, even if they enjoyed them previously. Playful activities can be successfully used with people with severe dementia. This may extend to activities of childhood, such as the use of dolls and beach balls. This approach is skilled, but can be achieved by rehabilitation workers when provided with the appropriate training.

Delivering effective interventions in treatment and care settings: pointers for practice

- A person-centred approach must be promoted at all times. This means having a full knowledge of the person or people you are working with and the lives they have lived in the past.
- Not only must activities be relevant to the past and present lives of the people who are to be involved, they must also be pitched at the correct level so that memory impairment is not emphasised and the person is still able to achieve what is being suggested.

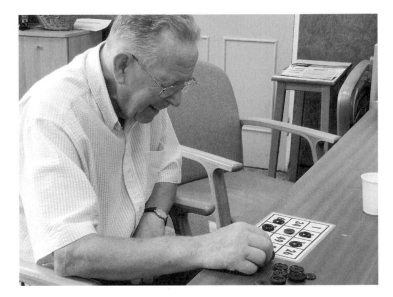

Figure 8 Activities must be relevant to the client's past and present life.

■ Not everyone enjoys group situations. This must be acknowledged in the planning of activities.

■ The importance of good communication with the client and their carers cannot be underestimated.

■ Good planning and co-working with other workers is essential. This includes giving full and accurate feedback to other staff.

■ You should try to help the person maintain their independence as much as possible, rather than trying to do everything for them. This can mean standing back at times and letting the person try to cope alone.

■ Family carers should be invited to continue to be involved, no matter where their relative is residing. Therefore, carers should continue to be involved when the person they have been caring for has entered residential care.

■ Conclusion

Rehabilitation workers are extremely well placed to support clients with memory loss and provide a range of interventions to assist them to cope in a range of different settings. An individual approach towards the needs of clients is an essential requirement and must underpin both general interactions as well as the undertaking of specific interventions.

■ Further reading

Buzan, T. (2003) *Master your Memory.* London, BBC Books. *This book describes a system to help improve memory which is based around visual imagery and associations.*

Memory loss

Carter, R. & Illman, J. (2005) *Use Your Brain to Beat Memory Loss: The Complete Guide to Understanding and Tackling Memory Loss.* London, Cassell Illustrated (pubs).

Mace, N.L. & Rabins, P.V. (2001) *The 36-hour Day: A Family Guide to Caring for Persons with Alzheimer Disease, Related Dementing Illnesses and Memory Loss in Later Life.* New York, John Hopkins Press Health Book. *This book provides a practical guide for families and carers of people with Alzheimer's and other other dementing illnesses.*

Oddy, R. (2003) *Promoting Mobility for People with Dementia.* London, Age Concern (pubs). *Examines a range of issues around dementia and memory loss, with a focus on the physical needs and environment including providing physical assistance to people with dementia.*

Mountain, G. (2004) *Occupational Therapy with Older People.* London, Whurr Publishers.

Perrin, T. & May, H. (2000) *Wellbeing in Dementia: An Occupational Approach for Therapists and Carers.* London, Churchill Livingstone.

Perrin, T. (ed.) (2004) *The New Culture of Therapeutic Activity with Older People.* Oxon, Speechmark.

Memory loss

Fatigue

Angela Knisely-Marpole & Hazel Mackey

Fatigue: what is it?

People often mean different things when they talk about fatigue, and the variety of meanings can be a source of confusion. The term *fatigue* can refer to a lack of energy, feeling exhausted after completing an activity, or an overwhelming desire to sleep. Fatigue is common. All of us have felt tired at some time in our lives, due to periods of stress, overwork, depression or lack of sleep. However, in some cases fatigue is both persistent and sufficiently severe to interfere with daily living activities. Chronic fatigue is distressing, and mental and physical stress adds to fatigue, creating a cycle that is difficult to break. This chapter will cover the various causes of fatigue and how you, as a rehabilitation worker, can help individuals to improve their quality of life, so enabling them to live a full and enjoyable life.

Persistent severe fatigue can be caused by many diseases and illnesses. Eighty per cent of people with multiple sclerosis complain of fatigue, and most say that fatigue is their most disabling symptom. Chronic fatigue syndrome (CFS) is gaining increasing recognition amongst health professionals as a cause of prolonged disability, particularly in young adults. Treatments for cancer, chemotherapy and radiotherapy are known to cause severe fatigue, as are malnutrition, anaemia, immobilisation, depression and pain. Post-operative fatigue is most often seen in people who have undergone thoracic or abdominal surgery. Usually, fatigue is worse during the first seven days following surgery, but may still be experienced after a month. Post-operative fatigue is linked to pain, psychosocial problems and limitation of activity. Additionally, fatigue is a well-known side effect of some medications, such as some anti-seizure medication and medication used to reduce anxiety. It is important to have a full assessment of the underlying cause of the fatigue in order to establish an appropriate rehabilitation programme. The assessment may involve medical practitioners, consultants or a multidisciplinary team, depending on the perception of the underlying cause.

Stop and think

A careful history is needed when individuals complain of fatigue. In rehabilitation the solution depends on the underlying problem. Read the following very different cases of two people presenting with fatigue and consider the ways in which the rehabilitation programmes may differ for the two cases.

Case 1. Rose is 37 years of age and has carcinoma of the right breast with widespread secondary growths. She is receiving palliative radiotherapy. She presents with exhaustion upon exertion and extreme shortness of breath when climbing the stairs.

Case 2. Derek is 63 years old. Following a road traffic accident, he suffered multiple fractures and spent a considerable period of time on bed-rest. He now feels weak and tired most of the time, and requires assistance to climb the stairs.

Both cases were referred to the rehabilitation team because of fatigue and difficulties climbing the stairs. Derek's fatigue was due to arm and leg weakness; an extra rail and a graded exercise programme might help. However, in Rose's case the problem was due to breathing difficulties and a stair rail will not provide the solution. Instead, the rehabilitation worker may be involved in adapting the environment so that Rose does not have to climb the stairs.

■ Symptoms of fatigue

Tiredness

Tiredness can vary enormously in its severity. In its strongest form it can totally disrupt the client's lifestyle because in every waking moment there is an intense yearning to sleep. Even though the client may sleep as much as sixteen hours a day, they still wake up feeling totally unrefreshed and want to go back to bed.

In a milder form, fatigue is like the after-effects of flu. The client feels relatively strong first thing in the morning, but by the afternoon their strength is at an end. The individual feels slightly below par for most of the time.

In an even milder form, tiredness becomes an inconvenience. The client may have to buy a louder alarm clock to make sure that they get up each morning, and they may find that by mid to late afternoon they are feeling low. By early evening they may have picked up again and feel reasonably alert until bedtime. This cycle of highs and lows is very common.

Weakness

Muscular weakness is often experienced, together with tiredness. When it is at its worst, actions such as standing, sitting and lifting light objects become extremely difficult and walking can be nearly impossible.

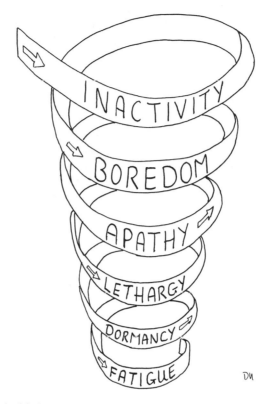

Figure 1 The spiral of fatigue.

In the more common milder form, the lack of physical strength makes life difficult in any number of small ways. Bottles and jars have to be opened by a helpful friend. Taps cannot be turned on and off, heavy pots and pans cannot be used, and even heavy clothing can sometimes present problems.

Pain

For many people, pain is one of the most distressing symptoms of fatigue. Pain may be constant, a dull background ache, or it may be intermittent and sharp, perhaps made worse by overactivity. The most common pain associated with fatigue is in the head, neck and/or back. It is very similar to a migraine headache and is often accompanied with extreme light sensitivity and nausea. Muscular pain is also very common, and may feel like a dull ache which escalates to a burning sensation after too much exercise.

Memory and concentration

Many people find that their ability to concentrate is impaired by fatigue. This in turn can affect memory and comprehension, all of which get noticeably worse when the individual is tired. Although these problems can be frustrating they are not usually signs of any permanent brain damage, and often lessen as general health improves.

Emotional difficulties

People with fatigue may experience depression and anxiety. Indeed, it can be very hard to sort out whether the symptoms of lethargy, muscle pain and poor concentration are due to depression or fatigue. Mood swings are widely recognised in cases of extreme fatigue and feelings of anger, loss and fear are common.

Breathing difficulties

Fatigue and difficult or laboured breathing often go together. Individuals describe their symptoms as feeling short of breath, not getting enough air, chest tightness and finding it difficult to move air.

■ The physiology of fatigue

People become fatigued for a variety of reasons. It may be that their illness makes moving very difficult; that their muscles are weak; or that they have an illness in which enduring fatigue is a symptom. Some people become fatigued for a different reason: lack of exercise and activity. Whatever the reason, it is important to tackle the issues involved before they result in the fatigue cycle (Figure 2).

If you went to bed for three weeks and did not get up or do any exercise, apart from using a bedpan and feeding yourself, certain changes would occur in your body, even if you were super fit to start with. When you eventually did get out of bed the following changes would have occurred in your body:

- Reduction in muscle strength.
- Reduced efficiency in heart functioning.
- Reduced will to exercise or move.
- Lowering in mood.

If this happens with just three weeks of bed-rest, imagine what would happen if you had been in bed for three months.

■ How to assist in the prevention of fatigue

You, as a rehabilitation worker, can do a lot to help prevent deconditioning and fatigue: it is easier to prevent it than to cure it. Try and encourage your clients to do some gentle movements themselves: it may just be rolling their shoulders back and forwards. The best way is to set a daily exercise plan for them to do.

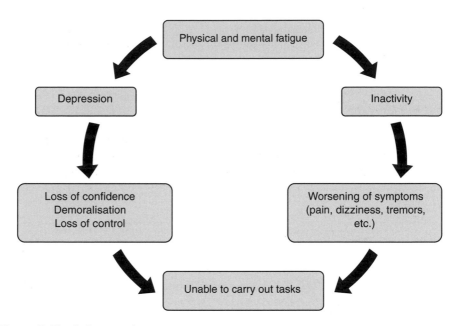

Figure 2 The fatigue cycle.

This does not need to be done all at once but can be split up into four or five sessions throughout the day. For example each of the following exercises to be done twice:

▪ Circling your feet.
▪ Pull your toes up and push your feet down.
▪ Tighten your thigh muscles and try to lift your heel off the bed.
▪ Bend your knee and straighten it.
▪ Move your leg out to the side and bring it back again.
▪ Roll your knees in and out.

These last three can be made easier by putting a tray under the heel to make a slippery surface.

▪ Pull your tummy in and hold it while breathing in and out.
▪ Sit on the side of the bed or a chair and slowly turn to look left and right.
▪ Roll your shoulders forwards and back.
▪ Lift your arms up, one at a time forwards and sideways.
▪ Reach behind the back and behind the neck.
▪ Bend and straighten your elbows.
▪ Keep your elbows bent at right angles, turn your palms up and down.
▪ Bend and straighten your wrist.
▪ Make a fist.

These can be included in activities of daily living: roll your shoulders before you get dressed, then use putting on a jumper for the exercise of lifting your arms up.

Fatigue

▪ Rehabilitation and fatigue

The solution depends on a thorough history being taken in order to identify the underlying problem. The client's needs will vary depending on his or her circumstances, and any rehabilitation programme will need to be customised. Rehabilitation workers can:

- Help people to recognise their condition.
- Provide positive encouragement by acknowledging limitations yet offering solutions.
- Provide support through active listening.
- Explore emotional stressors and facilities for support.
- Work with individuals to identify their current stamina levels and what type of rehabilitation programme is most suitable for them.

Balancing rest and activity

This is one of the most important messages that a rehabilitation worker needs to give to an individual with chronic fatigue difficulties. Too many people with chronic fatigue difficulties live on a rollercoaster ride of alternating bursts of activity with periods of doing nothing. They do too much one day, feel much worse as a result, and are then able to do much less for the next day or two. After resting they feel better and immediately try to catch up, do too much, and feel worse again.

Pacing

Pacing is a way of avoiding this problem. It means alternating limited time periods of activity, both physical and mental, with periods of good quality rest. Mental activity can be as tiring as physical activity, so activities such as sitting and watching television do not count as real rest. The aim should be for the client to stop doing an activity before getting exhausted, even if it means leaving something unfinished.

Each person will need to work out their own personalised programme of rest and activity. One way you may be able to help them to do this is to ask them to complete an activity diary for a few weeks. In this diary, all activities, timings, symptoms and feelings should be recorded. The simplest diary consists of a page a day with columns for time, activity, physical feelings and emotional feelings.

The diary will help you to sit with the person and plan out a programme of balanced rest and activity. When you discuss the diary entries with the client, you should be able to identify patterns, such as the 'rollercoaster' of doing too much, followed by doing too little. You will have a much better idea of what the right amount of activity is for the person, and you can then advise on a structure to the day, with targets set and spread out across the week. Consistency is vital, even if it means doing less at one point in the day in order to spread the energy levels over a longer period.

Prioritisation

When planning the programme, it is important to include the things that the person gains pleasure and satisfaction from. It may be useful to think in terms of energy supply as a limited budget. The client may have to prioritise the activities that are most important to them, or that they are able to do, and avoid doing others within their 'energy budget'. It is important to remember that you cannot make these choices for other people. Often, as a rehabilitation worker, we assume the client will want to concentrate on personal and domestic living skills, when they would rather use their energy to walk their dog, or go with friends to the local coffee shop.

■ Teaching relaxation techniques

The word *relaxation* can mean different things to different people. What we mean by relaxation techniques during a rehabilitation programme is learning the activities, skills and methods which let go of physical tension in the muscles. Deep physical relaxation and calm breathing will help the person with fatigue, as tensed up muscles use up energy that could be used elsewhere. It takes time and practice to learn how to do this and often, as a rehabilitation worker, you will be involved in teaching simple relaxation techniques.

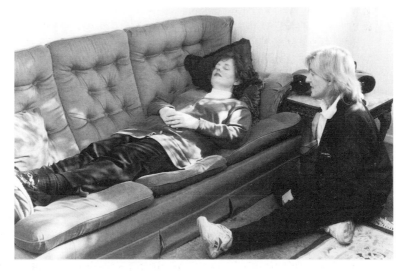

Figure 3 Rehabilitation worker helping a client to relax.

Fatigue

> **Box 1   A simple relaxation technique**
>
> Choose a time and place when you know you will not be disturbed. Encourage the person to sit or lie in a comfortable position, with support to the neck and arms.
> Relax your muscles
> Some people find that if they first tighten up the part they want to relax it helps them to recognise the difference between tension and relaxation. You can guide the person through the muscle groups of the body, encourage them to let the tension go, and leave the body feeling loose and heavy.
> Relax your breathing
> Teaching good breathing techniques and practising them regularly will encourage the person to feel less anxious. The aim should be to use all the lung capacity, letting the ribs and diaphragm do the work rather than just the top of the chest.
> Relax your mind
> Relaxation time is not for thinking about the shopping, or what to prepare for the next meal. It is important that the individual switches off from anxious thoughts and thinks about something peaceful and happy instead. You can help by talking through a peaceful scene or setting, concentrating on the details of sight, sound and smell. After relaxation allow the person time to stretch and gradually return to their normal state.

Graded activity

Once you have helped the individual to adjust to a level of physical and mental activity that they can manage each day, you may move them onto the next stage by gradually increasing their activities. 'Little and often' usually works well. The purpose of graded activity is to build the client up to a sustained and consistent level of activity on a daily basis.

Be careful that the client does not attempt to do too much too soon. People who have previously been very fit often expect to be able to return to their previous levels of activity quickly. However, if their body has lost condition, they will take some time to build up to their previous levels of fitness. There is also a risk that they will attempt to do too much when they are going through a good phase, to catch up on what they could not do when they were very weak. As a result, it is very important to be disciplined about incorporating rests into the graded activity, regardless of the symptoms.

Advise the individual to build appropriate periods of activity and rest into their pacing programme. If you are uncertain of where to start, ask a physio-therapist to work out a physical exercise programme for you to follow. Some people find it beneficial if one week they concentrate on a small increase in some physical activity and the next week on some mental or social activity (while maintaining the physical increase). It is important not to expect the individual to increase all of their activities simultaneously. Set realistic targets by talking with the individual, and evaluate them regularly. It is a good idea to focus on the client's particular areas of difficulty, or activities they have been avoiding.

The goals of the activity programme should be clear, specific and manageable (Cox, 2000). For example:

(1) To get out of bed at 8 AM every day.
(2) To go to the supermarket once a week.
(3) To walk for 15 minutes, three times per day.
(4) To rest for thirty minutes, four times per day.
(5) To have a friend visit twice a week.

Stop and think

Have you have ever exercised regularly, for example three or more times per week, whether it was in the gym, playing sport or jogging?
If you were reasonably fit and you hurt your back, how would you ease yourself back into regular activity?
What do you think would happen if you started strenuous exercise again before your injury had healed itself?

Energy conservation

If the individual continues to do things in the same way as they did before they were ill, they are likely to hit obstacles, become frustrated and give up completely on some tasks. As a rehabilitation worker one of your main roles is to advise on how to adapt techniques or the environment in order to encourage the successful participation in activity. You may be able to advise on pieces of equipment that would make the individual's life easier, or on general techniques.

Energy conservation is using the least amount of energy in the most efficient way to do a good job. There is no one way of doing a task that will be acceptable to all people. Before commencing a task, the individual needs to decide whether:

■ It needs to be done.
■ It can be given to someone else to do.
■ It can be made easier.

There are four ways of achieving energy conservation.

(1) **Elimination:** establishing whether all or part of an activity can be eliminated. For example by cooking a meal in the same dish in which it is to be served.
(2) **Changing the order:** energy can be conserved by carrying out activities in a different order, for example putting all lower garments over the feet, then standing to pull up, rather than standing to pull up each separate item.
(3) **Combining:** planning ahead can save energy, for example by collecting all articles together before starting a task, or planning for the next day's dressing when undressing, by keeping clothes within easy reach and leaving them in the order they are to be put on.

Fatigue

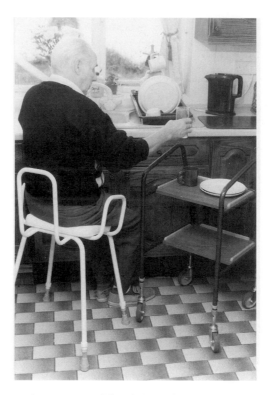

Figure 4 Client conserving energy whilst doing other activities.

(4) **Simplification:** usually there are ways of making each task easier to do, for example using convenience items, such as an electric tin opener, or ready-made meals, or quilts rather than blankets.

Memory cues

As a rehabilitation worker, there is advice you can give to the individual to help cue memory and to maintain cognitive function. More information is available in the previous chapter on Memory loss, in this book. The client should be encouraged to cut down on what they are trying to remember by using lists and notes which are carefully stored. Try to identify times when the client is more mentally alert and plan to do the more draining mental tasks then. Routines should be encouraged, such as always putting the house keys in the same place immediately after use. When concentration is needed distractions like noise from the radio or television should be cut out. To a degree, mental activity should be treated in the same way as physical activity. The brain needs as much exercise as the body. The individual should be encouraged to continue with mentally stimulating activities, such as reading or crossword puzzles, even if they find them difficult at first. Once again pacing is important.

Stop and think   Making life easier

Think about the positioning of furniture and equipment around your home, are they in the most labour-saving place?
Where is your cupboard containing the tea or coffee in relation to the mugs and the kettle?
Are the containers with the ingredients next to the kettle or are they in a high cupboard? In which case do you have to reach up, and move the containers to the work surface?
Is the soap powder kept near the washing machine or is it over the other side of the room?
Where do you keep the toiletries that you use in the bathroom? Are they on the washbasin or close to it, or are they on a shelf on the other side of the room?
How high are the coat hooks in the hall? Do you have to lift your arms above shoulder height to hang your coat up?

■ Fatigue and relationships

The physical and emotional toll of fatigue can put a great deal of strain on relationships between the client and their friends, family and work colleagues. Fatigue is often associated with depression, which reduces the ability and desire of the client to socialise. The physical burden of fatigue can mean that the client may only be able to spend very short periods of time socialising before they become tired again. It is easy to underestimate the amount of energy that socialising requires. Therefore, it is important to manage the social contact and interactions of the client. Social contact can be incorporated into the graded activities of the client. In the early phases of graded activity it is important to ensure that social contact is time limited, it takes place in a comfortable environment for the client, and periods of rest are built in afterwards.

Families and friends can find it difficult to fully appreciate the impact of fatigue. It is valuable to explain to them that the client only has a limited 'budget' of energy, and be clear about the need for the client to be able to stop whenever they need to, and set clear time limits around the interaction. See Section 4: Working with clients and carers to enable independence, for more information about carer support.

■ Conclusion

It is clear that chronic fatigue has the potential to affect virtually every aspect of an individual's life. Your challenge as a rehabilitation worker is to support the individual to maintain an optimum level of independence. This chapter has outlined the areas in which practical advice, rehabilitation programmes

Fatigue

and adaptive strategies may help. You play an important role as assessor, educator and adviser, and your knowledge of other support agencies can open up additional channels of support and encouragement to individuals and families learning to cope with fatigue.

■ Further reading

Burgess, M. & Chalder, T. (2005) *Overcoming Chronic Fatigue*. Constable & Robinson. *A guide that will help sufferers to learn how to break free from the vicious cycle of fatigue.*

Chalder, T. (1995) *Coping with Chronic Fatigue (overcoming common problems)*. London, Sheldon Press. *A self-help book which encourages fatigue sufferers to assess their own level of fatigue, discusses many everyday and common problems and offers practical solutions.*

Cox, D.L. (2000) *Occupational Therapy and Chronic Fatigue Syndrome*. London, Whurr. *Provides a great deal of information specifically about chronic fatigue syndrome, but also covers a range of treatment approaches which may be useful for other sources of fatigue.*

Fatigue and arthritis http://www.orthop.washington.edu/arthritis/living/fatigue/01

Fatigue in cancer http://www.cancersupportivecare.com/fatigue.html

HIV and AIDS www.aidsinfonet.org

National MS Society http://www.nationalmssociety.org/Sourcebook-Fatigue.asp

Payne, R. (2000) *Relaxation Techniques: A Practical Handbook for the Health Care Professional*. Edinburgh, Churchill Livingstone. *This book contains a practical introduction to 17 different relaxation techniques.*

Sharpe, M. & Wilkes, D. (2002) ABC of psychological medicine. *British Medical Journal*, **325**, 480–3 (31 August) also on bmj.com

Fatigue

Palliative care

Peter L. Hudson & Bob Spall

Introduction

This chapter focuses on key aspects of care delivery for the client who requires palliative care. While the focus of this chapter will be on home-based care delivery, much of the information will still be relevant for in-patient or residential care facilities for older people.

To exemplify several key points in this chapter the following case study will be referred to.

Case study   Mick (see Case study 4, p. 65)

Mick is a former miner who stopped working when the pits closed in the early 1990s. He stopped smoking two years ago. He is 55 and has chronic emphysema, but lives in a three-storey terraced house, which is at the top of a steep hill. He has difficulty getting a loud enough voice to talk to people. His wife, Esther, is a good support, but worries about his wheezing and inability to sleep. She is also concerned about his frequent coughing or choking during eating or drinking.

What is palliative care?

Palliative care is support that is offered to people who have a life-threatening illness that is not curable. The terms '*palliative*' and '*hospice care*' are now commonly used interchangeably. While many people currently receive palliative care because they are imminently dying, palliative care is not limited to this end stage of an illness. The World Health Organization and many palliative care institutions emphasise several core elements associated with palliative care:

(1) Care is focused on promoting physical, social, psychological and spiritual wellbeing.
(2) Impeccable symptom management is required.
(3) Support is offered not only to the client but also to his/her family.
(4) Care should be provided in accordance with needs and not be limited to the final stages of the illness.
(5) Bereavement support should be available.
(6) Palliative care clients and their families should have access to a multidisciplinary team.
(7) Where possible, access to 24-hour advice should be offered.
(8) Care should be provided in an environment chosen by the client.

◾ Who can receive palliative care?

Many people who receive palliative care have advanced cancer. However, palliative care should also be available to people with other life-threatening illnesses such as HIV/AIDS, some neuro-degenerative disorders (for example amyotrophic lateral sclerosis), and for people with advanced organ failure (for example Alzheimer's disease, lung disease).

Mick might be eligible for palliative care as he has significant lung disease, the symptoms of which may shorten his lifespan. However, a palliative care specialist or a doctor should confirm whether a client may meet the criteria for palliative care.

Stop and think   Does the client I'm caring for require palliative care?

If you believe that your client has a life-threatening illness and is not receiving palliative care, contact the client's registered nurse or doctor to confirm their eligibility.

◾ Where is palliative care offered?

Theoretically, palliative care should be available in a setting chosen by the client. If, for example, a palliative care client wants to remain at home, then appropriate resources should be put in place to support him or her. Many hospitals have access to health professionals with palliative care skills and most areas have designated palliative care beds either within general hospitals or via specific palliative care units, sometimes referred to as hospices. Increasingly, there has been a request for people within residential aged care facilities to be able to access suitably qualified palliative care health professionals.

Palliative care

If Mick is eligible for palliative care because his lung disease is so bad, he should be able to determine whether he would prefer to stay at home to receive care.

■ What is a multidisciplinary palliative care team?

Given the often complex needs associated with an incurable illness, access to a multidisciplinary team is important. While the specific make up of the team may vary, a typical team may comprise: registered nurse, doctor, social worker, volunteer, psychologist, pastoral care worker or chaplain, bereavement counsellor, rehabilitation worker and music/complementary therapist.

In the home the client's general practitioner (GP) is usually the person responsible for overseeing the medical care. Ideally, the registered nurse and other health care professionals work together in a coordinated way.

Mick may not need to access all the different members of the palliative care team. However, the range of services is important because needs may vary from client to client. If the rehabilitation worker believes that Mick may benefit from a volunteer or pastoral care worker, for example, the rehabilitation worker should liaise with the registered nurse or case manager.

Stop and think   Palliative care clients should have access to a multidisciplinary team.

Remember that no single health discipline or individual can adequately meet the needs of palliative care clients. A multidisciplinary team that works together in a supportive and coordinated way is the optimal way to provide best care.

■ Core skills and awareness for the rehabilitation worker

Caring for a client with a palliative illness can be quite challenging, given the physical, psychosocial and spiritual issues associated with confronting death and dying. While many skills and awareness of various issues are required, here are a few key areas for the rehabilitation worker to consider.

Communication skills

Optimal palliative care depends on good communication skills. Research studies have concluded the following:

(1) Expressing empathy and listening actively improves psychological adjustment.
(2) Comprehensive information provision about what to expect in the future promotes psychological wellbeing.

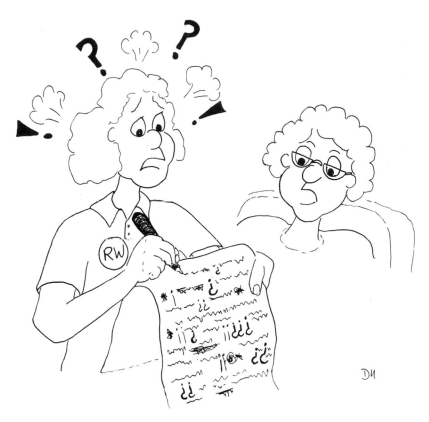

Figure 1 Rehabilitation worker struggling to make sense of a wide range of issues the client is talking about.

(3) An opportunity to discuss feelings with a health professional reduces psychosocial distress.

(4) Where pertinent, referral to health professionals who specialise in the management of psychosocial distress can have favourable outcomes.

(Adapted from National Health and Medical Research Council, Australia, 2003).

The following skills should be considered in any consultation with a palliative care client.

Supportive communication

■ Ask the person if he/she would like someone to be with him/her during the discussion.

■ Show regard and concern for the person by using appropriate verbal and non-verbal behaviour, including sitting attentively and facilitating the person's responses.

■ Use verbal and non-verbal behaviours which are appropriate to the person's age and cultural background.

■ Express empathy and listen actively.

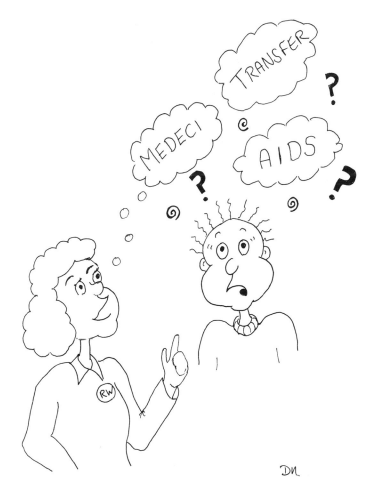

Figure 2 Rehabilitation worker using jargon and perplexing the client.

- Allow and encourage the person to express his/her feelings, such as crying, talking about concerns, fears, anger or anxieties.
- Handle embarrassing or disturbing topics directly and sensitively.

Delivering information in plain English

- Assess the person's understanding before providing additional information.
- Explain difficult terms and avoid medical jargon.
- Use explicit categorisation (provide information clearly grouped into specific topics).

Strategies to aid recall and understanding

- Actively encourage questions and seek understanding.
- Make use of simple diagrams and pictures where appropriate.
- Repeat and summarise important information.

■ Reinforce important information by using one or more of the following aids:
  ▫ writing down relevant information
  ▫ taping the consultation as needed and if wanted
■ Send a summary letter as follow-up.

Ongoing support

■ Assess the person's level of family and social support.
■ Provide the names and contact details of relevant persons or organisations to enable the person to obtain more information.
■ Refer to a specialist nurse or other professional for support as required.

(Source: adapted from Psychosocial clinical practice guidelines: providing information, support and counselling for women with breast cancer. Cited in National Health and Medical Research Council, Australia 2003)

Being clear about your responsibilities

It is important that you are clear about your specific role and responsibilities. This will help determine what tasks are relevant to the care of the palliative care client. If you are unsure please liaise with your manager.

Knowing when to refer to a health professional

Sometimes it can be particularly hard knowing when to refer to another health professional. Also, some palliative care clients build up a very good rapport with the rehabilitation worker and may prefer his/her input or advice to that of others in the team. This is illustrated by a comment of an American health care professional who had cancer and was on the receiving end of care for nearly five years before he died in the mid-1990s: 'I've had more pleasant conversations that were emotionally or psychologically healing with those people (nursing assistants) than I have had with the highest multi-degree medical professional' (Schmele, 1995).

It is important, however, to refer to a doctor or senior nurse if:

■ Physical symptoms are not controlled.
■ Psychological distress seems apparent.
■ Family members are demonstrating that they are finding it very difficult to cope.
■ The client is asking questions and you do not have the relevant training/knowledge to allow you to provide an informed response.

Being aware of the potential impact of your own thoughts about death and dying

Some health professionals may have a tendency to avoid personal issues concerning death and dying. They may put off making a will because they don't

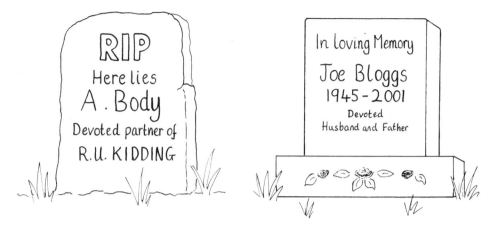

Figure 3 Perceptions of mortality.

want to have to discuss what should happen after their death, or may have an underlying superstition that it would be tempting fate. When asked if they would complete a form detailing their wishes regarding their own funeral arrangements (for example cremation or burial), some would prefer not to or would only see it as appropriate when they are much older. It may be assumed that death is a long way off so it is unnecessary to think about it as yet. To talk or think about death may be viewed as morbid, and this may be partly culturally determined. This kind of avoidance may make it difficult for staff to provide emotional care for palliative care clients.

In order to help get alongside and empathise with clients needing palliative care, it is helpful for rehabilitation workers to give some consideration to their own mortality. See the Stop and think box for some useful questions to ask. You may find it helpful to share your thoughts on these questions with a colleague.

Stop and think   Personal awareness of mortality

Reflect on the following questions:

- Do you fear dying before achieving specific goals in your life?
- If you had a serious illness and were told that you would die in about six months, what would you do with your life?
- Do you have fears about the process of dying, for example dependency, indignity?
- Think of three words that you associate with death.
- What does death mean to you? (for example death is 'final', belief in after-life).
- If you had a gravestone after you died, what epitaph would you like on it?

To illustrate the possible effect of a worker's views, imagine that a rehabilitation worker associated the following words with death: 'cheated', 'frightened' and 'unacceptable'. Then suppose that a particular palliative care client held similar views about death. One outcome might be that the rehabilitation worker can empathise with the client, but alternatively, entering into discussion with the client may be difficult because of being reminded of one's own anxieties and concerns. An extreme, but possible, effect might be a tendency to avoid the client. The important thing in this kind of scenario is to be aware of these thoughts and feelings and be able to discuss their possible impact on work with clients, for example in a supervision forum.

It is also important not to make assumptions about how an individual client may be feeling, for instance just because someone is religious, it doesn't necessarily mean that they are coping well all the time. It may be tempting to think, for example, that 'if I were in this client's situation I would be much more upset and angry'. It could be that by the time you are caring for the client, he/she has already worked through some of these emotions, or that the only way the client can cope is to block out or deny the full implications of being seriously ill.

Knowing when to seek help for the rehabilitation worker

It is also important that rehabilitation workers recognise that they may need some help themselves, in order to better deal with the role of supporting a palliative care client. In such circumstances the rehabilitation worker should speak with his/her manager or palliative care health professional (for example nurse or social worker). See Section 4: Teamworking and supervision for more information on how to obtain your own support needs.

The impact of receiving a palliative diagnosis

In order to be better equipped to care for the palliative client, rehabilitation workers should familiarise themselves with common issues that confront clients and their families when palliative care is required.

The impact on the client

When people are informed that they have a life-threatening illness that is probably not curable, they usually find this devastating. Many people worry about when they might die and how this will affect their family. Emotions will vary, but people commonly experience a mix of anger, frustration and shock. They may be thinking 'Why me?' and attribute blame to someone, or feel that they are being punished and it is too early to die. The important thing to note is that there is no 'normal' or correct way for people to react. However, if you perceive that a client is significantly distressed, anxious or depressed please seek his/her permission to liaise with an appropriate health professional.

The impact of palliative care on the family

Research has clearly shown that when a person is diagnosed with an incurable illness this news has a major impact on the family unit. Family members may worry about whether their relative will experience pain and how he/she will cope with such disturbing problems. Typically, family members want to know how to provide comfort to their relative, how to provide emotional support and how to care for themselves.

▪ Family-centred palliative care

Why is family-centred care important?

Family-centred care means that support should be provided not only to the client but also to his/her family. Family, in this context, refers to those people, whether they are relatives or friends, who are considered to be key people in the client's life. Research has also shown that many family members who take on a caregiving role may be confronted with negative psychosocial implications. For example, some family caregivers may become socially isolated, have their finances affected and suffer some degree of psychological discomfort. If the family is better supported there is less likelihood of negative outcomes. Some caregivers actually find the experience rewarding, even though it is very challenging. The client may also feel comforted knowing that their relatives or friends are also receiving comprehensive guidance and support. Another observation that highlights the importance of family-centred care is that many of the complaints made by relatives (to health professionals) following a client's death seem to relate to issues of poor communication.

Esther, Mick's wife, would require information about what palliative care is and what support might be available.

What are the challenges of providing family-centred palliative care?

Providing support to families is not without its challenges. Here are some examples of common issues that confront health professionals.

- **Family dynamic challenges:** some families do not communicate well. When there is disharmony in families and different needs it makes it very difficult for the rehabilitation worker to meet family needs. For example, if there are rifts in families, arrangements may have to be made so that certain family members never visit at the same time. If the client is on a ward there may be arguments between different family members and staff about who should be informed first about any deterioration in the client's condition. The husband of one of the author's clients was dying in a hospice and the children from his first marriage, whom he had not seen for 30 years, visited. This caused a lot of distress for the various parties involved.
- **Communication process challenges:** concentration is impaired when we are stressed, and this may make assessing family needs difficult, as families

may not be able to absorb information or adequately express their needs. It is also very hard to prepare and support families if there is open denial of the disease progression. Furthermore, for many lay people, talking about death is extremely difficult. Sometimes collusion may occur, for example staff and family members are aware of the seriousness of the client's condition, but the client has not been told. This poses particular difficulties for open communication. Also, we know that most family caregivers do not want to bother health care professionals and view their own needs as secondary to those of the patient. An issue that staff do not seem to ask about routinely relates to the client's sexuality or sexual needs. When asked, clients often refer to a need for intimacy and closeness and regard this as more important than sexual intercourse.

▪ **Health system challenges:** many health professionals do not receive formal tuition on how to assess family needs. Also, resources may be so compromised that it is difficult for palliative care services to be able to comprehensively assess needs and ensure the continuity of care.

What are the key strategies for providing family-centred palliative care?

▪ **Determine key family members:** with limited resources it may be very difficult to comprehensively meet the supportive care needs of all family members and significant friends. Therefore, start with the primary family caregivers. Ask the clients who they regard as the key people in their life. Sometimes staff may need to advocate for the needs of the most significant family members, as other relatives (who may not have been involved much in the client's care) might try to take over and dictate what should happen.

▪ **Consider the need for a structured family meeting:** well-conducted family meetings, facilitated by a suitably qualified health professional can be a useful means of assessing client and family needs.

▪ **Provide written information to complement verbal information:** verbal guidance alone is not enough. The strategic administration of key written resources is vital. Many clients and families will not retain information that is only provided via the spoken word.

▪ **If respite services are available these should be offered.**

▪ **Document family issues:** key family member needs must be included alongside the client's needs in documented and evaluated care plans.

▪ **Assess the family's satisfaction with care delivery:** regular assessment of family needs is vital as needs change from day to day.

▪ **Provide honest answers:** answering questions related to death and dying is not particularly straightforward. Research has consistently identified, however, that families of palliative care clients want honest answers.

▪ **Involve members of the multidisciplinary team:** no sole practitioner, or indeed discipline is able to meet all the needs of palliative care families.

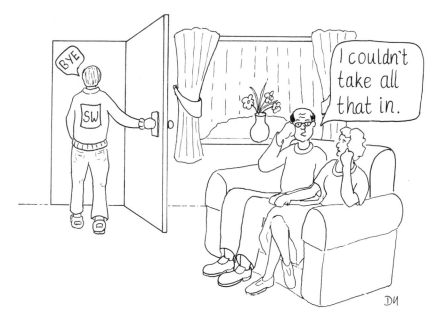

Figure 4 Social worker overwhelming the family with information.

■ How do clients and families cope?

There is a great degree of variability in terms of how clients and families cope. People respond to potentially stressful circumstances in different ways and the way they cope may vary from day to day. Some people will be more expressive about their emotions and others may appear less forthcoming. It is important to note that there is no universally accepted correct way to cope. So the strategies one person employs may not be beneficial for the next person and vice versa.

It shouldn't be assumed that emotional distress is inevitable and normal and therefore does not require attention. A key role of rehabilitation workers is to inform their manager, or the client's nurse or doctor if they perceive that a client or family member is finding it so difficult to cope that it is negatively affecting their psychological wellbeing. Some signs that a client may be distressed include:

- Continuing feelings of hopelessness and despair.
- Feelings of worthlessness, for example guilt about being ill and a burden to others.
- Suicidal thoughts, especially if the client has a specific plan worked out.
- Anxiety and apprehension as indicated, for example, by an inability to relax, tension headaches or panic feelings (that is intense fear associated with physical discomfort such as palpitations).
- Appearing anxious and worried when talking about experience of deaths in family members or friends.
- Very concerned about other difficulties, for example health of other family members.

Palliative care

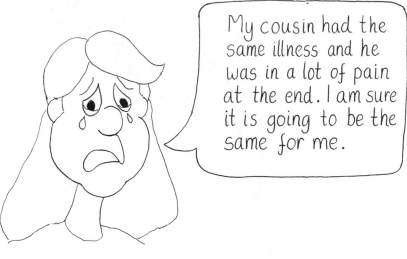

Figure 5 Negative assumptions about illness and dying.

■ Not fully understanding his/her illness and making false, negative assumptions, for example that symptoms will worsen and be less treatable as death approaches.

■ Strong regret about unfulfilled goals in life, or guilt about things he/she has done.

■ Frequent reference to a long-standing estrangement in the family.

■ Struggling to attribute meaning to, or make sense of his/her life.

Some of the above could also be indications of distress in family members. Other causes for concern in family members include: showing a high level of strain in connection with caregiving; deterioration in their own health; interpersonal problems in the family, which in turn might limit the amount of support available for caregiving; high anxiety about how they will cope when the client dies; and a high level of dissatisfaction and anger with the client's current care from professional staff, which is out of proportion to any problems in the actual quality of care. The latter may be part of what is referred to as anticipatory grief, in which the family member is experiencing a range of emotions before the client has died (in this case, anger and maybe guilt).

A useful question for Mick and Esther is: 'What are your biggest concerns at the moment?' This will help determine the key issues and who within the multidisciplinary team might be best to assist.

■ Common ethical and legal issues

Ethical and legal issues sometimes arise when providing palliative care. While it is not your role to manage these issues, if they arise it is vital that you are aware of them so that you can refer on to the appropriate health professional. Furthermore, the client or family may raise these issues with you, so being prepared for these matters is useful. The usual issues around client confidentiality also apply. Medical information about the client should only be given to those authorised to receive it. The client's care manager should have access to these details.

Issues of prognosis and truth telling

Collusion was referred to earlier (under Communication process challenges). Some family caregivers worry about their relative knowing the implications of his/her diagnosis. It is not uncommon for family members to say: 'Please don't tell her she has a life-threatening illness, she won't cope with that news' (see Figure 6). In such circumstances it is important to check carefully the client's understanding of her condition. Sometimes she may 'know' or suspect what is wrong and that it is serious, even if a formal explanation has not been given. In most situations suitably qualified health professionals can address this issue with relatives by pointing out that many people want an opportunity to pre-pare for their death and that there is a cost associated with such collusion, for example the client having no opportunity to put affairs in order or to say goodbye to close family members. Family caregivers can also be advised that clients have a right to information about their medical condition and if they are inappropriately denied being told that they have a life-threatening illness, then this is unethical. Given the importance of having accurate medical informa-tion, a doctor or nurse should be involved in such discussions with clients and relatives.

Decision making when the client is no longer competent

Some clients choose to arrange for a friend or family member to be legally responsible for them in case their decision making becomes impaired. Increas-ingly, clients are being encouraged to document their health care wishes in advance.

Desire to die statements

Some clients with advanced disease make desire to die statements such as 'I wish it could all end today'. The rehabilitation worker should inform the relevant health professional about such comments, as further exploration of the reason behind such statements should be initiated.

■ Spiritual and cultural care

In most situations clients will at some point explore spiritual or existential impli-cations associated with confronting their life-threatening illness. Spirituality is

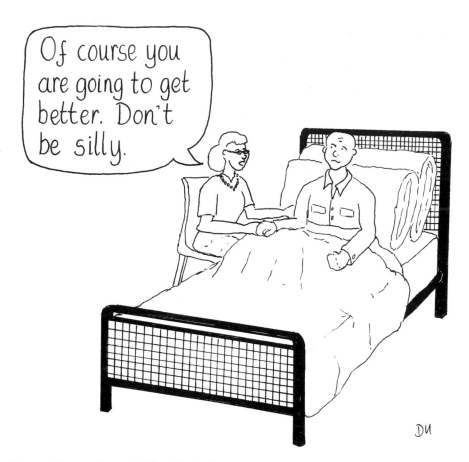

Figure 6 Prognosis and telling the truth.

not necessarily specifically associated with religious practices and usually relates to matters about life's meaning, values and belief systems. The client and family caregiver should be offered access to a chaplain/pastoral care worker to explore spiritual issues, although any member of the team should be prepared to listen to a client or family member who wants to talk about spiritual matters.

We all have some practices and beliefs in our lives that stem from our cultural backgrounds. Palliative care clients and their family caregivers should be provided with culturally specific care. It is inappropriate to assume that because a person originally came from another country that they will act in a certain way. A typical question that should be asked is 'Are there any cultural or religious issues that we need to be aware of in order to provide optimal care?' If a client or family caregiver does not understand English and important health care discussion needs to occur, then a suitably qualified interpreter service should be arranged.

■ What constitutes a good death?

While people may differ from time to time in what they consider to be the optimal attributes of a good death, there are some main features that most people strive for. They include:

- To know when death is coming, and to understand what can be expected.
- To be able to maintain a sense of control.
- To be afforded dignity and privacy.
- To have control over pain relief and other symptoms.
- To have choice over where death occurs (at home or elsewhere).
- To have access to information and excellent health care.
- To have access to spiritual and emotional support as required.
- To have access to palliative care.
- To have control over who is present and who shares the end.
- To be able to issue advance directives which ensure wishes are respected.
- To have time to say goodbye.
- To not have life inappropriately prolonged.

(Adapted from Hockley & Clark, 2002.)

The term 'appropriate death' has also been used, and refers to a style of dying that is adaptive and unique to each specific person. This will relate, for example, to personality and how people have coped with previous life crises. It could be argued that people die in the same way that they live. People are likely to make sense of the experience of dying in the light of previous life patterns, for example one person may view it as 'a resignation' while another may view it as 'a challenge' (Samarel, cited in Wass & Neimeyer, 1995).

A health professional with relevant experience should ask Mick and Esther if they have particular concerns or wishes in relation to end of life care.

Care for the client and family when death appears imminent

Knowing when a client may be approaching imminent death can be difficult. Recognising when a client with cancer is imminently dying is usually easier to determine than for clients with other life-threatening illness. Families need to be made aware that for some clients death may occur more quickly than expected; for others, the dying process may be more prolonged than expected. However, immediately before death (within hours to days) several of the following symptoms and signs may be present:

- Extremities become cold due to lack of blood flow.
- Changes in respiratory patterns (Cheyne-Stokes breathing).
- Not responding to verbal and/or physical stimuli.
- Uncharacteristic or recent restlessness and agitation.
- Retained upper airway secretions.
- Rapid pulse or low blood pressure.

(Australian Government Department of Health and Ageing, 2004.)

Palliative care

If the rehabilitation worker notices any of the above signs then the relevant health professional should be contacted.

Esther should then be advised if Mick appears to be imminently dying, and have an opportunity to discuss the implications of this.

Care following a client's death

Confirming that death has occurred

Some rehabilitation workers may be in a situation where a client dies when they are providing care. While a rehabilitation worker cannot legally pronounce death, being aware of the following signs is important, particularly so that appropriate information can be given over the phone to a health professional if the death has occurred at home.

Esther may want to be informed about these specific signs in advance, to help her prepare for Mick's death but the information should not be forced upon her.

The signs of death include:

- Absence of pulse.
- Cessation of breathing.
- Pupils fixed and dilated.
- Body becomes pale.
- Body temperature decreases.
- Muscles and sphincters relax.
- Urine and faeces may be released.
- Eyes may remain open.
- Jaw may fall open.
- Trickling of fluids internally can be heard.

(Source: Adapted from Ferris et al. 2003, p. 609)

If death has occurred, advise family members that there is no rush. Advise them that it is acceptable to embrace, kiss, hold hands and talk to their relative. If death has occurred at home then telephone a registered nurse and/or doctor to arrange for medical confirmation of the death. The funeral company should also be notified. Some people choose to have their deceased relative bathed and redressed. Some carers like to dress their relative in favourite clothing. Depending on the precise role and skill level, the rehabilitation worker may be involved in this aspect of care.

Bereavement support

Ideally, if a client has been receiving palliative care then some bereavement support should be available. The rehabilitation worker should advise the family as to what is available and how to access the support.

Esther should be informed that it is normal to experience a range of emotions and she may even feel physically unwell. She should also be informed that there is no exact timeframe for when the emotional impact of grief subsides. It may

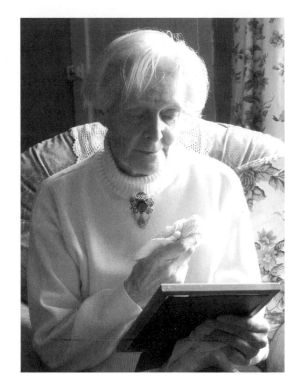

Figure 7 Bereaved partner.

be helpful to provide written information on normal reactions and the support available.

Self-care strategies for the rehabilitation worker

An important first step in self-care is being able to recognise sources of stress. These include:

- Personal factors, such as being a perfectionist and having high expectations of oneself. This might involve an unhelpful personal philosophy such as seeing one's own role as the relief of suffering for all clients/relatives and result, for example, in seeing clients or their relatives outside normal working hours.
- Various problems relating to the work role. Role overload refers to having too much to do in one's job. Role ambiguity occurs when there is no general agreement about what you are expected to do (the need for clarity was referred to earlier) and role conflict happens when there is conflict between the various aspects of one's roles in life, for example professional versus personal.
- Problems relating to interactions with clients and families (which was mentioned earlier). An example of this would be when the rehabilitation worker

identifies with a client or member of his/her family. If, for example, the client reminds you of your dead father with whom you had a very good relationship, you may give this client extra attention and find it difficult to be objective about his needs.

- Problems relating to interactions with colleagues. This may occur if the roles of team members become blurred and they do not fully understand each other's role. Another example would be having to relate to a manager with a dictatorial style.

There are many signs of stress that could indicate the need for more self-care. Examples are: taking the stress of work home and being unable to switch off, difficulty in sleeping; changes in appetite; tension, with difficulty in relaxing; and increased use of alcohol. Also, there can be a strong sense of failure that you have let some clients down because they were distressed and did not die a 'good death'. At the extreme end, workers can become burnt out, that is, totally physically and emotionally exhausted, and are unable to work effectively with clients or their families. A very stressed nurse once bravely admitted to one of the authors that he felt a sense of relief when a client died because it was one less person to care for.

Box 1   Self-care

- Try to maintain a balance between work and home life, for example ensure enough time for family, friends, interests and hobbies.
- Make time for specific ways of relaxing, for example relaxation via the use of imagery, listening to music.
- Develop ways of mentally disengaging from work, for example one nurse imagines leaving work baggage at the ward door when she goes off duty, another worker plays loud music during the drive home.
- Don't set yourself impossible standards: a 'good enough' rehabilitation worker is better than one who is stressed out due to being unable to meet high ideals.
- Attend palliative care training and do further reading, in order to gain a sense of competence.
- Accept that rehabilitation workers may grieve following the death of a client. Consider attending a client's funeral, particularly if you knew him/her well and had a good rapport.
- Try to ensure that you have at least one form of regular, formal supervision, for example one-to-one clinical supervision, peer supervision in a group. This enables time to reflect, for example on the difficulties of the work.
- Obtain support from your informal peer network. Other staff doing a similar job to yourself are in the best position to understand your job stresses and provide support.
- From time to time remind yourself of the positive, rewarding aspects of palliative care work.

Self-care is very important when working with palliative care clients and their families, as the work can be very stressful. Box 1 gives some suggestions. The second point (relaxation via guided imagery) can be something simple like imagining a favourite, peaceful place and trying to make use of all the senses to imagine all that you can see, hear and smell. Many staff find that adopting an appropriate personal philosophy can be very helpful. One such philosophy, which has been suggested to help young medical students who are finding it difficult to work with dying people is: 'Your turn will come and it may be sooner than you think. What can you do today, when it's not your turn, that you hope that someone will do for you tomorrow when it may be?'

■ Conclusion

Supporting clients who require palliative care and their families can be extremely challenging for health care workers. Confronting the end of life raises many issues of concern for clients and their family and friends. However, it is clear that providing good quality care helps many people deal with this difficult period of their lives. While providing palliative care can be difficult for rehabilitation workers it can also be extremely rewarding and may help workers enhance their own life skills. Remember, good communication with clients, families

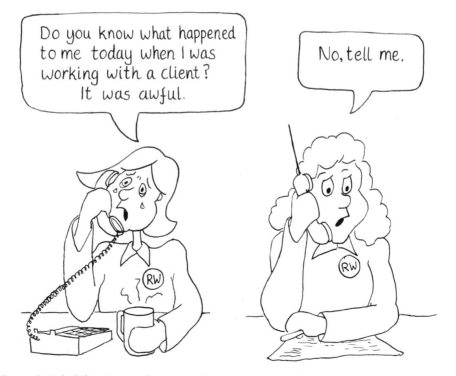

Figure 8 Rehabilitation workers providing peer support.

and other health care workers is imperative. A team approach lessens the load for all.

■ Further reading

Websites

http://www.growthhouse.org/palliat.html *An excellent resource on a wide range of palliative care issues, including pain management, communication, grief and bereavement. Includes useful links to other websites.*

International Association for Hospice and Palliative Care http://www.hospicecare.com/manual/IAHPCmanual.htm *The manual includes some useful sections on principles and practice of palliative care, ethical issues, symptom control and psychosocial aspects.*

National Council for Hospice and Specialist Palliative Care Services http://www.hospice-spc-council.org.uk/informat.ion/abcofpc.htm *Useful links to articles, for example on communication, carers, bereavement, the last 48 hours and pain control.*

Other publications

Addington-Hall, J. & Higginson, I. (eds) (2001) *Palliative Care for Non-Cancer Patients.* Oxford, Oxford University Press. *Provides a comprehensive account of palliative care for people with a non-malignant disorder.*

Australian Government Department of Health and Ageing (2004) *Guidelines for a Palliative Approach in Residential Aged Care.* Canberra, Australian Government Department of Health and Ageng. *Very good guide for all health professionals working in aged care settings.*

Doyle, D., Hanks, G., Cherny, N. & Calman, K. (eds) (2003) *Oxford Textbook of Palliative Medicine.* Oxford, Oxford University Press. (Paperback edition published in 2005.) *This is a useful reference book (1270 pages) and includes chapters on rehabilitation, communication, emotional problems in clients and family members, stress in professional caregivers and the contribution of various health professionals (occupational therapists, physiotherapists etc.).*

Ellershaw, J. & Wilkinson S. (2003) *Care for the Dying: A Pathway to Excellence.* Oxford, Oxford University Press. *Provides an overview of common issues faced by dying people and offers a useful framework for multidisciplinary care planning.*

Ferris, F.D., von Gunten, C.F. & Emanuel, L.L (2003) Competency in end-of-life care: last hours of life. *Journal of Palliative Care Medicine,* **6,** 609.

Hockley, J.M. & Clarke, D. (eds) (2002) Centre for policy on ageing. In: *Palliative Care for Older People in Care Homes.* Milton Keynes, Open University Press.

Hudson, P. (2003). Home-based support for palliative care families: challenges and recommendations. *Medical Journal of Australia,* **179**(6), S35–37. *Short account of home-based care issues and strategies for optimal support.*

Hudson, P. (2004). *Supporting a Person who Requires Palliative care: A Guide for Family and Friends.* Melbourne, Palliative Care Victoria. *Guidebook for family/friends of a person with a life-threatening illness. Includes strategies for self care. Email* info@pallcarevic.asn.au *for more information.*

Lemieux, L. (2004) Sexuality in palliative care: patient perspectives. *Palliative Medicine* **18**, 630–7. *A report of a study of the meaning of sexuality to ten palliative care clients in Canada. Emotional connection to others was seen as important, and more so than physical expressions of sexuality. The article includes observations on barriers to expressing sexuality in hospital and hospice settings.*

National Health and Medical Research Council (2003) *Clinical Practice Guidelines for the Psychosocial Care of Adults with Cancer. Offers evidence based strategies for optimal psychosocial support for people with a cancer diagnosis.*

National Institute for Clinical Excellence (2004) *Guidance on Cancer Services: Improving Supportive and Palliative Care for Adults with Cancer. The manual.* London, National Institute for Clinical Excellence. (Web address: http://www.nice.org.uk/page.aspx?o=110007). *A document which outlines core strategies for palliative care.*

O'Connor, M. & Aranda, S. (eds) (2003) *Palliative Care Nursing: A Guide to Practice.* Melbourne, Ausmed Publications. *Useful book outlining nursing care strategies, but much of the information is relevant to other health care workers.*

Rumbold, B. (2003) *Spirituality and Palliative Care.* Melbourne, Oxford University Press. *Book which explores spiritual care issues and strategies.*

Samarel, N. (1995) Chapter 4 The dying process. In: H. Wass & R.A. Neimeyer (eds) *Dying: Facing the Facts* (3rd edn). Washington D.C., Taylor & Francis, 92–3.

Schmele, J.A. (1995) Perceptions of a dying patient of the quality of care and caring: an interview with Ivan Hanson. *Journal of Nursing Care and Quality*, **9**(4), 31–42.

Steinhauser, K.E., Christakis, N.A., Clipp, E.C, McNeilly, M., McIntyre, L. & Tulsky, J.A. (2000) Factors considered important at the end of life by patients, family, physicians and other care providers. *Journal of the American Medical Association*, **284**(19), 2476–82. *This article reports on the results of a large American survey conducted over a few months in 1999 and identifies a range of issues thought to be important, including preparation for death, achieving a sense of completion and being treated as a whole person.*

Palliative care

Section 4
Issues

- Working with clients and carers to enable independence
- Lifelong learning
- Teamworking and supervision

Working with clients and carers to enable independence

Claudia von Zweck & Maureen Coulthard

Introduction

Carers perform an essential role in enabling the independence of people of all ages. They provide ongoing assistance, without pay, for the large majority of care provided within the home of family members and friends who are in need of support, due to physical, cognitive and/or mental health issues. Carers may also play a major role in providing assistance to individuals who are residents of long-term care facilities or have been admitted to a hospital. Rehabilitation workers therefore need to recognise carers as partners in their work with clients towards attaining intervention goals.

This chapter provides a profile of carers, explores the carer–client relationship and the role of the rehabilitation worker with carers. Strategies are outlined that promote effective working relationships between the rehabilitation workers, clients and their carers. The case study below will be used to illustrate the key points and concepts in the chapter.

Case study   Evelyn

Evelyn is 70 years old, living in a single-storey flat. She has partial hearing loss in both ears. Evelyn has been becoming increasingly forgetful over the past five years. Her daughter, Merryn, who lives in the same suburb, is her main carer. Merryn drops around before and after work every day and takes Evelyn home to her house at weekends, although she has her own family to care for as well.

■ Who are carers?

As we move through the various stages of our lives, any one of us may be called upon to provide care for a family member, friend or neighbour in need of assistance. Often, adult children are called upon to provide assistance to their ageing parents to enable them to remain in their own home. Others may be spouses, partners, family members, neighbours or friends who provide care for a loved one suffering from an illness or disability. Carers may also be the parents of children with physical, mental or emotional illness. In some cases, young children are called on to care for their parents.

Caregiving is a common activity, particularly among middle-aged and older adults. Approximately one quarter of persons over the age of 50 living in Canada and the USA provide assistance to an older person. Many older people are both providers as well as recipients of caregiving. In the UK, it is believed that nearly one in every ten people is involved in providing care for a relative or friend.

Caregiving tasks are often combined with many other activities. The majority of carers in Canada under the age of 65 work outside the home and many aged between 45 and 54 live with a spouse and children. Carers therefore face many competing demands for balancing family, work and caregiving roles.

Stop and think Has the need for carers changed over the years?

The health care environment has changed, and there is increased demand for carers to provide assistance in private homes or supplement the caregiving provided by professional staff in hospitals and facilities. Earlier discharge from hospital and limited home health services result in increased demand for caregiving in the home. Increased survival rates of premature babies, clients who have suffered a catastrophic injury or illness and those with chronic conditions also contribute to increased demands for family and friends to step into the carer role.

■ The client–carer relationship

The client and carers as a family system

Together with the client, carers form a family or community of people living together or in close contact who take care of one another. The individuals within this family unit or community assume different roles and responsibilities. Each family is different and their uniqueness must be respected. Care of the client therefore cannot be considered in isolation of his/her own family and/or community of carers.

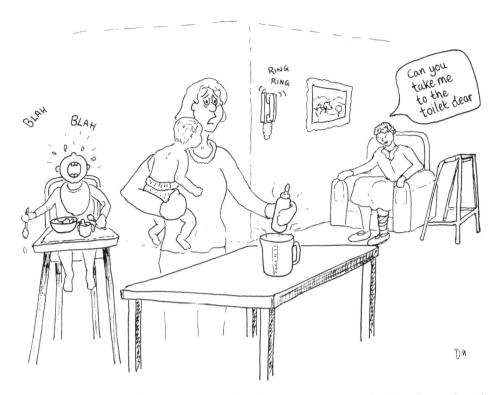

Figure 1 Carers may face many competing demands to balance their family, work and caregiving roles.

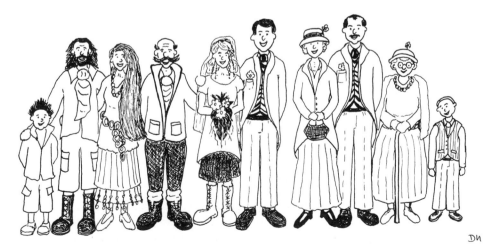

Figure 2 Family uniqueness must be respected.

Role changes associated with caregiving

There are far too many situations in life where caregiving demands among family members are suddenly and drastically altered. Family members can be submerged into carer roles without warning or time to acquire skills needed to meet caregiving demands. When a family member or friend becomes ill and requires assistance with caregiving, it changes the relationship between the carer and client. Think of a young couple involved in a tragic car accident that leaves the husband with quadriplegia. The relationship and caregiving demands for that couple will be changed forever. Another example is a teenage daughter who is struggling to provide care for her mother recently diagnosed with multiple sclerosis. Adjustment to fulfilling a carer role is an evolving process, particularly when caring for individuals with deteriorating conditions. Each progressive loss requires an adjustment by both the carer and the client.

The impact of the client–carer relationship on client outcomes

Optimal client functioning occurs within a supportive family and community. While health services may change for the client over time, the family remains constant and must be supported in order to provide the stability needed for the ongoing care of the client. Clients and carers need to feel confident about their ability to be successful in carrying out their responsibilities. Rehabilitation workers can help the client and carers by helping them to understand

---

Box 1   Recognising the signs of elder abuse

It is important that as a health care provider you recognise signs of potential abuse. Keep your eyes open and know how to respond. In many areas it is mandatory to report suspected abuse situations to the appropriate authorities in your region. Indicators of potential abuse include:

- Unattended health problems, such as dehydration, malnutrition, untreated bed sores or poor personal hygiene.
- Physical injuries to the client, such as bruises or fractures.
- Unsanitary or unsafe conditions in the home.
- Sudden change in client behaviour.
- Agitation, detachment and low self-esteem of the client.
- Refusal of the carer to allow visitors to see the client alone.
- Client report of maltreatment.
- Inappropriate and/or inadequate client clothing and/or necessary assistive devices (for example glasses, hearing aids, dentures).

their role, developing their ability to problem solve and make decisions about care issues, and providing access to the information and resources they require. This empowerment process promotes positive caregiving and works toward the prevention of unwanted outcomes of care.

The manner in which the carer and client interact may either prove beneficial in facilitating the desired results, or hinder the outcomes of care. Positive involvement, interest and support of carers can be an invaluable resource to the client. Social supports are very important in reducing stress about illness or disability for the client. Carers therefore may become a vital support for the emotional needs of the client. On the other hand, extreme carer stress or unwanted responsibilities for caregiving may result in situations where the carer abuses the client physically and/or emotionally. Theft or misuse of the client's money or property may also occur. Unfortunately, such abuse is not rare. Studies from Canada, Australia and the UK estimate that as many as one in ten older people have experienced some form of abuse.

The impact of caregiving for the carer

When health issues arise, clients require time and assistance to adjust to their altered abilities and may fear loss of control and independence. Carers wish to care for their loved ones in the best way possible, but may feel unprepared and nervous about their new role. Both the client and the carer need the opportunity to grieve for the loss of their former relationship with the client. Expectations on the carer to support the client and perhaps assume the former responsibilities of the client may interfere with this grieving process.

Carers can receive great satisfaction and joy from caring for their loved ones. Without sufficient skills and assistance, however, the effects of caregiving for the carer can be significant. Carers may face loneliness and social isolation and have less time and resources for friends, family and other social networks as they become more involved in caregiving. Family and friends may also have difficulty dealing with the grieving processes faced by the client and the family, and may avoid the client and carer as a result.

While carers need acknowledgement of their work, a client may not have the emotional or cognitive capacity to show appreciation to the carer. Sometimes the carer may be blamed for problems experienced by the client and others, particularly if the client has limited insight or denies problems.

The stress of caregiving may lead to issues such as disturbances of sleep, depression and physical illness. Financial costs may arise as a result of lost wages due to the time required for carers to be away from their paid work to provide care. The carer may also be faced with substantial out-of-pocket expenses for items such as medication, medical supplies, mobility equipment, home adaptations and respite care. In addition to the day-to-day costs, the carer may be concerned about the future care of their loved ones. Carers may wonder about how they will cope over time and what will happen when they can no longer provide care.

Stop and think

Reflect on the relationship between Evelyn and her daughter Merryn. Think about the type of role changes Evelyn may have experienced as result of her increasing memory problems. Explore the impact of Evelyn's illness on her daughter.

■ What is your role as a rehabilitation worker?

As a rehabilitation worker, you will contribute toward enabling the client and carers to become competent in meeting their caregiving needs. In this role you must consider the ability of carers to provide assistance, and the priorities and values of the client and the family, to plan how you will deliver your services.

Promoting client-centered caregiving

It is very important that the client has an active role in identifying and achieving goals. Participation in activities that are meaningful to the client promotes positive health outcomes and can lead to greater life satisfaction. Increased dependency, lack of confidence and/or depression may result if clients are denied this opportunity for active involvement.

Understanding carer roles

An individual client may be supported by a number of carers. Rehabilitation workers should be aware of the motivation, attitude and expertise of different carers in order to appropriately involve and assist them in addressing client needs. Different carers have different preferences for their role and level of involvement in the care of the client, based on previous experiences, priorities and values. It is important to respect a carer's desired level of involvement. Not every adult wants to, or is able to be a primary carer for ageing parents. Often a carer may not even recognise the contribution they are making. Sometimes a friend or neighbour may feel that they are contributing very little, when in fact they have made a significant impact in the caregiving process.

A carer may assume or include one or many of the following roles:

- **Listener:** provides an opportunity for the client to share feelings and experiences.
- **Helper:** cares for the day-to-day needs of the client, for example associated with personal care, housekeeping and home maintenance.
- **Therapy provider:** assists the client with intervention programmes to meet therapy goals.

- ■ **Information provider:** assists the client to seek out information to identify and evaluate options for care.
- ■ **Enabler:** uses/creates opportunities for clients to successfully meet their own needs using their own skills and knowledge.
- ■ **Decision-maker:** makes decisions with and/or on behalf of the client.
- ■ **Negotiator:** helps to resolve differences between others.
- ■ **Advocate:** takes action to help others to understand client needs/views.

Structuring positive caregiving experiences

Rehabilitation workers can assist individual carers to provide care so that it will be a positive and successful experience. The carer needs to remain objective and non-judgemental. Individual differences, such as cultural values, race, religion, language, income status, gender and sexual orientation must be considered and respected to maintain an effective relationship between the client and carer.

It is important to understand that not all help is considered useful by the client. The client needs to have the right amount of help at the right time. Help is considered most useful by the client if the carer is proactive, positive and offers assistance rather than waiting to be asked. The client must be able to trust that the carer is committed to work collaboratively to establish and achieve mutually agreed goals. It is also important that the carer and client are both able to work together to identify and deal with any power issues that arise. Caring should never convey a sense that the client is inferior, incompetent or inadequate. As well, the carer should avoid imposing assistance or advice when the client clearly is not ready or willing to accept such assistance. The carer can undermine the confidence of the client if the assistance provided takes control away from the client, prevents active client participation, or fosters a sense of indebtedness to the carer. Consider the case of overbearing parents who do not allow their children to try new activities for fear of them failing. Such carers deny the client the opportunity to develop strengths and skills to enable independence.

Providing information

Rehabilitation workers may assist clients and carers to obtain information they require for informed decision making regarding the client's care. Such information can be obtained from a number of sources, such as libraries, health and community resource centres and the Internet. However, not all information sources are reliable. The rehabilitation worker may assist the carer and client to seek out knowledgeable individuals and expert sources to ensure the best information is used for making decisions.

Rehabilitation workers may also need to share information with carers about the client to enable them to support the client and maintain a healthy environment for other family members or health providers. In sharing such information, the need to protect the confidentiality of client information must be given primary consideration. Client consent must be obtained before any client information is shared with carers.

Supporting the carer

Rehabilitation workers need to support carers and assist them to understand the impact of their relationship with the client on the outcomes of care. Carers may be juggling multiple roles and, as a result, experience considerable stress when caregiving is added to their responsibilities. This is especially challenging for young carers when they have limited experience and judgement to draw upon for the caregiving role. Young carers may require extensive assistance with organising and prioritising caregiving tasks. They may also require education about risks to the client and to themselves, associated with their caregiving.

Carers may not recognise the symptoms of stress stemming from their multiple roles (see Figure 3). The rehabilitation worker may observe situations that suggest carer stress and have opportunity to provide assistance or suggest respite resources before the quality of care is negatively impacted. Common signs of carer stress include:

- Anger with the client.
- Denial about the effects of the client's illness or disability.
- Anxiety and depression.
- Exhaustion.
- Lack of concentration.
- Emotional outbursts.
- Sleeplessness.
- Other health problems.

Stop and think

It is important that the rehabilitation worker recognises signs of carer stress when they occur. Consider the daily demands for Merryn and suggest potential sources and signs of stress that she may experience.

Many carers experience guilt if they feel anger or resentment towards the client. Carers should be encouraged to find opportunities to express their concerns and feelings appropriately. It is important that carers understand that it is acceptable to seek help from others. You may be able to support the carer by providing information about support groups and activities in the local area.

The degree of stress felt by carers is often associated with their sense of competence in dealing with the challenges of caregiving. It is also impacted by opportunities for rest and respite from their caregiving roles. Too often people neglect their own needs as they devote their time and attention to caregiving. Regular use of community programmes, such as meals on wheels can reduce the workload for the carer and provide needed respite. Carers are often unaware of relief or respite programmes in their community until they have reached a crisis situation. Acknowledging the need for relief and arranging for such support may help prevent a difficult situation that can become abusive for the client or the carer.

Both the client and carer should be involved in discussions around planning for respite care. Carers may need assistance from the rehabilitation worker to recognise when it is necessary to stop caregiving and seek assistance. The rehabilitation worker may also need to help the client to understand the need for respite services.

Stop and think

Are you aware of the respite services in your area? Do you know the referral process to access such services?

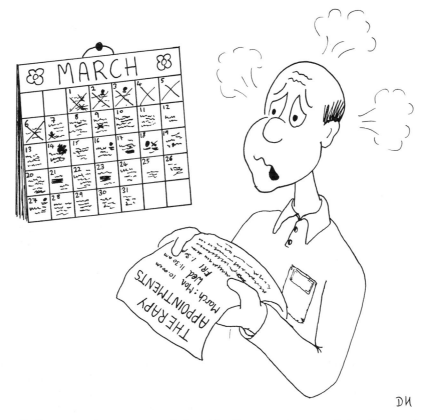

Figure 3 Carers can become overwhelmed by the commitments of the client and their own family.

■ Re-enablement strategies for the carer and client

Re-enablement strategies assist rehabilitation workers, carers and clients to achieve positive working relationships.

Promoting effective communication

You can assist the carer and/or client to use effective ways to communicate. Clients with a sensory loss, such as declining vision or hearing abilities may experience unique difficulties with communication. This may result in frustration for both the carer and the client. You can address potential issues before they become a problem. Interventions may be as simple as cleaning glasses, replacing a battery in a hearing aid or having regular eye exams to have prescriptions changed. Providing the client with adaptive devices such as large print books or a phone with large number pads may also be helpful. Carers may be unaware that their actions may be frustrating for the client, for example an instruction or request made from across the room to the individual with a hearing impairment will result in frustration to both the client and the carer, as it will not achieve the desired results. See Section 3: Communication, for more guidance on appropriate ways to communicate with the carer and client.

Creating/using enabling opportunities

Clients should be encouraged to do as much as possible for themselves within the limits of their abilities and endurance. You may need to help the carers understand the importance for the client not to be isolated or considered differently within their family and community. You can assist carers to work with the client to identify appropriate opportunities to participate in activities that are important to them.

The extent to which clients can actively participate in meaningful activities depends on a variety of factors, such as their age, maturity, cognitive, emotional and physical health. You can assist the carer to build on the client's strengths to create opportunities for them to engage in activities that are best suited to the client, the environment and level of care required.

Therapy programmes may be designed to assist clients to develop the physical, social, cognitive and/or emotional skills needed to gain greater independence in activities that are important to them. You may be involved in helping carers to gain an understanding of the client's needs, abilities and goals, as well as methods of therapy intervention. In helping the carer with therapy activities, you must respect family time and be aware that therapy goals and activities should be incorporated as much as possible into a typical daily schedule. It may be too overwhelming for the client and family to find yet another hour in the day to address specific therapy programmes.

You may help the carer make changes to the caregiving environment to promote safety and facilitate care. For example, removing rugs may prevent falls, or reducing distractions such as a loud television may help the client to concentrate and participate in a care activity. Referral to appropriate health professionals may be necessary to obtain assistive devices that may help the client gain greater independence or safety.

Other strategies that can be used by the rehabilitation worker to enable client participation include:

- Modifying care activities to match skills and abilities of the client more effectively.
- Breaking down care activities into smaller tasks to identify opportunities for the client to participate in part of the activity.
- Developing a schedule of caregiving tasks to ensure priority activities for the client and family are addressed. A well-established routine provides stability and can help balance activities for both the client and the carers. The schedule should include rest breaks for the client and carer. Activities such as listening to music, regular exercise and reminiscing with photos and stories can promote relaxation.

Carers may underestimate the impact of the client's illness or disability for participating in particular activities. This may have serious consequences if it puts the client and/or others at risk, for example if a senior with impaired balance is encouraged to climb stairs to access the bathroom, or an individual with early signs of dementia wishes to continue driving a car. You need to avoid being critical of the carer who is denying or minimising what is believed to be a serious problem (see Figure 4). Instead, you need to provide information to improve the knowledge of the carer and then, together with the carer, look for shared concerns as a starting point for discussing options for the client.

Managing challenging behaviours

Sometimes it is necessary for the carer to seek assistance in managing difficult client behaviours. Often clients with cognitive or emotional difficulties can be especially challenging. You may be able to help identify triggers that appear to be associated with a client's negative behaviour. For example, you may notice that the client becomes agitated in noisy or distracting environments. You can then work with the carer to structure the caregiving activity and environment in the best way to meet the client's needs and abilities to promote positive behaviour. In the above scenario, it may be possible to make changes to reduce environmental stimulation by lowering the lighting and decreasing background noise. Alternatively, the rehabilitation worker can introduce regular rest periods in the client's schedule and/or assist the carer and client to modify the activity to avoid frustration and over fatigue. You may also work with the carer to set limits and expectations for behaviour and help the client and carer to understand and respect these limits. When outbursts do occur, the carer should be taught to manage the situation without antagonising the client. The carer should use techniques to soothe the client and defuse emotionally charged situations. It may be

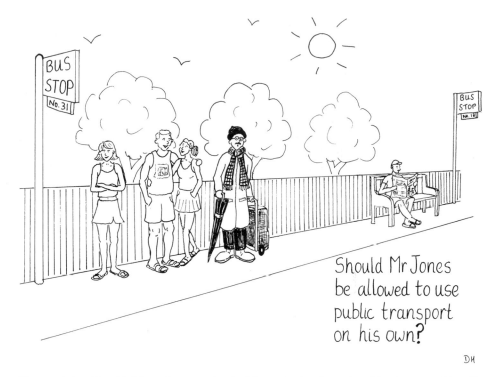

Figure 4 Avoid criticising the carer's decisions. Instead work with them to identify appropriate solutions for the client.

helpful, for example, to speak in soft tones, use humour and/or distract clients by drawing their attention to a more favourable or acceptable activity.

Facilitating informed decision making

Clients should be involved as much as possible to make well-informed decisions that meet the needs of both the client and carers. In situations where the client is unable or unwilling, the carer may be required to make decisions on behalf of the client. The rehabilitation worker can assist the carer by ensuring the client's needs and desires are considered and by providing education and resources needed to make decisions. Carers may also sometimes overstep their role in their haste to provide what they consider to be needed assistance, and make decisions on behalf of clients who have the ability to make their own decisions. The rehabilitation worker can foster client decision making by focusing the carer on meeting the needs of the client and validating attempts of the client to participate in the process.

The rehabilitation worker can assist everyone involved in decision making to be open to consider options and encourage the client and carers not to draw conclusions based on inadequate or incomplete information. Sufficient information should be sought out to make decisions that best fit the circumstances of the time and situation. Where possible the long-range needs of the client

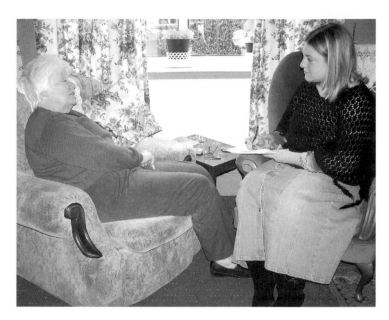

Figure 5 Rehabilitation worker discussing issues with a carer.

should also be considered. It may be necessary, however, to acknowledge that appropriate choices made at one time may no longer be appropriate or valid in the future, as the circumstances in the caregiving experience evolve.

Promoting positive negotiation skills

Undoubtedly, at some point in the caregiving relationship, the client may face differences of opinion with carers. It may then be necessary for carers to negotiate with the client, or act as a mediator to help resolve differences between the client and other individuals. The rehabilitation worker can assist the carer to address differences in an effective manner. A wise agreement needs to be reached that does not damage the long-term relationship between the client and the carers.

The rehabilitation worker should promote the following principles for dealing with differences of opinion:

■ **Goal:** the use of negotiation to promote cooperation, support and attain client and family goals, and maintain the integrity of the long-term caregiving relationship.
■ **Approach:** communicate in an open, friendly, honest and respectful manner. Avoid a confrontational approach. Do not undermine or dismiss input from the individuals involved. The focus of attention should remain on the issue or problem, separated from opinions regarding individuals and their personalities.
■ **Process:** take time to understand all aspects of the issue. View the issue from the perspective of the other party. Look for areas of agreement as

a starting point. Acknowledge differences of opinion. Consider areas where compromise may be possible.

Fostering constructive advocacy skills

The carer may be called upon to advocate for the rights and services of the client. Helping others to understand a different view of an issue through advocacy can be a challenging role for the carer. To be effective, carers need to work with the client to be well informed and knowledgeable regarding the issues of contention, mechanisms that can influence change, as well as the goals of the client and family. Carers may also require information and assistance with understanding existing systems of care for the client. They may be uncomfortable with having to actively assert their views and opinions. You may assist the carer by promoting linkages with support groups and networks that can assist with building the carer's required knowledge and expertise.

Stop and think

Consider the future for both Evelyn and Merryn. What will happen as Evelyn's cognitive status declines and Merryn is responsible for increasing amounts of decision making and financial management? Explore potential future considerations for Evelyn. Discuss how you as a rehabilitation worker could assist them to make informed decisions about their future plans. Identify other individuals who could be of assistance to Evelyn and her mother at this time.

■ Conclusion

Carers provide an integral support to the client by assisting in a wide range of roles. You need to work effectively with carers to attain desired outcomes of care. Carers face many challenges in carrying out roles they may have little knowledge or training to perform. By promoting effective communication, creating enabling opportunities, facilitating informed decision making, promoting positive negotiation and fostering constructive advocacy, you can empower carers and the client to assist them to meet their priorities for successful caregiving.

■ Further reading

Websites

Carers Australia www.carersaustralia.com.au/ *Provides a range of information and resources for carers, as well as links to a number of other national and international sites to support carers.*

Working with clients and carers to enable independence

Caring about Carers www.carers.gov.uk *This is the UK Department of Health website designed to support carers and carer organisations.*

Cranswick, K. (2003) Caring for an ageing society. Retrieved 30 September 2004 from www.statcan.ca. *This report uses data from the General Social Survey of 1996 and 2002 to examine the topic of caregiving in Canada. The report addresses questions related to the characteristics of informal care providers and seniors receiving formal and informal care.*

Family Caregiver Alliance. Caregiver's guide to understanding dementia behaviours. Retrieved 30 September 2004 from www.caregiver.org *This free caregiver guide is one of many resources available on the website of the Family Caregiver Alliance.*

Law, M., Rosenbaum, P., King, G., King, S., Burke-Gaffney, J., Moning, J. et al. Family-centred service fact sheets. Retrieved 30 September 2004 from www.fhs.mcmaster.ca/canchild *The CanChild Centre for Childhood Disability Research website contains valuable information and research regarding family-centred health services, including this series of fact sheets.*

Seniors Resource Centre of Newfoundland and Labrador (2004) Looking beyond the hurt: a service provider's guide to elder abuse. Retrieved 30 September 2004 from www.seniorsresource.ca/beyond.htm *A free downloadable handbook for health providers on elder abuse recognition, intervention and prevention.*

Other publications

Canadian Association of Occupational Therapists (1998) *Living at Home with Alzheimer's Disease and Related Dementias.* Ottawa, Canadian Association of Occupational Therapists. *This manual provides references, information and resources to assist carers with their role in caregiving with persons with dementia.*

Canadian Association of Occupational Therapists (2002) *Enabling Occupation: An Occupational Therapy Perspective.* Ottawa, Canadian Association of Occupational Therapists. *This publication describes a conceptual framework and process model for client-centred practice.*

Dunst, C., Trivette, C. & Deal, A. (1998) *Enabling and Empowering Families: Principles and Guidelines for Practice.* Cambridge, Brookline Books. *This publication outlines a social system perspective of enablement and outlines principles and strategies for enabling families as carers.*

Nolan, M., Lundh, U., Keady, J. & Grant, G. (2003) *Partnerships in Family Care.* Buckingham, Open University Press. *This book considers how family and professional carers can work together more effectively to provide high quality care to help people to remain independent in their own home.*

Lifelong learning

Sandi Carman

Introduction

The purpose of this chapter is to equip you with a range of options to help you to continue your own lifelong learning. Lifelong learning is a common phrase that people use to cover all types of learning activity. Significant learning will influence your future attitudes and behaviours, thus having a 'lifelong' impact. It is never too soon or too late for learning.

Becoming a lifelong learner requires the right attitude. The way that you learn is up to you and very much depends on your personal preference and lifestyle. If you make the most of every opportunity you will be surprised at how many times during the day you learn things without realising it.

Your learning and the quality of care you provide to your clients are very closely linked. Section 1: Teaching for rehabilitation highlighted a number of approaches you may use to support learning for your clients. This chapter is designed to help you identify your own learning needs and approaches. Many of the obvious ways of applying learning are discussed in this chapter. After reading this chapter you will understand more about the way people learn and what different methods to use. You can use the skills you develop in this chapter to help your clients by learning different ways of promoting good health and understanding the individual learning preferences your clients may have.

How do we learn?

Kolb & Fry (1975) looked at the way we learn through experiences and identified four stages that individuals need to go through to apply the learning to practice. If learning is to be effective you need to go through each stage of the learning cycle. You can start at any stage in the process. However, the whole

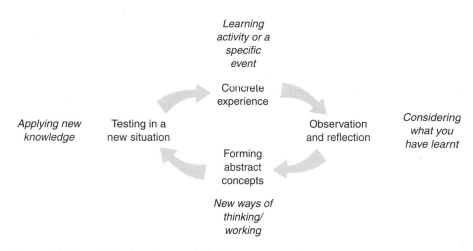

Figure 1 Kolb and Fry learning cycle (Kolb & Fry, 1975).

process should be seen as a continuous upward spiral which is always developing, rather than a flat circle. This learning process has been criticised as being too simplistic to reflect the complexity of learning. However, it can be viewed as a basic framework for learning activities and may help you understand how you learn.

Stop and think

Spend some time studying the Kolb cycle and think about which parts of the cycle reflect the way that you learn. You may be at a number of different stages in the cycle depending on the learning activity.

Although it has some critics, the learning cycle is a useful framework to understand how your learning can develop your attitudes and behaviour though the use of reflection and changes in practice.

The first part of this chapter will cover some of the different ways of learning, how to access learning opportunities and how to record your learning activity in a personal development portfolio. The final part of the chapter describes how to set objectives, prepare for your appraisal, and how you can identify your learning needs using a personal development plan.

▪ Accessing learning opportunities

It is important to recognise your own responsibility for your learning and to make the most of every opportunity. However, your manager can help you clarify your

Lifelong learning

learning needs and assist with preparing your personal development plan. To do this you normally start with an appraisal (sometimes called a *development review* or *personal performance review*). This is your opportunity to review your achievements over the last year, discuss with your manager your objectives for the next year and identify how your learning can support this.

Step one: preparation for the appraisal

When you undergo your appraisal, the following guidance on roles and responsibilities may help.

Your role:

- To update and maintain your portfolio.
- To participate fully in your review meeting by:
  - Preparing thoroughly
  - Contributing to the setting of targets and objectives, based on the organisation's objectives, business plans and your role
  - Identifying personal development objectives
  - Providing upward feedback on support given
  - Follow-up actions agreed at the review meeting

Stop and think

Before you go into your review meeting, do a short self-appraisal to help you plan what you want to cover in your appraisal. Consider the following questions:

(1) What do you feel you have achieved since your last review?
(2) What staff development have you undertaken?
(3) How has your work and personal development benefited as a result of these activities?
(4) What prevents you from doing your job as well as you would like?
(5) What measures can you take to overcome these difficulties?
(6) What measures can others take to help you overcome these difficulties?
(7) What do you think should be your objectives for the next twelve months? Look at a copy of your department's business plan or manager's objectives. This will give you an idea of some of the key areas you may wish to focus on.
(8) What training and development support do you feel you may need to help you achieve your objectives?
(9) What are your longer-term objectives or career aspirations in one, three and five years?

Your reviewer's responsibilities:

- To plan and prepare for your review.
- To agree an appropriate time and place for the review.

- To conduct an objective review of performance to jointly review and evaluate impact of training and development.
- To agree future objectives based upon the organisation's objectives, business plans and your role.
- To identify any training and development needs.
- To discuss your review and future objective with their line manager.
- To ensure that there are 'no surprises'.
- To follow up on the actions agreed at review meeting.

Step two: the appraisal

Make sure you have the appraisal in a quiet room with no interruptions. Remember this is your time to discuss your development needs and career aspirations. Use the time well and listen carefully to any constructive feedback or advice from your manager. At the end of the appraisal you should have agreed some draft objectives for the next year. Aim to have these written in a final format about two weeks after the appraisal and make sure that both you and your manager have a copy.

Step three: objective writing

Writing your objectives is sometimes the most difficult part of the appraisal process. It may be worth following these simple stages when you are planning

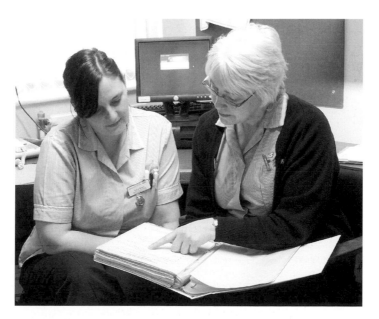

Figure 2 Staff member appraisal with supervisor.

them:

(1) During your review discuss with your line manager 'key areas' for your objectives. These may include a mixture of:
   (a) Personal objectives (for your own development)
   (b) Professional work objectives
(2) Write out the objectives using the Objectives Template (see Figure 3).
(3) Check that they are SMART (see Box 1 below).
(4) Finalise your objectives with your line manager.

It is important that you both agree on your objectives. This may involve a bit of negotiation because sometimes individuals have different expectations.

Some organisations have a competency framework to help guide individual learning and development to support the needs of the organisation and service delivery. The framework will list the essential skills and knowledge required for you to be fully competent to carry out your work role. In some cases this framework will replace the objective setting process. Your learning needs will be identified by comparing your existing skills and knowledge with those identified in the framework. This information will form your personal development plan.

Within the National Health Service (NHS) this process is being developed through the NHS Knowledge and Skills Framework. This means that everyone working for the NHS will have a competency outline that matches their job description. This will describe the types of skills and knowledge that individuals will be encouraged to develop. If you match all of the competencies then you know that you have all the skills to do your job well.

Step four: personal development planning

Finally, your objectives need to be turned into a personal development plan. Once you have agreed your objectives you need to assess the skills and knowledge you have to achieve these. Your personal development plan is used to determine the areas where further education or development would enhance your performance to help you achieve your objectives.

Box 1 SMART objectives

Specific: does it say precisely what has to be done in order for you to succeed?
Measurable: how will the results be measured? How will you know you have got there?
Achievable: is it challenging and can you do it? Have you taken into account all the possible factors and constraints?
Relevant: does the objective feed into the organisation's objectives? Is it relevant to your job role?
Timebound: do you have a timeframe for the completion of the objective?

INDIVIDUAL OBJECTIVE SHEET

Name: .... Objective Number: .... of ....

Department:... Date: ....

Objective (statement of objective)

Targets/Action plan (an outline implementation plan of what you have to do by when)

Success criteria (how will you know when you have carried it out successfully?)

Resources needed

Anticipated constraints

Notes on attainment (complete during/at the end of year)

NOTES

- Please photocopy this original and use one copy of this sheet for each objective

- In total, you will normally have no more than 6 objectives

- Aim for a mix of objectives between service – organisational/culture – people management

- Agree jointly between manager and job holder

Please photocopy these pages where applicable

Figure 3 Objective template.

A personal development plan should:

- Describe the areas for development that have been identified.
- Include the action required to meet these areas for development.
- Identify the support and resources needed in order to fulfil your plan.

> **Box 2** Tips for completing your personal development plan
>
> ■ Don't over complicate your development objectives. Break them down into manageable chunks which are easily measurable.
> ■ Try to avoid long timescales. This can hinder you as you may lose sight of what you are seeking to develop.
> ■ Be very open-minded about your learning activity. Don't expect all of your learning to come from training courses.
> ■ Identify how you have learnt best in the past and use this as a means of guiding your learning in the future.
> ■ Be realistic about what you can achieve.
> ■ Review your progress regularly and keep your records up to date.
> ■ Talk to your colleagues and manager about your own personal development needs, they can often spot things that you probably can't.

A plan should take into account the diverse range of learning activities that can support development; these are listed in detail later in this chapter. Whichever activities you choose, there must be clear learning or development outcomes. When making decisions about your development it is often useful to talk through the different options available to you. Your manager, supervisor and training department can provide help and guidance. Remember, some mandatory training is also an important part of maintaining your skills (for example moving and handling, fire lecture).

A personal development plan can help focus your learning and enables you to chart your progress. It is worth setting aside some time every month to review your plan and check your progress.

▪ Levels of learning

Your learning has to be relevant for your current skills and ability. Don't worry if everything seems too hard or advanced, over time this will become easier as you learn more. Some organisations have access to staff who are specialists in teaching English and maths (sometimes called 'skills for life' or 'basic skills') to support people who have not had the opportunity to develop these skills fully at school. This is your opportunity to seek assistance in a confidential forum. If you feel unable to talk to your manager about these opportunities then try your union representative or look out for locally run courses.

Many formal learning activities now carry some sort of academic qualification or accreditation. This is a useful way of getting your work recognised and may help you to get the qualifications you need for your next career opportunity. If you are daunted by the size of a full qualification, in many cases you can work towards a qualification by completing one module at a time. Usually, you can

PERSONAL DEVELOPMENT PLAN

Name: .... Role: .... Dept: ....

Line Manager: .... Date: .... Next review date: ....

Personal objective from appraisal	Development need and action to take	Resources/costs	Timescale	How will it improve objectives and appraisal individual, team and organisational performance?
Summarise your objectives from section 8	What development activity do you need to do to achieve this objective, i.e. shadowing, coaching, training course, reading	How much time will this take to achieve? Which people will you need to have access to? How much will it cost?	When will you have achieved this by?	How will this contribute to the trust's aims? How will this contribute to your department aims?

Figure 4 Personal development plan.

do this over a few months or years. The amount and frequency of work is up to you, but having a clear plan will help you keep on track.

■ Ways of learning and learning styles

This section identifies some of the many different ways of learning. As you read through this section, consider some of the methods you have used in the past and which ones you found most useful.

Training courses and study days

The most obvious and most common mode of learning is through attending training and education courses, either provided by your employer or educational institutions. Attending a course provides the opportunity for focused learning, enables you to switch off from your normal work tasks and allows you to network with other people who may have similar roles and interests to you.

Shadowing

It is vitally important to consider other ways of learning and to make the most of every opportunity. During your time at work make a particular effort to watch and learn from your work colleagues. If you need more information why not ask to shadow another member of staff. Ensure that you set clear objectives for the shadowing period and use the time to question your practice and reflect on how you can improve client care.

Some organisations have a formal shadowing scheme, where you can ask to shadow an individual from other organisations. This is an excellent way to gain new ideas and provides a useful way for you to review your practice.

Action learning

Action learning involves bringing together a group of people to work together for an agreed length of time to undertake a task. In doing this they learn together through an environment of questioning, understanding and reflection. The unique nature of the group enables work and learning to take place simultaneously.

Action learning sets often form part of a wider educational programme that enables team members to develop their learning in a group situation. From each learning set you will usually have a couple of development actions to be undertaken before the next meeting. This could be reading an interesting article or just talking to someone about an aspect of their role.

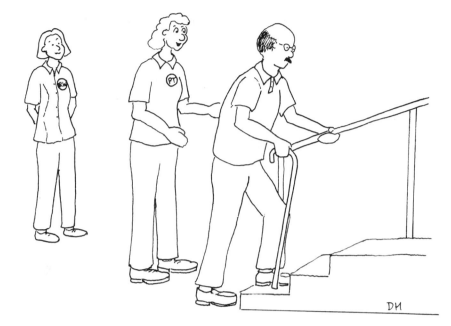

Figure 5 Work shadowing.

By joining an action learning set you will be together with a group of about six other people who all want to learn from undertaking the task and sharing ideas and experiences. The success of the learning sets depends on the facilitator and the group as a whole. Make sure you have something to contribute, listen to other people and try not to dominate the proceedings. A good facilitator will enable everyone to contribute to the discussion.

Videos/DVDs/films and radio

There are many videos, DVDs and films around that can help with your learning; these are also a very useful mechanism for learning with your clients. The ability to rewind and review sections you don't understand is invaluable. You may wish to sit with your client and discuss the contents of the programme. As well as helping their understanding of the condition this opportunity will also enable you to build rapport with your client.

There are ways that improvements in technology will help your lifelong learning. Within the National Health Service the majority of acute hospital beds have interactive bedside units which enable patients to make and receive phone calls and include a screen on which patients can watch television, look at public health information and videos. Understanding the content of these videos not only helps with your learning but enables you to provide a consistent message to your patients. You will also be able to help them answer any questions or queries about the video.

Lifelong learning

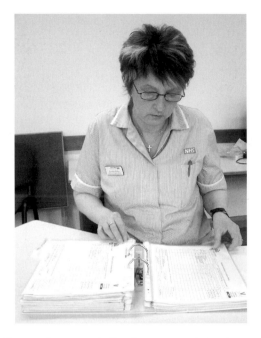

Figure 6 Rehabilitation worker completing her personal development portfolio.

E-learning

E-learning is a term used to describe any learning delivered through a specially designed computer software package. These can come on CD ROMs or be available on the Internet. They are useful because they allow you to do short bursts of learning when you get the time. This is especially true with Internet-based packages because you don't need to be in the same place every time you study since the material is available wherever you have computer access.

The disadvantages of these packages are clear. If you don't understand a question or statement then who do you ask? In some cases the package will have an email or telephone help desk enquiry line. This is useful, but doesn't help if you need an immediate answer and are unable to use the phone. Some organisations use e-learning packages in a classroom situation, where a teacher or facilitator is present, which gives you the best of both worlds.

The wider use of e-learning has enabled the development of many e-learning packages, covering areas such as computer skills, fire, health and safety awareness, or communication skills. Not everything can be delivered through e-learning, but it is a useful way of getting a message across to a number of people in a cost effective way. For example, some ambulance services use e-learning so that drivers can learn while they are waiting on standby in their vehicles. The paramedics use laptops with pre-loaded learning packages which can be easily shutdown when an emergency call is received.

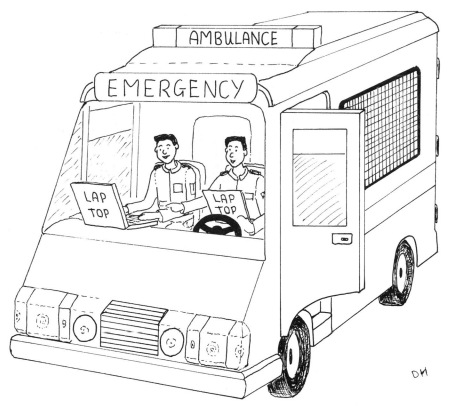

Figure 7 Ambulance drivers involved in e-learning on the job.

Coaching

Coaching is a way of improving your performance on the job. Your coach is usually an individual who has a knowledge and understanding of the process you need to learn. In many cases this may be your line manager or supervisor. A good coach should be looking at your needs, reviewing your awareness levels and planning a joint approach. After the event or sessions you should both evaluate the process and confirm the learning outputs.

Coaching is something you may already undertake with your clients during treatment sessions, without realising it. Often you will be working though a process that is familiar to you but new to your client. Coaching is different from mentoring, as it tends to be hands-on and involves direct support, advice and guidance.

Mentoring

A mentor is someone who can assist you in working through any work or career issues. Their role is not to tell you what to do, but help you gain insight into

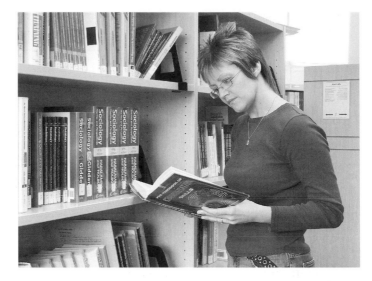

Figure 8 Rehabilitation worker engaged in self-directed library based learning.

what you need to do. They may do this through gentle questioning or acting as a sounding board. A mentor is usually someone other than your line manager. They act as a guide, adviser and counsellor and will often be someone who is established in their field. Talk to your manager about finding a mentor. You may find a mentor within your own organisation, through a professional association, or through special schemes that have been set up to provide mentorship.

Journals and newsletters

Many journals tend to be quite academic. If you like this style of writing your local library will be able to help you identify the journals that relate to your area of work. You may also find that a number of publications, newsletters, leaflets or briefing notes are available within your department. Ask to be put onto these mailing lists, although don't expect to have time to read everything. The key is to be selective and focused with your reading and concentrate on specific areas which align to your personal development plan. That way you will be able to recognise a real difference from your reading and not get overwhelmed by the task.

Role models

This is the easiest but most interesting way of learning: people watching. Look carefully at the people you think do a good job, or are respected in their field. What mannerisms are they using? How do they conduct themselves in difficult situations? What attitude do they have to work? What methods do they use to approach patient care? Many of these questions can be answered simply by observing the individual. But why not take this one step further? What about asking if you could spend some time shadowing that individual and get to understand their style better?

Learning styles

It is quite common to use a number of different methods to learn about a topic; this is known as blended learning. Depending on how you prefer to learn you could combine your learning experiences. If you are not sure how you learn, a number of questionnaires have been designed to help you identify the way that is most appropriate for you. The most popular of these is Honey & Munford's (1992) Learning Styles Questionnaire (LSQ) which identifies four different learning preferences:

- Activists learning by doing.
- Reflector: learning by observing and then thinking about what has happened.
- Theorist: learning by understanding the theory behind the actions.
- Pragmatist: learning by seeing how to apply the concepts in the real world or in your own life.

No style is better than any another and it is suggested that a good learner should be able to vary their learning preference depending on the circumstances. You can do the LSQ survey on-line at www.PeterHoney.com to determine your own preferred learning style. The LSQ should not be used to identify your only way of learning, but can be used as a guide to help you along the way. Don't be persuaded to think that learning can only be undertaken in a set way. Use whatever method works best for you.

Using a number of different ways to learn is called blended learning. You may want to choose a specific theme for six months and then look at the best way of identifying what you need to learn. This may be through a combination of shadowing, reading and attending a short course, for example.

■ Why bother?

With our busy lives it is often hard to find time to commit to learning.

> 'I don't have time for training, my clients come first'
> 'I've done this job for 15 years there is nothing you can teach me'

Does this sound familiar? If these are your views then congratulations for even getting this far into the chapter. Maybe you are starting to understand why learning is important for everyone at every stage in their career. If these are the views of your colleagues then this chapter will give you some key arguments to challenge them and recognise why ultimately they can have a detrimental effect on client care.

Lifelong learning

It is the easiest thing in the world to say 'I don't have time'. Everyone has time, the difference is how you decide to prioritise that time. Many people have numerous pressures on their time, both within work and outside, for example caring for elderly relatives or children. One of the first steps to good time management is to say 'no'. Think about all of those extra jobs or projects you agree to, then run out of time. The next step is to plan small chunks of time to spend on your development. Try talking to your manager about completing your normal work an hour early for one day a week and using that time to sit and spend some time on your development. Not every manager will be willing to do this; usually because of the demands of the workload. Remember, you may need to be flexible in your requests and be willing to come to a compromise solution. Why not try working at home? Ensure that your family are aware of the time you need to work on this. As a minimum try an hour per week, or if you prefer more then dedicate an evening or part of the weekend every few weeks. Breaking down your study into small chunks will make it more manageable. You will be surprised by how much you can get done over a six-month period.

Health and social care practice is changing daily; we have a responsibility to our clients to ensure we are using the most up-to-date treatment methods. This means we should be committed to the principles of lifelong learning. If you are a member of a professional organisation you will probably find your code of conduct expects a level of continued learning throughout your career. Not maintaining and developing your skills and knowledge will have a detrimental effect on the service you provide to your clients.

Personal development portfolios

A personal portfolio is your collection of achievements, objectives, learning undertaken, etc. The way that you organise this is entirely up to you. Over time you will find a format that works for you. A number of professional organisations (for example the College of Occupational Therapists or the Chartered Society of Physiotherapists) provide standard templates that may give you a useful starting point. Your own employing organisation may have a portfolio template that you can use. If you are unable to access any of these a simple A4 folder with dividers will suffice.

Box 3 Suggested sections for the content of your personal development portfolio

Curriculum vitae
Job description/personal details
Learning and development activity
Appraisal and objective information
Reflective practice

Curriculum vitae

This is a summary of your personal details, employment history and achievements. The format of this can vary. If you want some ideas why not ask one of your work colleagues to share their CV with you. Many books look specifically at the design and layout of your CV. Initially, you could just jot down your previous jobs, which schools you have attended and any qualifications gained. Don't worry if these are few; many people are now looking for people with the right attitude rather than specific skills. When writing your CV, rather than just listing your jobs, look at what you have achieved or learnt in that job and summarise it in a few sentences. This will make more sense to a prospective employer, especially if they don't know the organisation you previously worked for, or if you have an unusual job title.

Job description/personal details

It is useful to keep a copy of your current job description. Make sure that your job description matches the job that you do. If not, then discuss it with your line manager during your appraisal review.

Learning and development activity

This section is a record of your achievements and skills. You may want to include education details, courses/study day records, group/activity details. Don't just make this section a collection of your certificates. Write a short summary about the courses and how you have implemented any changes from the learning gained.

Appraisal and objective information

In this section you can keep the paperwork used in your appraisal. You may wish to keep previous years' paperwork as well but it is your choice. Store your personal development plan here, but remember to update it when you have undertaken some learning activity.

Reflective practice

One of the ways of ensuring that you get the best from your learning is to reflect on the activity and look at how you can make changes as a result of the experience. This is called reflective practice. Reflection alone is not sufficient for development, as this focuses more on the process than the outcomes. Reflective practice focuses on outcomes and possible changes in practice.

Lifelong learning

Schon (1991) has written a lot about the benefits of using reflective practice, particularly after an incident or event. In itself, reflective practice can be used as a useful learning tool. You may wish to reflect on a specific learning activity or just an event that has happened during the day. Reflecting on an event is a useful opportunity to ask for feedback from your work colleagues. This will help you understand how different people perceive an event and will assist your learning. Often a situation can appear clear-cut to one person but ambiguous to the other.

To become a reflective practitioner you need to look at what you would have done differently with the benefit of hindsight. It may help to write this down in the form of a learning log or critical incident diary. Recording and reflecting on what you have done is probably one of the most important parts of any learning activity. Writing that up and adding to your personal development portfolio is a useful way of demonstrating learning.

You can apply reflective practice principles to learning. Once you have undertaken any learning why not apply the 'so what?' question and reflect on the event: Consider:

> What difference will your learning make to you and your clients?
> How will you change the way you work as a result of the learning?

Write the answers to these questions in your learning log. The format is up to you; in its basic form a learning log could include the most important thing you have learnt and three reasons why that is important. This method will also give you the opportunity to reflect on how your learning has impacted on your client care.

If you enjoy this style of learning why not develop this into a critical incident diary. In this case you select a specific incident and describe the nature of the incident; look at the questions this raised; look at what happened afterwards; make notes on how, given the same opportunity again, you would do things differently; and finally, look at how this experience can be used as a learning opportunity. Put a bit of time aside every month to work through your portfolio and update it. When you apply for another job this will be an invaluable resource for filling in your application form. If you are still unclear about what to include, talk to other members of your team and ask how they keep their portfolio.

■ Conclusion

It is vitally important not to view learning in isolation. Almost every moment of the day carries a learning experience. The key is to ensure that you are always receptive to change and learning new things. Sometimes the new information will challenge your traditional way of thinking and therefore prevent you from accepting or recognising new or important information. Keep an open mind, be willing to review and challenge all new information and make your own decision about the relevance of that information.

Lifelong learning

■ Further reading

Honey, P. & Mumford, A. (1992) *A Manual of Learning Styles.* Maidenhead, Honey.

Hornby, M. (1998) *Thirty-six Steps to the Job You Want.* London, Prentice Hall. *This book provides a practical guide to career development, giving many good tips about getting that right job.*

Kolb, D.A. & Fry, R. (1975) Towards an applied theory of experiential learning. In C.L. Cooper (ed.) *Theories of Group Processes.* pp. 33–58. London, John Wiley. *The original information on the learning cycle. Worth a read.*

Megginson, D. & Whitaker, V. (2003) *Continuing Professional Development.* London, Chartered Institute of Personnel and Development. *A practice and comprehensive guide to support your development, which will help you at any stage in your career.*

Schon, D.A. (1991) *The Reflective Practitioner: How Professionals Think in Action.* Aldershot, Ashgate Publishing. *A detailed text, but provides an excellent overview of reflective practice and how this benefits your service.*

Teamworking and supervision

Susan Nancarrow

Introduction

People who choose to work in the helping professions generally spend a lot of time giving to other people. In fact, people are often attracted to the helping professions for altruistic reasons. The title of this book 'Enabling independence' reflects your role in creating opportunities for other people to make the most of their own abilities. However, often, little thought is given to providing you with the support that you need to go into situations that can be demanding and challenging, with people who you may not always get along with.

The purpose of this chapter is to help you to identify and access the types of support that you are likely to need in your role as a rehabilitation worker. That means being able to access the right sort of supervision and training when you need it; understanding your relationship to your team; and being in a team that has the right structures to enable you to do your job. It acknowledges that at some stage in your career as a rehabilitation worker, you are likely to be both a supervisor and a supervisee, and explores both of these roles and relationships.

What is a team?

A team is a group of people who come together to share a common purpose or a task, and who depend on the input of each other to succeed. Like teams of footballers who cooperate to score the maximum number of goals, rehabilitation teams work together to try to achieve common goals that are based around the requirements of the client.

Enabling someone to remain independent in their chosen environment normally requires the skills and input of a range of different types of workers. Some of the workers may only provide input for a short period of time, whereas others

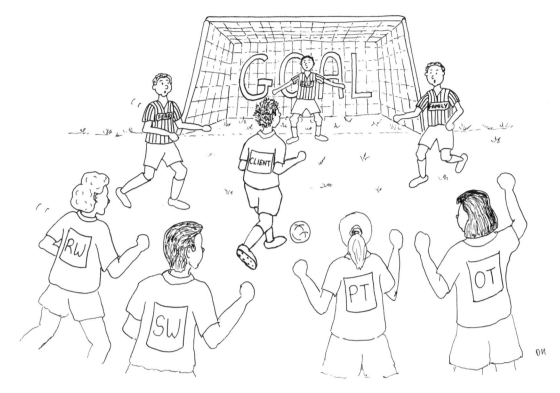

Figure 1 Teamworking to achieve a common goal.

may have longer-term involvement with the client. The workers may all belong to the same service and return to the same office, which makes sharing information about the client relatively easy. Alternatively they may come from a number of different organisations, in which case, sharing information is more complex. The team might work together in the client's home, in a community based facility, or sometimes in a dedicated part of a hospital. In any case, these people come together to form a team to try to get the best outcomes for the client.

The way that the team works together is influenced by a range of different factors, including the client's goals and needs; the number and different types of workers involved in the care of the client; the place where the care is provided; team management; and the types of communication strategies the team has in place.

Consider the differences between working with clients in an in-patient facility, like a hospital, compared with their own home. In a hospital, there are normally a number of patients in a single ward. Unlike people's homes, hospitals are purpose built to care for sick people. They have wide corridors to make it easy for staff and patients to move around, and facilities like hoists and rehabilitation gyms to aid recovery. Rehabilitation workers will probably have relatively easy access to medical, nursing and allied health staff, and, in fact, you are likely to see these people regularly in your everyday work. You will probably learn new techniques by watching other people, and others will learn from

> ## Box 1   Identifying the team
>
> Consider one of the clients that you work with. Take a piece of paper and draw an image of the client in the middle of the page. Then around that client, make a note of all of the health and social care needs that are likely to be met by someone other than their family (for example, rehabilitation, cleaning the house, meal preparation, gardening, dental and medical support). Beside each need, list all of the different workers that meet those particular needs of the client (for example, dentist, GP, meals on wheels, community health services).
> Now consider the following points:
>
> - Are there any areas where the services might overlap in the provision of care to the client?
> - Are any of the client's needs not being addressed?
> - Does any one person, or service have a role in coordinating all of the services received by the client?

you. When you need input from another member of staff, you can normally find someone nearby to ask. If there are issues that the whole health care team need to resolve, team members can normally get together quite easily to talk about them.

Now think about working in the client's home. Your clients may live a long way apart, which means that you need to allow time to travel, and you may only be able to see two or three clients a day. Every home will be different. Instead of two-metre wide corridors with hard floors, you may be working in a house that has narrow, carpeted hallways, steep stairs, a kitchen and bathroom that were not designed with rehabilitation in mind, and a barking dog at the front door. The fact that you have to travel to see each client means that you may be a long way away from the rest of your team. Your main means of accessing support may be by telephone. You might be required to do tasks that have been delegated to you by another worker. In the hospital, the people that you work most closely with are likely to be other hospital staff. In the client's home, you will encounter a more diverse range of people, including the client's family, people from different agencies such as meals on wheels, the client's GP, home help, and postal and garbage services.

These two scenarios raise quite a number of important and different issues for teamworking and supervision. In the hospital setting, a lot more 'informal' or accidental supervision takes place, whereas in the home setting, it is possible that a rehabilitation worker may go for some days without having contact with another member of staff. Community based settings, such as outpatient facilities or day centres bring different types of team management and supervision issues again. The different settings of care highlight the following important questions about teamworking and supervision:

- How do team members communicate with each other about the client's goals and progress?

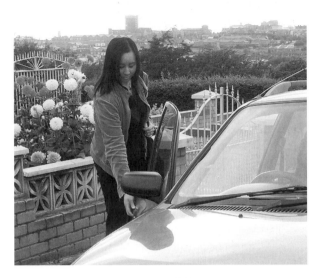

Figure 2 Rehabilitation worker leaving a client's home.

- How does the team communicate day-to-day issues about their work?
- How do team members access technical and professional support?
- How do staff learn new techniques and share these with other team members?
- What are the safety considerations for staff working in different settings and how are these addressed?
- How do you deliver your intervention if you do not have access to high tech or specialised equipment?
- Who are the different people and agencies that you are likely to encounter when you are working with the client, and how do you manage these relationships?
- How do you ensure that there is no duplication in the services or types of care received by the client?
- Who do you need to consult about different aspects of client care?

There are no right or wrong answers to these questions, and teams can use different and innovative approaches to addressing these issues. Some of these questions will be answered in this chapter.

Stop and think

Reflect on your own workplace and attempt to answer each of the above questions as they relate to your own job.

Teamworking and supervision

Different types of teams and teamworking

A number of different approaches to team organisation have been developed to address the questions raised above. First, it is important to clarify some of the common terms that are used to describe teamworking in rehabilitation. These are *multidisciplinary* and *interdisciplinary* teams.

- A *multidisciplinary* team is a group of workers from different disciplines who work side by side, each bringing expertise to problems separately. These teams undertake separate assessments, set discipline specific goals, and there is little coordinated planning or provision of the services.
- An *interdisciplinary* team is a group of workers from two or more disciplines who coordinate their expertise to provide care to patients. They meet regularly to exchange information about the client, to develop the treatment plan and cooperate in its implementation. The focus of interdisciplinary care is on common problem solving. Interdisciplinary care recognises the core contribution of each profession and allows a blending of different components of professional input to reach client goals. It is seen as being more holistic than multidisciplinary care. There is a growing body of evidence that interdisciplinary teamworking has better outcomes for clients that multidisciplinary working, and there is an increasing trend in re-enablement for the use of interdisciplinary teams.

It is important that all of the appropriate team members are involved in decision making about the client assessment and intervention. There are a number of different ways of organising teams to meet the needs of the client. If you go back to the first Stop and think box in this chapter, you will see that a client can be involved with a number of different individuals and organisations, which can be confusing for the client, and may lead to the duplication or overlap of services.

Traditionally, clients with multiple health and social care needs who need to be seen by a range of different practitioners would undergo a separate assessment by each one. This approach has a number of disadvantages. It means that the client is required to repeat the same information to many different people, which is time consuming for the client, and an unnecessary waste of practitioner resources. It also means that the practitioners are unlikely to have access to the same or consistent information, particularly if they use different assessment tools.

There are two common ways of managing clients with complex care needs, although the terms used to describe them, and the way they are implemented will vary a great deal across different services. These are the use of a *single assessment processes* and *case management*. One of the goals of these approaches is to provide coordinated care. In other words, they try to reduce the amount of duplication of services and prevent gaps where the client's needs are not met.

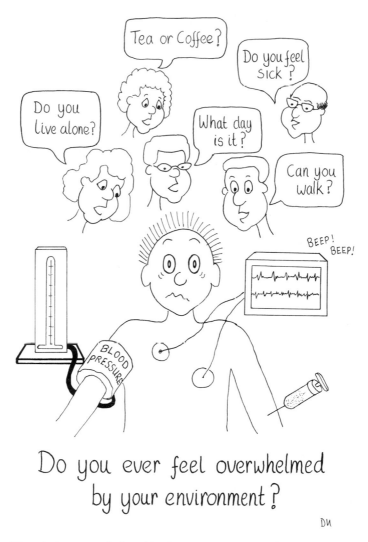

Figure 3 Client being overwhelmed by too many assessments.

Single assessment process

As the name implies, the single assessment process involves the use of a client assessment tool that uses a holistic approach to gauge the needs of the client. The assessment will normally incorporate an examination of the physical, social, psychological, environmental and care support needs and status of the client. It may be applied by one trained practitioner who will use the tool to gain a general oversight of the health and social care needs of the client. Alternatively, different types of workers may complete specific parts of the same tool. The completed assessment will be used to determine the service needs of the client, in consultation with the team members. Normally, all members of the team will have access to the assessment, so they can see the information that has been collected about the client, and do not have to repeat the information collection. The assessment should be reviewed in the same way as described in Section 1: Agreeing and reaching goals.

Case management

Another way of streamlining the use of a number of different services is to allocate a case manager (sometimes called a key worker or primary worker). The case manager is one member of the multidisciplinary team who takes the responsibility for coordinating the care of the client, and is the main contact for everyone else who works with that client. The case manager takes responsibility for reviewing, monitoring and modifying the care plan, coordinating the discharge, and ensuring that all of the appropriate services are in place at all stages through the episode of care. Sometimes the case manager may be responsible for coordinating, or undertaking the single assessment.

Sharing client information

When you are working with a client in the community, your team may include a number of people from outside the service that you work with, including the client's GP, their carer or family members, and other services such as home help. Because these people are involved in the care of the client, however indirectly, you are likely to have to communicate with these people. Often, your communication will be fairly straightforward, although, on occasion, it can become fairly complex, and sometimes challenging. Good communication between team members is important to prevent the client being bombarded with the same questions by multiple practitioners; to ensure that there is no duplication or unnecessary overlap in the care provided to the client; and to ensure that the client is not receiving different treatments that may be dangerous if given in combination. Good communication also helps to ensure that all members of the team are working towards consistent client goals.

There are a number of different ways of sharing client information with other members of the care team:

- **Shared client notes:** with shared client notes, all members of the team will keep written notes about the client using a system that allows the information to be seen by other team members. This might involve completing a paper file that is stored in a safe place in the client's home. Some services use computerised client records that can be accessed by a number of different service providers. This could be completed at an office, or might use portable computers to manage the information which is stored in a central place.
- **Case conferences:** this normally involves a meeting of the client, and everyone who is involved with the care and support of the client. This could include family members or carers, as well as staff from the range of

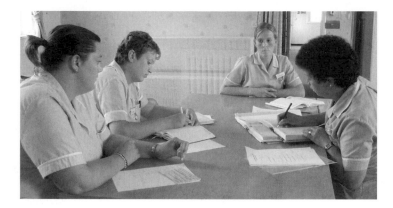

Figure 4 Team members at a case conference.

different organisations that will be delivering the care. Case conferences may take place at different stages of the episode of care, but are most typical at the beginning of care, to agree goals and negotiate roles and responsibilities of the different stakeholders.

▪ **Log books:** if your team works from the same office, and staff go back to that office daily, or at least regularly, a log book can be a useful way to keep the rest of the team informed about changes to particular clients. A log book will normally be used by all of the members of the team to record which clients they saw, to give a brief description of the intervention they delivered, and to leave important information for other team members about changes to the status of the client. For instance, you might use the log book to notify the physiotherapist that a client is ready to be discharged from their care.

▪ **Joint visits:** one way of sharing information about clients and client care is to deliver that care with other members of the team. Joint visits are not always appropriate because it means that the team members need to be available at the same time. You also need to consider the physical space that is available in the client's home. It may be a bit intimidating for the client if ten different staff members suddenly file into their bedroom. However, joint visits are a good way for a small number of staff (normally not more than three) to identify shared client needs and develop a coordinated approach to addressing those needs.

▪ **Team meetings:** these are often used by staff members who work together to share information about a particular client. The disadvantage of this approach is that it does not include staff who work for other teams.

▪ **Letters:** it is normal practice to write a letter to the referring practitioner, and generally the client's GP to keep them informed about the outcome of an assessment or the progress of care. Technology means that sometimes this is now done by fax or email. Where a large number of people are involved in delivering care, it is impractical to communicate with all of the

Teamworking and supervision

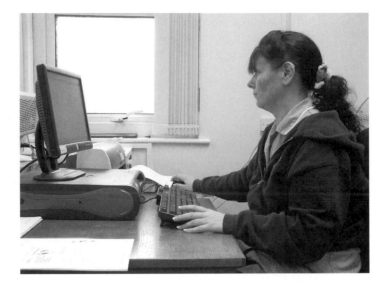

Figure 5 Support worker sending an email.

team members by letter, so other methods of communication are often used.

■ **Telephone**: telephone communication is not useful when you need to share information with a lot of people, for the obvious reason that you will need to repeat the same information many times to all of the members of the team, and it does not create a written record. Telephone communication is most valuable when you need to notify one or two key personnel about an issue relating to the client, or you need urgent assistance. For instance, if you notice that the client needs a new prescription, you may telephone their GP to ask for a repeat, and you might also contact the case manager (if there is one). You would document the telephone calls in the written client file.

■ **Huddling:** the informal meetings that you have with team members as you meet them walking down the corridor, in the kitchen or cloakroom, have a name: management experts call those meetings 'huddling'. Cricketers and footballers regularly use huddling as a way of deciding immediate team strategies when they are on the field. Huddling is useful for passing on quick pieces of information verbally and as you think of them, but does not mean that the information will necessarily be recorded or remembered. Some organisations use regular, organised huddling as a way of passing on useful information quickly.

Client confidentiality

When you are sharing information about a client, it is important to be aware of the confidentiality policies of your organisation and your health care system.

You need to be clear about who has the right to access information about the client, and ensure that the client is aware of the people with whom the information will be shared. Any identifiable client information should be held in a secure place and treated with respect. Be careful not to accidentally breach client confidence by leaving files unattended. Ensure that you are not inappropriately overheard discussing a client, and be wary of computer security.

Most countries have legal requirements that guide the confidentiality of personal information. Part of being a competent practitioner is having an awareness of the confidentiality information. Your organisation should be able to provide you with easy access to information about the confidentiality requirements that you need to adhere to, and this should form part of the induction to your team.

■ What makes a good team?

No matter how large or small the team, a number of basic principles can help the team to ensure smooth teamworking, and that the client receives the best quality care.

- An effective team has clearly defined objectives that are agreed, understood and followed by all members of the team.
- Good teams work together to ensure that there is client-centred goal setting and joint decisions about the interventions and evaluation of the interventions.
- All team members need to be involved in making decisions that influence the team and feel that their input is heard and valued.
- Team members need to be clear about their own role and function within the team, as well as the roles of the people they work with. This includes having an understanding of their supervisory support and lines of accountability. Each member of the team should be aware of their limitations, and know when they need to access more support.
- Team meetings are important for the outcomes of the team. Regular team meetings lead to greater innovation in patient care, and teams that meet at least once a week are more likely to introduce new innovations than teams with fewer meetings.
- Teams that include a mix of different types of workers (nurses, doctors and therapists) are more likely to discuss a range of different options for delivering client care, which improves the quality of the care delivered.
- Teams should use a common language. Team members can be excluded by the use of professional jargon and abbreviations, so it is important to work together to develop clearly understood terms to ease communication.

Team leadership is particularly important. There has been a lot of research into what makes a good leader. Essentially, a good leader is someone who will represent the team; help the team to work together well; establish trust with external services and stakeholders; facilitate conflict resolution; promote appreciation of team members' contribution to the team; encourage flexibility; develop the capabilities of team members; and encourage collective learning about ways to work together.

Stop and think   Is your team working as effectively as it could?

Does your team have clear vision and goals?
Can you name your line manager?
Does your team have regular, scheduled meetings?
Do you feel comfortable raising issues that are important to you at your team meetings?
Do you know who to contact if you have a question around specific clinical issues relating to a client?
Does your team have regular input from a number of different types of professional groups or workers?
Do you have systems in place for monitoring your effectiveness?

(1) as an individual worker
(2) in improving patient care
(3) in achieving team goals

Are these systems checked, monitored and updated on a regular basis?
Do you have systems to share information about the care of particular clients that you are managing together (such as case conference meetings; common notes; a log book at your team base)?
Does your team work from the same physical base or office?

Team dynamics

Imagine a football team that was just made up of goalkeepers, or one where everyone thought that they were the captain of the team. A team where everyone has the same set of skills or competes to do the same job is unlikely to be very functional. An effective team is one that draws together people with diverse strengths, skills and abilities who work towards achieving the same goals. If you look back at the first Stop and think box in this chapter, you will see that each team member has an important and different role to play in client re-enablement.

In the rehabilitation setting, team diversity is introduced in a number of different ways:

■ Multidisciplinary and interdisciplinary teams bring together practitioners from different professional backgrounds such as doctors, nurses, therapists and rehabilitation workers. Each different group brings their own perspective to the management of the client.
■ Individual personalities play an important role in the way that the team functions together.

▪ The way the team is organised and managed, as well as the stage of the development of the team, will impact on the team dynamics.

You are probably already aware of the contribution that having a number of different types of practitioner groups adds to your team. Now think about the different personalities of each of the people you work with and the way this impacts on your team. Think about people in terms of their attention to detail; ability to finish tasks well; creativity and the new ideas they bring to the team; problem solving skills; leadership skills; and communication skills. Psychologists have developed tools to look at the different personality traits, motivating factors, skills and attributes that people bring into their workplace. Sometimes these tools are used as a way of developing their teams and identifying particular strengths of individuals. They can also be used for career planning and increasing your self-awareness. You will find a link to some of these tools in the further reading section at the end of this chapter.

The way your team is organised will impact on the way you work together. For instance, a team that has good leadership, regular meetings and a process that allows everyone to contribute their ideas will generally function far more effectively than a team that rarely meets and where all the decisions are made by the manager without consulting staff or service users. The physical location of your team is also important. If your team does not share a common office, then it is very difficult for you to meet regularly to share information and ideas. The style of management and supervisory arrangements within your team will also impact on the way that your team works together.

The stage of development of your team is important for teamworking. If you have ever been involved in the development of a new service or team, you will know that it takes some time to work out where the team is going, who is responsible for doing specific jobs and how the team members work together. The four commonly described stages of team development are:

▪ **Forming:** this is the stage where the group get together and test out their ideas and relationships with each other.
▪ **Storming:** it is normal for new teams to experience some conflict between group members and some resistance to working together as a team to achieve the desired goals. This is called the storming phase.
▪ **Norming:** following the storming phase the team will start to develop a clear structure and become more cohesive. A supportive structure starts to develop.
▪ **Performing:** the final stage of team development arises when the team members work together as one unit to achieve the goals of the group. Individual roles have developed to a stage where they clearly fit the task at hand.

Researchers have shown that it can take up to eighteen months for a health care team to reach the performing stage.

Teamworking and supervision

Stop and think   Team roles

Consider your team and your role within your team.
What stage of development do you think your team is at (forming, storming, norming or performing)?
What skills do you bring to your team?
List three colleagues in your team who have different roles to you. What skills to they bring to the team that are different to your own skills?
Are there any areas where your skills and roles overlap?

■ Supervision

So far, this chapter has talked about the way that teams work together. The team is one very important component of the support that you will need to do your job as a rehabilitation worker. However, every worker will have their own specific support needs.

You are likely to require different types of supervisory support for the various aspects of your role, and it is unlikely that all of these roles will be fulfilled by a single person. For instance, you are likely to require support both from an organisational perspective, which includes aspects of your work such as the hours you work, your relationship with other members of your team, holidays, the team goals and objectives. But you are also likely to require different levels of support around the technical or clinical aspects of your role. This may come from a single, dedicated person with expertise in your particular field, or if you are working across professional boundaries, it may be necessary to identify a number of different people from whom you can access specific support. For instance, you may require frequent advice from a physiotherapist and occupational therapist if you are a generic rehabilitation worker working across a number of different professional boundaries. But you may occasionally require the input of, for example, a dietitian and a social worker to advise you and support you regarding specific clinical or technical aspects of the work that you are delivering.

You will also need management support to help you develop your role in line with the needs of the job and your own personal development needs. Your team will have a manager who is responsible for ensuring that the whole team works together to achieve the objectives of the service. As a result, your manager is ultimately responsible for addressing the needs of a number of workers. Your manager is unlikely to have technical expertise in all of the different areas in which you are likely to work. Supervision can be used to fill these roles, and can be tailored specifically to meet your own workplace needs.

Why is good supervision important?

Good supervision is vital for rehabilitation workers for two main reasons. First, you need to receive support so that you can give of yourself to provide the best care you can. Second, it is important to have good supervisory structures in place to protect you and the client.

Matching your own needs to the needs of the client

Working in a helping profession means giving a lot of yourself. Working with vulnerable people means that you will take on a number of different roles. At various times in your job you might be called on to be a teacher, counsellor, listener, therapist, friend, colleague, tradesperson, manager or supervisor. These roles demand a number of different skills and emotions, which can be difficult to deliver if you are in any way physically or emotionally vulnerable yourself.

As a worker in a helping role, there is often an expectation that you need to be seen to be emotionally neutral in order to be professional. As a human being who brings a range of different experiences and expectations to the job yourself, it can sometimes be challenging to deliver professional, client-centred care. Your ability to deal with these situations will come, in part, from your own experience and maturity. However, there are times when you will need external support to help you cope with your job and deliver the most appropriate service; supervision may help you achieve this.

Stop and think   Meeting your supervision needs

Try to recall a time when you attended work after having some personal difficulty, such as experiencing some emotional distress or feeling physically unwell.
Who did you tell?
How did it impact on your work?
How did you balance addressing your own needs with those of your clients and colleagues?
What supervisory structures did you have to support you?
What supervisory structures could have helped you more?

What is supervision?

Supervision is an interaction between two people, where one person is given the role of supporting the other to become more effective at doing their job. Sometimes the supervisor has some responsibility for overseeing the performance of the supervisee. Most people will have experience of being supervised at some stage in their career, although we are given little preparation for this role. A smaller, but significant number of workers will also be supervisors, and are often inappropriately prepared for this role as well.

> **Box 2** Developing a supervision support map
>
> This exercise will help you identify the different types of support you have in your job, and the support needs that you have.
>
> Write your name or draw an image of yourself in the middle of a blank sheet of paper. Now think about all of the different types of support you get that help you do your job, including professional support, personal support, moral support and learning. Don't forget to include the support that you get from people outside your job, including your family, friends, lecturers or teachers, even a priest. You might want to sit down with a colleague and do this exercise together. You could swap your 'support-maps' and see if you can identify any areas that the other has missed.
>
> Now consider the following questions:
>
> ■ Are you getting enough support?
> ■ Are you getting the type of support you want?
> ■ Are there any gaps in your support?
> ■ Are there any gaps in your support network?
> ■ What could you do to start to fill those gaps?
>
> If you have identified some gaps in your level of support, make a plan to show how you are going to meet at least one of these in the next month.

Traditionally, supervision has been seen as a relationship that is largely controlled and determined by the supervisor, with relatively little input from the supervisee. However, you can take some responsibility to ensure that you receive the supervision that you need and to establish your own support systems. It is unlikely that a single supervisor is going to be able to meet all of the needs that you will encounter in a rehabilitation setting. You also have the day-to-day supervision needs of someone to resolve conflicts and voice your concerns about the direction of the team. It is important to identify the different types of needs that you have and consider who the best person or people are to help you meet those needs.

To a certain extent, every worker has a responsibility for reflecting on their own practice. Some people call this self-supervision. If you adopt the principles of reflective practice and use that as a way of monitoring and reviewing your own progress then this will help you to constantly improve your practice. (See previous chapter on Lifelong learning.)

Supervisory contracts

To get the most out of your supervisory relationship, whether you are the supervisor or supervisee, you may want to consider setting up a supervisory contract. A supervisory contract helps you to clarify and put in writing the goals and expectations of both people regarding the supervision relationship. The types of things you might include in your supervisory contract include:

(1) The ground rules for your supervisory relationship. For instance, where will you meet, when and how often? You should also negotiate how you will access more frequent supervisory meetings if either of you need them.
(2) What you hope to achieve from your supervisory relationship.
(3) Any fears or concerns around the working relationship.
(4) How you will monitor and review your supervision relationship. You may want to set aside a small amount of time on a regular basis just to check how well your supervisory relationship is going.
(5) What processes you will go through if the supervision relationship fails to work for either or both of you. For instance, what will you do yourselves, and who will you go to next?

What makes a good supervisory relationship?

■ You should feel comfortable with your supervision process, be involved in the process, and be able to accept and discuss feedback with your supervisor.
■ You should have clear objectives around how you do your work with your clients.
■ You should have a clear understanding of what is expected of you in your role, and know how this will be evaluated.
■ A good supervisor will encourage you to think in new ways.
■ Your supervisor should be accessible at times when you need support.

You also have to take on some responsibilities as a supervisee. You cannot expect your supervisor to be a mind-reader, so ask for help when you need it. If you have a good supervisory relationship you will feel comfortable asking for help. Your supervision relationship is designed to give you feedback and support, so try to be open to the feedback you receive and not defensive. You do not necessarily need to agree with all of the feedback your supervisor gives you, and if you do disagree with some feedback, attempt to discuss this calmly. If you have set up a good supervisory contract, it will sometimes be appropriate to give your supervisor feedback about the supervision process. Ensure that you do this in a calm and non-aggressive way.

Being a good supervisor

It is likely that at some stage in your career as a rehabilitation worker, you will be required to supervise other staff. This may range from supervising students who are on placements with your team, newly qualified staff, up to entire teams or service networks. You may even decide to develop your career as a manager. Yet few staff who work in the helping professions actually receive formal training in supervision or management. We often expect that we will have the innate skills to be able to supervise other people without this training, and put high expectations on ourselves to do it well.

As a supervisor, it is important to keep in mind your experiences as a supervisee, to make sure that you make the experience as beneficial as possible to your staff and team members. In fact, the starting point for being a good supervisor is being able to be a good supervisee. When you become a supervisor, it is still important that you have supervisory support structures for yourself.

As with the rest of your role as a rehabilitation worker, your role as a supervisor requires that you perform a number of different functions:

- Teacher
- Counsellor and adviser
- Manager
- Technical expert

The attributes of a good supervisor include:

- Flexibility: able to use or understand a wide variety of approaches and methods.
- Able to see the same situation from a variety of angles.
- Capacity to manage and contain anxiety (their own and the supervisee's).
- Open to learning. Just because you are the supervisor it does not mean you have to have all the answers all the time.
- Sensitive and aware of the wider contextual issues that affect the supervisor–supervisee relationships, and the supervisee's work setting.
- Anti-oppressive practice (able to manage power).
- Humour, humility and patience.

Often, people in the helping professions will have developed a number of the interpersonal skills to help them in the supervision process. It is important to remember that supervision is not about giving 'therapy', it is about providing support.

■ Are you competent to practise?

Before you were offered your job, your employer should have ensured that you had some of the basic requirements that demonstrate your competence to practise in your workplace. The standards for competency vary for different types of workers, and between each country, state or region, and sometimes across different employers. The most commonly used measures of competence are things like your basic qualification, membership of a professional association and state registration. For example, in order to be able to work as a physiotherapist in Australia, you need to have a physiotherapy qualification from a recognised tertiary institution. Some employers also require you to have a criminal records check. In the UK all health/social care/rehabilitation staff must have a CRB (Criminal Records Bureau) check prior to commencing work.

You may also be required to have your own insurance to protect your client if something goes wrong. Again, this will vary between workplaces and countries, but you should check with your employer to make sure that they have insurance cover for you, or whether you need to obtain it yourself. You must take the responsibility for ensuring that these things are up to date and appropriate for your current workplace.

It can be a bit more difficult to determine the competence of rehabilitation workers who are not required to have a degree or diploma, and who do not require formal regulation or registration. In some cases, your employer may require that you have a vocational qualification, such as a certificate from a technical college or college of further education. In the UK, National Vocational Qualifications (NVQs) are a way of providing formal recognition for skills that the worker has developed in their job. However, some rehabilitation workers have learnt their skills from having many years of experience on the job and do not have any formal qualifications. This can present difficulties if you want to change jobs, because it is very difficult for a new employer to gauge your level of experience or expertise without some formal certification of your level of skills and ability. Sometimes you might even experience difficulties working with other staff who do not understand your role or expertise, and who feel that you may be encroaching on parts of their work. Unfortunately, without recognised formal qualifications, it can be difficult to convince other people or employers that you are competent to do your job and, at the moment, there are no easy ways to overcome this bias.

Staying competent

No matter what your basic level of training or experience is, it is important that you constantly revise and update your skills to ensure that you are delivering the best, most effective care. Some professional groups have compulsory systems, such as accreditation, to demonstrate that they are maintaining their skills, and without which they may be restricted from practising. However, there are a number of different ways to keep your skills up to date.

The previous chapter on Lifelong learning describes a number of possibilities for continuing your learning. One of the most common and easiest ways to learn is through on-the-job training. You can also take formal courses; attend conferences; read newsletters, books and journals that relate to your work; join a journal club; access resources from the Internet; or become a member of a special interest group that is relevant to aspects of your work. It is important to be critical of the quality of the information that you access. For instance, the information in books can be out of date, and the information published on the Internet is not always from credible or reliable sources.

Your appraisal should describe the ways that you intend to maintain and update your skills so that you have some way of gauging your progress within your workplace. If you are a reflective practitioner, you should also be constantly reflecting and revising the way that you work, based on your interactions and feedback with clients and other staff members. The previous chapter on Lifelong learning gives more information about how to be a reflective practitioner.

> ### Box 3   Being a competent worker
>
> ■   Do you have sufficient training to do the job that is being asked of you?
> ■   How are you keeping your knowledge up to date?
> ■   Do you have the appropriate legal protection in place to do your job?
> ■   You need to be aware of your own personal and professional boundaries, and know when it is appropriate to ask for help, or say 'I am not comfortable doing this'. When this happens, you need to know who to contact to provide you with the best help and support.
> ■   Are you aware of the policies and guidelines in your workplace about client safety, moving and handling, client confidentiality?

■ Conclusion

In order to do your job effectively, you need the appropriate levels of training and support. If you do not have the appropriate types or levels of support, or you feel that you are not adequately trained to perform your job, it is important that you bring this to the attention of a senior member of your team or organisation as quickly as possible. Teamwork and supervision are two-way processes and you should have some control over the way you interact, both as a team member and a supervisee. Every interaction will be different, and every team will have different dynamics. Being aware of your own support needs, and your own role within a team should enable you to function effectively within these relationships.

■ Further reading

Website

Pyschometric tests: http://www.psychometrics.com/onlinetest/ *This link provides access to a wide variety of psychometric tests to help you determine your role within your team and examine team dynamics.*

Other publications

Hawkins, P. & Shohet, R. (2003) *Supervision in the Helping Professions* (2nd edition). Maidenhead, Open University Press. *Primarily designed for social care practitioners, this book provides useful information for supervisors and supervisees.*

Ovretveit, J. (1993) *Coordinating Community Care: Multidisciplinary Teams and Care Management.* Maidenhead, Open University Press. *This is one of the relatively early descriptions of community based teamworking and approaches to organising multidisciplinary working.*

Teamworking and supervision

Tight, M., Morton-Cooper, A., Palmer, A. (eds) (1999) *Mentoring, Preceptorship and Clinical Supervision: A Guide to Clinical Support and Supervision.* Oxford, Blackwell Science. *This book is specifically designed for nurses, but provides valuable information for all health and social care practitioners about supervision.*

Index